Third Edition

Fitness Management

A Comprehensive Resource
for
Developing, Leading, Managing, and Operating
a
Successful Health/Fitness Club

Stephen J. Tharrett, M.S.
Dallas, Texas

James A. Peterson, Ph.D., FACSM
Monterey, California

ISBN: 978-1-60679-215-5
Library of Congress Control Number: 2012934339
Book layout: Studio J Art & Design
Front cover design: Studio J Art & Design
Front cover photos: (row 1) Stephen Tharrett, BananaStock, Jupiterimages; (row 2) Fuse/Thinkstock, Brand X Pictures, Creatas; (row 3) iStockphoto/ Thinkstock, Pinnacle Pictures, ©2007 Jupiterimages Corporation; (row 4) IT Stock, Pixland, Stephen Tharrett
Photo of Stephen Tharrett (back cover): Alyssa Tharrett

Healthy Learning
P.O. Box 1828
Monterey, CA 93942
www.healthylearning.com

This book is dedicated to my family. To my wife, Denise, who has stood by me for 35 years, providing support, inspiration, patience, and love. To my children, Alyssa and Travis, for their love and support and for teaching me so much about what is required to be a leader. Finally to my father, John Tharrett, who passed nearly two decades ago, an individual who was my hero growing up. While this project was a labor of love, I could not have done so without the unconditional love provided by my family.

S.T.

This book is dedicated to every individual who has helped make the joy of exercise a reality for another person.

J.P.

Dedication

Acknowledgments

I want to acknowledge all of the incredible people in this industry who have shared their passion and wisdom with me about the business of operating a successful health/fitness club.

First, I would like to thank the leaders and peers who served with me for 21 years at ClubCorp, including Robert Dedman Sr., Richard Poole, Bob Johnson, Doug Howe, Frank Gore, Murray Siegel, and Steve Plakotoris, each of whom it was my honor to work with, and who gave me the opportunity to learn and grow by freely sharing their knowledge and love of the business.

Second, I would like to acknowledge the incredible members of the ClubCorp athletic and tennis committees, over 40 strong dedicated and passionate leaders. Each of these special people (particularly the committee leaders, including Gordon Collins, Billy Freer, Tommy English, Nony Michulka, Rich Andrae, Jill Bauman, Vicki McGrath, Frank Martin, Mike Saldivar, Pam Koch, Jim Swieter, Teresa Thomason, and Bill Johnston) never hesitated to share their wisdom or heart.

Third, I would like to express my appreciation to the over 5,000 employees who worked in the athletic and tennis arena at ClubCorp, including my wonderful assistant, Michele Arnette, who, without knowing it, taught me the real "in and outs" of the business.

Fourth, I would like to thank my colleagues and friends at the Russian Fitness Group, a group of dynamic and talented professionals, with whom I had the honor of working for nearly three years during my tenure as the company's CEO and managing director from 2008 to 2010. I want to extend a special thanks to my executive team at RFG, including Alla, Alexey, Dima, Irina, Julia I., Julia K., and Roman. I also want to give a special thanks to Yana, who acted as my guardian angel during my three years in Russia, and Olesya, who served as my executive assistant, translator, teacher, and friend.

Lastly, I would like to acknowledge the industry leaders who have been so open and willing to share their knowledge and insights about the industry. Frankly, there are so many individuals to thank in this regard that I cannot begin to mention everyone who has impacted my professional life in a positive manner. On the other hand, I would like to personally thank those individuals who have served as role models for me during my extended tenure in the industry. With over 2,000 years of collective experience, these exceptional industry individuals are a true reflection of the nature of the industry. The list of those individuals to whom I am eternally grateful in this regard includes people such as Rick Caro of Management Vision, Norm Cates of the Club Insider, Frank Napolitano of GlobalFit, Spencer Garrett of Pierpont Racquet Club, Rob Goldman of the Columbia Association, Gary Klencheski of Fitcorp, Mitch Wald of the Maryland Athletic Club, Carl Porter of the Michigan Athletic Club, Gale Landers of Fitness Formula, Steve Schwartz of Tennis Corporation of America, Tim Rhode of the Maryland Athletic Club, Jill Kinney of Club One, Red Lerille of

Red's, Rudy Riska, who spent more than four decades as the executive director of the Downtown Athletic Club in New York, Jim Gerber of Western Athletic Clubs, Annbeth Eschbach of Exhale, and Robert Chaiken and the esteemed members of the Faust Group, as well as the countless other individuals with whom it was my honor and pleasure to serve during my involvement with the industry. In addition to the aforementioned industry leaders, I would also like to give very special thanks to John McCarthy, former executive director of IHRSA, who has been a mentor over the years and provided valuable insight into the writing of this book. Finally, thanks to the entire team at IHRSA, particularly Hans Muench, for their incredible efforts in advancing the industry over the past two decades.

I also would like to acknowledge the wonderful and talented people involved in other aspects of the industry who have shared a wealth of information with me over the years. In particular, I would like to thank Andy Richters of Matrix Fitness and formerly of Star Trac, Gary Klein of Keiser, Bob Taggert of T2 Fitness, Mike Zinda of Life Fitness, Stan Peterman formerly of Quinton, Ken Germano of the Medical Fitness Association, Dr. Cedric Bryant of ACE, Hervey Lavoie of Ohlson Lavoie, Richard Brunner of Michigan State, and Brian Davidson, formerly of Life Fitness. Frankly, space does not permit me to list everyone who has been a trusted friend and business associate over the past 20 years. It goes without saying that their assistance has been invaluable.

A special thanks to Dr. Dee Edington, former dean of the School of Kinesiology at the University of Michigan and director of the Wellness Research Center at the University, and Dr. Tom Sattler, former professor at the University of Illinois at Chicago, for their mentorship over the years. A very special thanks to my co-author, Jim Peterson, former director of sports medicine at StairMaster Sports/Medical Products, Inc. and a retired professor of physical education at the United States Military Academy at West Point. Over the years, Jim has helped set a professional course for me to follow, and has always been there to provide a helping hand. Finally, special and heartfelt thanks to my daughter, Alyssa, who provided immense assistance in pulling together the materials for this book.

Unfortunately, I am sure I have missed more names than I have mentioned. On the other hand, hopefully, all of the wonderful and talented people with whom I have been blessed to share this journey are aware of how grateful I am for the positive impact that they have had on my life. One key point is inescapable … we are all in an incredible business!

S.T.

Special thanks to Kris Heath, Kristi Huelsing, and Angie Perry as well as the rest of the creative team at Healthy Learning, for their invaluable assistance on this project.

J.P.

This book is designed to serve three distinct target populations. One group is the upper-level undergraduate and graduate students who are seeking to embark on a career in the fitness, health, racquet, and sport club industry. Another are young professionals who are already working in the industry and who are seeking information and insights that can help them expand their professional horizons and possibly move into management. Finally, the book is intended for seasoned industry professionals who want to know more about areas in which they may not have as much experience or knowledge as they would like to have.

As you read this book, keep in mind that the fitness, health, racquet, and sport club industry is currently in its adolescence and slowly approaching maturity. As the industry has matured and expanded over the years, the demand for professionals with both strong business acumen and a passion and understanding of the dynamics of the industry has become paramount to health/fitness club owners and investors. Sixty years ago, this industry was in its infancy, developed, operated, and pushed forward by entrepreneurs who had a passion for fitness and what they were doing. Circumstances forced these industry pioneers to focus on surviving first and creating an industry second.

Over the past four decades, as the industry has begun to mature, many of the dynamics of the club business have changed. For example, over the past decade, financial markets have and will continue to invest in the industry. Concurrently, major industry figures are creating national and international health/fitness club companies and franchises. This maturation process has resulted in a shortage of leaders and managers who can take the industry to the next level, and help it to continue to grow profitability on an ever-changing playing field. Much of this situation can be attributed to the fact that the industry has not established (at this point at least) a formal educational process for bringing professionals into the industry.

Over the years, one of the most pressing issues that other health/fitness club owners have brought to my attention is the critical need for a reliable mechanism for sharing the information that is needed to help better develop the future business leaders for the industry. This book is my attempt to help address that void. I have chosen to write it as a means of sharing with the readers the wealth of knowledge and passion that I have garnered from 30 years of working with the most incredible people in the industry. In reality, this book presents the insights and wisdom of industry leaders who collectively have over 5,000 years of experience in the industry.

This book is separated into ten distinct sections, based on the skill sets needed to succeed as a leader and manager in this industry. Part I introduces the reader to the fitness, health, racquet, and sport club industry by touching on the history of the industry, the current practices and trends in the industry, and the attitudes and attributes of the consumer who chooses to be a member

Preface

of a club. Part II focuses on health/fitness club membership, starting with a discussion of the differences between a member and a consumer, and progressing into the marketing and sales practices necessary to succeed in the business.

Part III provides an overview of member retention and the process of utilizing great service and great programming to create memorable member experiences. Part IV reviews the administrative business functions of the industry, beginning with the formation of a legal business entity, progressing to the financial standards and processes, and concluding with an examination of the key issues involved in buying, leasing, and selling a club. Part V looks at the employee side of the health/fitness club business, starting with a detailed overview of the people-related requirements, and concluding with a discussion of the essential aspects of leadership within the industry.

Part VI addresses the facility and equipment side of the business, covering topics ranging from facility design to equipment selection. Part VII details the key operational issues within a health/fitness facility, beginning with an overview of the risk management practices in the industry and progressing through the most essential operating practices for both front-of-the-house and behind-the-house club operations.

Part VIII addresses the emerging international market by providing an in depth overview of the health/fitness club markets in Asia, Europe and Latin America. Part IX offers a picture of what the future may hold for our industry. Part X presents case studies of unusual management experiences, ranging from customer and member-related scenarios to employee and big business scenarios. Each case study provides an overview of an unusual or unexpected business event and the actions taken by the respective clubs and their leaders.

This book also features several appendices that contain examples of various operating policies and practices that can be implemented within a health/fitness facility from day one.

In conclusion, our primary goal in writing this book is to expand the horizons of its readers and provide them with a valuable resource that can help them in their professional development. If the publication of this book has a positive impact on the key issues attendant to the fitness, health, racquet, and sport club industry, then the effort involved in writing it will have been more than worthwhile.

S.T.

INTRODUCTION TO THE HEALTH/FITNESS CLUB INDUSTRY

Legends of the Iron Game, Bill Pearl Enterprises

Part One

- Chapter 1: The Health/Fitness Club Industry: Challenge and Change
- Chapter 2: The Physical Activity Beliefs and Behaviors of Americans and Their Implications for Health/Fitness Clubs
- Chapter 3: Consumer Attitudes Toward Health/Fitness Clubs That Affect Their Reasons for Joining and Staying

1

The Health/Fitness Club Industry: Challenge and Change

Chapter Objectives

The primary objective of this chapter is to present an overview of the culture of the health/fitness industry. The chapter begins by reviewing the industry's history in order to provide insight into the cultural roots of the industry. This discussion is followed by a section that features a more in-depth look at the modern history of the industry (from 1970 forward), with particular emphasis on the state of the industry as of 2010. The chapter concludes by offering a review of likely industry trends that will occur over the next decade.

The Early Years (Pre-1980)

The first officially recognized fitness club, referred to at the time as a gymnastics club, was established in 1811 by Frederich Ludwig Jahn. Based in Germany, the club was originally called a Public Turn Platz. Shortly thereafter, it became known simply as Turnverein. Turnverein was developed to provide men and boys with an organized social environment in which they could prepare themselves physically to protect their country. Turnverein offered organized group classes, using Indian clubs, dumbbells, ropes, and a variety of equipment that is currently common to many gymnastic and fitness clubs. By the 1850s, approximately 150 Turnverein had been developed around the world, with the first American Turnverein opening in 1848 in Cincinnati, Ohio.

In 1847, the famous French strongman, Hippolyte Triat, opened a club in Paris, which he called "Gymnase Triat." Gymnase Traiat was the first club to sell shares to the public as a means to raise the necessary funds to develop and operate the club. Gymnase Triat was also one of the first club facilities to offer music in its exercise classes (in this case, group barbell classes), and to view the membership experience as akin to a form of entertainment.

In 1848, the first U.S. health club, a Turnverein club, was established in Cincinnati, Ohio. Shortly thereafter, the Boston YMCA opened its doors (1850).

The first officially recognized fitness club, referred to at the time as a gymnastics club, was established in 1811 by Frederich Ludwig Jahn.

Hippolyte Triat's gymnasium club (circa 1840s)

A decade later, the initial private athletic clubs in the U.S. began their operations. The first of these was the Olympic Club in San Francisco, which started in 1860. Subsequently, a mere eight years later, the New York Athletic Club opened its doors to members. These pioneering clubs had their roots in an industry culture that emanated from male-oriented social and sport clubs and institutes of physical culture. Interestingly enough, while women were not part of this male-dominated club culture, they were actively engaged in promoting exercise, as evidenced by Catherine Beecher's book entitled, _Housekeeper and Healthkeeper_, which was published in 1870.

These early athletic clubs (Olympic Club, San Francisco; New York Athletic Club, New York; Los Angeles Athletic Club, Los Angeles; Lille Athletic Club, France; Athletic and Cycling Club of Saint Petersburg, Russia; the Athletic Club of Florence, Italy, etc.) were developed to foster both social and business relationships and to promote a culture of physical activity. Each featured facilities that provided an environment for actively pursuing social networking and engaging in sport activities.

In 1894, Louis Durlacher, more commonly known as Professor Attila, opened one of the first commercial health/fitness clubs in New York City, Attila's Athletic Studio and School of Physical Culture. Professor Attila had opened his first club in Europe decades earlier, which targeted providing training to Europe's kings, queens, and dignitaries. Attila's N.Y. studio went on to become one of the most famous of its type in the U.S., and upon his death in 1926, the club was turned over to his protégé, Sig Klein. Klein built on the reputation of Attila's studio when he opened his own gym in 1927, which he called Sig Klein's Studio of Physical Culture. Klein's studio subsequently operated for over five decades in mid-town Manhattan.

Professor Louis Attila's Athletic Studio and School of Physical Culture

In the mid-to-late 1800s, two significant milestones occurred in the fitness industry that would change the way people exercised in gyms and athletic clubs. The first breakthrough was the development of exercise machines by Gustav Zander of Sweden. Dr. Zander believed that machines could provide a more efficient and effective means of training athletes and ordinary citizens. Starting in the 1850s, Zander started developing exercise machines that employed levers, springs, pulleys, and weights. By the 1870s, he had created a total of 27 distinct pieces of exercise equipment, which he later featured in the first studio he opened in the U.S., in New York in the 1880s.

The second significant event was the development of variable-resistance pulley equipment by Dudley Allan Sargent. Sargent, director of the Hemenway Gymnasium and an assistant professor of physical education at Harvard, developed the first pulley-driven variable resistance machines in the 1880s. Eventually, he developed over 30 pieces of equipment that had names such as the abdominal pulley system and chest pulley system. At one time, over 50 pieces of his equipment were located in the Hemenway Gymnasium at Harvard.

By the early part of the 20th century, the type of athletic club operated by Professor Attila in the 1890s became even more prevalent, with noteworthy growth in many of the larger urban markets including New York, Boston, Chicago, Los Angeles, and Philadelphia.

During the early 1900s, the primary concern of many men who might otherwise be interested in joining a health/fitness club was the pursuit of feats of strength and physique. During this particular time period, several pioneers, such as Eugen Sandow, Bernarr Macfadden, Alan Calvert George

Hackenschmidt, and Professor Attila, became the leaders and spokespeople for the growing field of physical culture. Bernarr Macfadden conducted traveling road shows with his family during the late 1890s and earlier part of the 20th century to promote physical activity. In 1899, Macfadden published a journal, called *Physical Culture* (a magazine that subsequently was published for 50 years), which provided a public venue for promoting the benefits of physical activity, physical culture, and proper nutrition. A few years after starting *Physical Culture*, Macfadden inaugurated a second publication addressing physical culture, *Beauty and Health for Women*. During that same general time period, Eugen Sandow also developed a chain of schools of physical culture, which were designed to instruct others on the art of physical-culture training.

In response to the publicity generated by Macfadden, Sandow, and others, gyms began to arise that provided an environment for individuals to pursue activities (e.g., weightlifting, gymnastics, and acrobatic arts) that focused on physical development. In 1902, the Milo Barbell Company was formed by Alan Calvert. Calvert's company provided the emerging "gym" industry with a new form of mass-produced, weight training equipment, which further helped to advance the relatively new cultural phenomena of exercising in a club. These physical culture gyms appealed to a relatively small audience of men whose fitness and sports goals differed considerably from the individuals who joined the socially oriented athletic clubs. Among the earliest efforts in this regard was a facility developed by John Fritze, who opened a gym in the 1930s in Philadelphia, PA, called Germantown, which was then followed on the West Coast by one built by Vic Tanny, which opened in 1939.

By the 1940s, the development of these "bodybuilding and weightlifting" gyms had come into vogue. One of the most renowned was Leo Stern's in 1946, followed shortly thereafter by Eastman's in 1947, and Harold Zinkin's in 1948. Relatively small, these original gyms offered memberships for around $60 annually. In 1947, Vic Tanny permanently changed the landscape of the club fitness industry when he opened the first club dedicated to serving middle class Americans. Tanny's gyms provided an alternative to the "bodybuilding gyms" that heretofore had dominated the club landscape. By offering middle-class men and women an attractive and affordable workout environment, Tanny's gyms introduced American consumers to a different club environment, one that included mirrors, carpet, chrome equipment, saunas, and pools. Over the next two decades, Vic Tanny's gyms went on to become the largest chain of clubs in the world, with annual revenue of $24 million ($176 million in 2010 dollars).

By the early 1950s, additional gyms had sprouted up across the west, including Bill Pearl's in 1953. During the early 1950s, a legend in the club business, Ray Wilson, established his first health club chain, American Health Studios. Over the next two decades, Wilson opened eight distinct health club chains, including American Health Studios, Silhouette Figure Salons, Club International, Trim and Swim Health Clubs, and European Health Spas. Wilson is credited with being the first person to introduce alternate-day club access for men and women, wherein men worked out on Tuesdays, Thursdays, and

> In 1947, Vic Tanny permanently changed the landscape of the club fitness industry when he opened the first club dedicated to serving middle class Americans.

Saturdays, and women used the club on Mondays, Wednesdays, and Fridays. Understandably so, Vic Tanny and Ray Wilson are considered the founders of the modern fitness club industry.

Two equipment innovations of special consequence (for the health/fitness club industry) occurred during the 1950s. One was the invention of the first prototype of the Universal Gym (i.e., a multi-station, weight training machine) by Harold Zinkin, a former Mr. California and regular at Muscle Beach. Zinkin created the first Universal Gym in the late 1950s in a back room of his Palm Avenue gym in Fresno, California. During this same time period, the second equipment innovation to change the course of the industry was the introduction of the Quinton treadmill, a state-of-the-art aerobic exercise machine that was embraced as a useful tool by the medical community, as well as the fitness community.

In the 1950s, the basic passion and enthusiasm for fitness that existed in such club facilities as Klein's, Stern's, and Pearl's, and in large chains, such as Vic Tanny's and Ray Wilson's, were introduced into almost every household in America. This movement from gym to home was driven by renowned fitness industry legend Jack LaLanne. Using the new (at the time) medium of television to reach out to millions of Americans everywhere with his gospel message of "get up, work out, and feel better," LaLanne brought the benefits of physical conditioning into the American consciousness. The Jack LaLanne Show, which started in the early 1950s and continued until the 1980s, brought physical activity to televisions nationwide. In the process, LaLanne created a demand for knowledge about the pursuit of physical activity.

The movement from gym to home was driven by renowned fitness industry legend Jack LaLanne.

Subsequently, Jack LaLanne's name was licensed by Ray Wilson, a process that created Jack LaLanne European Health Spas, which evolved into the largest chain in America during the late 1960s. In the late 1970s, Jack LaLanne European Health Spas were sold to Health and Tennis Corporation, which over the next few decades, in turn, became Bally Total Fitness.

During the 50s and 60s, the equipment found in most fitness centers consisted primarily of free weights (York), free weight benches (York or homemade), stationary bicycles, self-propelled walking machines (treadmills), vibrating belts, and pulley machines. During the 1960s, the health/fitness industry received a huge boost from the roll-out of the Universal Gym. The original Universal Gym was a multi-station machine, whose system of weight stacks and pulleys brought resistance training to the masses by offering a relatively safe, easy, and fast approach to training.

The next decade witnessed the dawn of the modern health/fitness club industry, sparked by both scientific efforts to investigate the need for and the benefits of exercise and marketing research that opened up a new segment of consumers for the industry. During the late 1960s and early 1970s, a new type of health/fitness facility originated—the racquet club. Some of the earliest examples of this genre included Kings Court, Minneapolis, Minnesota; Mel Gorham's Court Club in Pacific Beach, California; the Midtown Tennis Club in Chicago, Illinois; and the Racquetball and Sports Clubs of Atlanta.

**Nautilus became
the standard piece
of equipment for
health/fitness
facilities and began
appearing in almost
every gym, YMCA,
athletic club, and
racquet club in the
United States.**

While the athletic clubs and the gyms that were previously popular continued to grow, it was the introduction of the racquet club that brought an entirely new audience to the industry. These racquet clubs consisted mainly of individually owned businesses that were operated by people who had a passion for the pursuit of racquet sports and physical activity. These facilities primarily consisted of indoor tennis courts, racquetball and handball courts, swimming pools, and small fitness centers. During this period, two industry-related associations formed—one representing indoor tennis clubs (National Indoor Tennis Association) and one representing racquetball clubs (National Court Club Association). Nearly a decade later, in 1981, these two associations were combined to form the International Racquet Sports Association (IRSA). Concurrent with the growth of racquet clubs was the continued expansion and evolution of gyms and club chains, such as Jack LaLanne's European Health Spas, Holiday Health Spas, Scandinavian Health Spas, Ray Wilson's Family Fitness Centers, and the predecessor of Bally's, Health and Tennis Corporation, which was formed in 1962.

During the late 1960s and the decade of the 70s, five landmark events occurred that would forever change the landscape of the health/fitness industry and push it into its modern period beginning in the 1980s. The first notable occurrence was the development of Nautilus machines in the early 1970s by Arthur Jones, an unconventional eccentric who was at the forefront of an effort that questioned many of the standard prescription guidelines for training. Based on the principle of variable resistance, these resistance machines took the young industry by storm. For the first time ever, average Americans had equipment that they could use to muscularly condition themselves in a relatively short period of time. In the process, Nautilus became the standard piece of equipment for health/fitness facilities and began appearing in almost every gym, YMCA, athletic club, and racquet club in the United States. The popularity of this equipment led many racquet clubs and athletic clubs to convert one or more of their racquet courts into a "Nautilus Center," for which they charged additional fees to access the equipment.

The second milestone event was the introduction of the Lifecycle. Initially developed by Dr. Keene Dimmick, Ray Wilson subsequently purchased the rights for the Lifecycle from Dimmick, and shortly thereafter retained his first sales person, industry legend Augie Nieto. Under the entrepreneurial leadership and spirit of Wilson and Nieto, the Lifecycle become the first commercial, electronically operated stationary bicycle. The Lifecycle, by providing a user-friendly, fun way to perform cardiovascular exercise, helped advance the relatively young industry by motivating people to engage in stationary cycling.

The third significant event was the work of Kenneth Cooper, MD, who conducted groundbreaking research on the benefits of aerobic exercise. In his bestselling book, *Aerobics*, Dr. Cooper introduced the world to an easy-to-complete way to quantify the aerobic impact of physical activity and to the medical and health benefits of aerobic activity. Dr. Cooper's research and his resulting book produced a surge of interest in both exercise and health/fitness clubs that would springboard the industry into the mainstream of public life.

The fourth significant event of this period was the introduction of "aerobic dancing" by Jackie Sorenson and Jazzercise by Judi Sheppard Misset. These two women introduced the concept of group exercise, based on music and choreography, to the general public. These two programs became a driving force in the evolution of the fitness industry and the beginning of the industry's acceptance of women as an important audience for fitness.

The fifth and final noteworthy development involved the efforts of the American College of Sports Medicine (ACSM). ACSM, a renowned professional association of sports medicine, medical, and exercise science specialists, led the way in developing and disseminating the first set of nationally recognized guidelines for exercise testing and prescription. First printed in 1975, these guidelines would subsequently serve as a benchmark for all health/fitness professionals for prescribing exercise and assessing fitness.

In addition to the aforementioned trailblazing factors, two other individuals also had a substantial impact on the industry in the 1970s—Arnold Schwarzenegger and Richard Simmons. A former Mr. Universe, Schwarzenegger became the face of Gold's Gym (and later World Gym). Subsequently, through movies, such as Pumping Iron, he introduced an entirely new generation of people to the benefits of weight training. Concurrently, Simmons, with the introduction of his market-savvy videos, such as *Sweatin to the Oldies* and *Dance Your Pants Off*, became a fitness icon to millions of stay-at-home women. All told, over 20 million copies of Simmons' energizing and entertaining exercise videos have been sold to date.

As a result of the collective confluence of the previously noted developments, events, and individuals, the advent of the modern health/fitness and sport club industry occurred. During this significant period, the racquet-club industry grew quickly. At the same time, several new types of health/fitness clubs were introduced to the marketplace, including the Sports Training Institute of New York (facilities that offered a blend of physical therapy, personal training, and membership); Cardio Fitness Centers in New York City (corporate fitness centers that were staffed by exercise physiologists who had at least a master's degree); and Lucille Roberts women's only clubs.

The Modern Period (1980-2000)

The 1980s

In 1981, the International Racquet Sports Association (IRSA) was formed by the merging of the National Court Club Association and the National Indoor Tennis Association. The formation of IRSA represented the first landmark event of the modern era. The early founders of IRSA, Rick Caro, Norm Cates, Curt Buesman, and others, had no idea at the time that the association they created in 1981 would go on, under the leadership of its founding director, John McCarthy, to become the leading voice for the health/fitness industry and would serve as a compelling factor in the emerging recognition of this industry as an essential part of the American culture.

In 1981, the International Racquet Sports Association (IRSA) was formed by the merging of the National Court Club Association and the National Indoor Tennis Association.

According to early research conducted by IRSA, there were a total of approximately 6,200 clubs in 1982. By the end of the decade, eight years later, that number would rise to 13,854 clubs, servicing approximately 21 million Americans or 7.4 percent of the total population. This figure represented an increase of over 100 percent in the number of health, fitness, and sport clubs (Figure 1-1) over the eight-year period from 1982 to 1990. The 100 percent plus growth in the number of health/fitness clubs during the 1980s and the corresponding growth in the number of health/fitness club users (up to approximately 21 million) were fueled by several landmark activities, as well as the continued popularity of health/fitness facilities that was sparked by the landmark events of the 1970s.

Comparatively speaking, the 6,200 clubs that existed when the decade of the 1980s began and the 13,854 clubs that brought the decade to a close represented a real mix. For one thing, the racquet and tennis clubs began to diversify, creating fitness centers out of existing racquet courts (the beginning of the multipurpose club), as more consumers expressed an interest in engaging in cardiovascular and resistance training. Individually owned and operated health/ fitness clubs, commonly called "mom & pop" clubs, sprouted rapidly. Many of these clubs incorporated the term "Nautilus" in their commercial name as a means of attracting a wider audience. During this time period, Bally's became

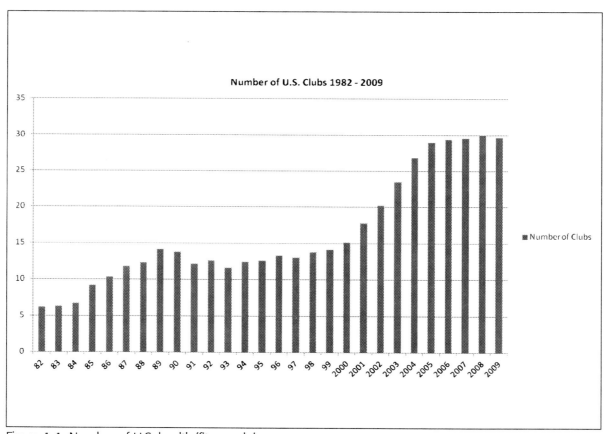

Figure 1-1. Number of U.S. health/fitness clubs

the industry leader, through its consolidation of many of the smaller chains (e.g., Holiday Health, Scandinavian, etc.).

In the process, Bally's became the face of the industry, much to the dismay of IRSA, which focused on representing health/fitness clubs that were committed to operating in a prudent, ethical manner. The emergence of Bally's was seen as both a positive and negative for the industry. On one hand, Bally's brought consumers to the industry; on the other hand, Bally's generated a degree of negative publicity on occasion because of its aggressive business practices.

In addition to commercial health/fitness clubs, the 1980s saw the emergence of the corporate fitness center industry. Because research showed that employee-based fitness programs brought a return for the company, many corporations began to actively integrate on-site heath/fitness facilities into their employee offerings. One of the first was the Pepsi Center in Purchase, New York, under the leadership of Dr. Dennis Colacino. Eventually, corporations such as Exxon, Monsanto, and Johnson and Johnson became the benchmarks for this new segment of the industry during this period.

The 1980s saw the emergence of the corporate fitness center industry.

Cardio Fitness of New York, which initially arose in the late 1970s as a result of the enterprising endeavors of Dr. Jerry Zuckerman, was the first club chain in the 1980s to focus its efforts on offering its clients the opportunity to achieve scientific and medically based cardiovascular fitness, targeting corporate executives. Another institutional entry during the 1980s was the Fitness Company of New York, which was developed on both a scientific and corporate health model of fitness. The Sports Training Institute (STI) of New York, founded in 1975 by Dr. Michael O'Shea, was the first club group to bring a personal training model to the market. While STI eventually closed, its organizational structure and approach would become a model for the entire industry and one of the landmark events of the 1980s. Subsequently, club chains, such as Ray Wilson's Family Fitness Centers in California and 24 Hour Nautilus in Northern California, became major players in the low-dues dollar business segment of the industry. In later years, they joined together to become the largest organizational player in the industry—24 Hour Fitness.

Tennis Corporation of America (TCA), originally founded by Allan Schwartz as a tennis club, became a leading operator of both tennis clubs and sports clubs. The Midtown Tennis Club, TCA's first club, which was opened in 1969, was the largest indoor tennis club at the time. Several other highly regarded industry-based companies, including Fitcorp of Boston, a corporate fitness-based company, and Club Sports International of Denver (now known as Wellbridge), an operator of high-end sports clubs, were also established during this period. About this time, women's-only clubs began to flourish, with chains such as Lucille Robert's and Living Well Lady. As the 1980s came to a close and the number of clubs had reached in excess of 13,000 facilities, the diversity of club offerings had expanded to include such facilities as pure racquet/tennis clubs, multipurpose sports clubs, fitness clubs, YMCAs, and corporate fitness centers.

As the number of clubs grew in the 1980s, so did the number of members who used the clubs and the manner in which they used them. While no accurate estimate of club patronage was available in 1980, by 1987 the industry was able to estimate that it served 17 million members, who on average used the club 72 times a year (about 1.4x a week) (Figures 1-2 and 1-3). The research also indicated that out of the 17 million members, approximately 30.6 percent (5.3 million) could be considered core members (i.e., individuals who use a particular club at least 100x a year) (Figure 1-4). This figure indicated that about one-third of all members actually were participating at their club at least twice a week.

The rapid growth in the number of clubs and members during the 1980s was fueled by both documented data that supported both the need for and the value of engaging in physical activity on a regular basis and the impact that targeted programming had on popular culture. An outpouring of new research continued to show the "exercise is medicine" connection. Study after study linked regular exercise with a reduction in cardiovascular disease, as well as almost every other health-related disorder, including diabetes, high blood pressure, cancer, and obesity. While such data definitely played a role in helping bring more people to the clubs, a more likely factor in that regard was the introduction of programming that emphasized the trends of the popular culture.

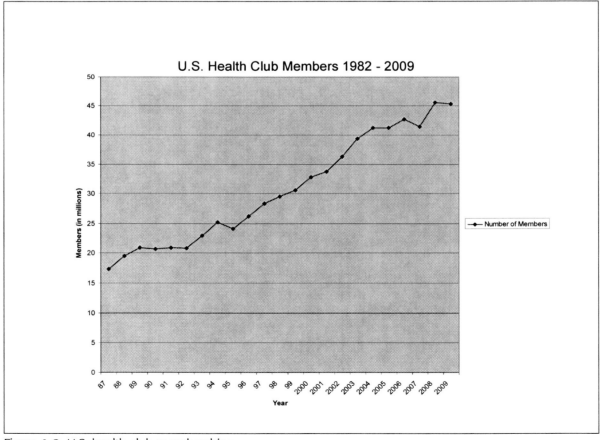

Figure 1-2. U.S. health club memberships

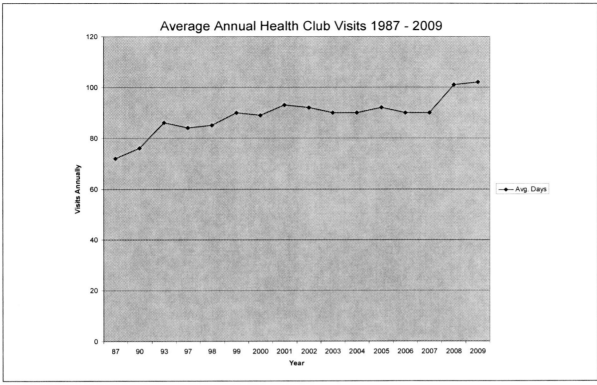

Figure 1-3. Average member visits annually

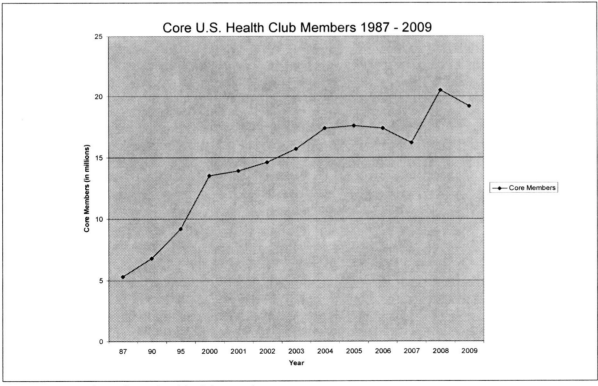

Figure 1-4. Number of core health club members

The rapid growth of aerobics introduced an entirely new market to health/ fitness clubs— women.

Programming innovations were a main factor in club growth in the 1980s. The biggest program trend to influence the industry and a landmark event by itself was the explosion of aerobic group-exercise classes (commonly referred to as "aerobics"). The rapid growth of aerobics introduced an entirely new market to health/fitness clubs—women. The primary appeal of aerobics to women was its dance orientation and, arguably more importantly, its socialization of exercise. Jacki Sorensen and her aerobic dancing program, along with Judy Misset and her Jazzercise offering, took the country by storm, both introduced around 1969. These popular exercise modalities were soon followed by high-impact aerobics and then low-impact aerobics, which were popularized in the mid-1980s by Jane Fonda in her best-selling book, *Jane Fonda's Workout*, as well as shortly thereafter in a series of books and videos that collectively sold over 20 million copies. The movie "Perfect," with Jamie Lee Curtis, also helped to popularize the "aerobic dance" craze during this period. By the end of the 1980s, aerobic dance classes were bringing more people to clubs than any other activity.

In the mid-1980s, personal training became a program trend in the industry, particularly on the east and west coast. Concurrently, racquet sports also played a significant role in the growing movement by facilities to become more program driven. The 1980s also saw the industry make a strong push toward raising the professional credibility of its instructors. In that regard, the American College of Sports Medicine undertook the preeminent role in the effort to certify health/fitness professionals. Joining ACSM in the effort were organizations such as the American Fitness and Aerobics Association (AFAA), The American Council on Exercise (ACE), The International Dance Exercise Association (IDEA), and the National Strength and Conditioning Association (NSCA). In response, each of these organizations offered educational and/ or certification programs to support the growing demand by the industry for qualified health/fitness professionals.

Another significant occurrence in the 1980s was the rapid growth of a new factor in the health/fitness industry—fitness equipment manufacturers. While Nautilus continued to flourish as a manufacturer and distributor of resistance training equipment, new competitors arose to serve the emerging market. For example, during this period, Eagle, later to become Cybex, became a significant player in the resistance equipment business. Joining Cybex were companies, such as BodyMasters, Paramount, and Universal. On the cardiovascular side of the equipment equation, Life Fitness, founded by Augie Nieto of Lifecycle fame, led the way. Through the introduction of the Lifecycle, the Liferower, and later the Lifestep, and the Lifetreadmill, Life Fitness took the lead in the manufacture and sales of cardiovascular equipment. StairMaster was another successful equipment manufacturing company that originated in the 1980s, under the visionary leadership of Randy Peterson and Nicholas Orlando. StairMaster evolved from the landmark creation, manufacturing, and marketing of the StairMaster—the first mechanical stairclimbing machine. It could safely be argued that the StairMaster was the industry's signature product during the 1980s and might have been the most popular form of cardiovascular training equipment in the United States during this period. The success of Life Fitness and StairMaster led other companies, such as Trotter, Unisen, and Precor, to enter the fitness equipment industry. During this decade, the motorized treadmill was even further popularized by companies such as Quinton and Trotter and later blossomed under the efforts of companies such as Precor, Unisen, and Life Fitness.

The 1990s

At the beginning of the decade, a total of 13,854 clubs were operating in the United States. By the end of the decade, that total had grown to approximately 16,000 clubs, an overall increase of 15 percent (Figure 1-1). Concurrently, the number of club members increased by 36 percent from 21 million members at the beginning of the decade to 33 million by the end of the decade (Figure 1-2). During this period, the number of core members in health/fitness clubs increased by 100 percent, from just less than seven million to nearly 14 million. Interestingly, the average club member at the end of the decade used the club on average 89 times a year, up from an average of 72 times a year 10 years earlier (Figure 1-3). In a similar vein, the percentage of Americans who were members of clubs grew from just over seven percent of the total population of the United States at the beginning of the decade to 13 percent of the population at the end of the decade. All of the aforementioned data indicates that the industry grew more in terms of both the number of members using clubs and how frequently these members used the clubs, rather than being simply a by-product of the proliferation in the number of clubs. In other words, demand was growing faster than supply, a positive indicator for the continued growth of the industry.

> In the 1990s, the number of core members in health/fitness clubs increased by 100 percent.

A significant change in the market demographics of the average club member also occurred in the 1990s. During the growth period of the 70s and 80s, the typical member of a health/fitness club was a male between the ages of 18 and 34, with an annual income under $50,000. As the industry progressed during the decade, however, the demographics of club members changed. The primary market for membership became individuals who were older (35 to 54), as well as more affluent ($50,000 to $75,000). By the end of the decade, the average age and household income of prospects continued to climb. At that point, a member was most likely to be between 35-54, equally likely to be male or female, and likely to be someone making in excess of $75,000 annually.

The aforementioned demographic swing, along with the new focus on family, would cause significant changes in the industry during the decade. It should be noted that during the 1990s, the total amount of retail spending in the industry had grown from around $6.5 billion in the early 1990s to $11.6 billion by the end of the decade, an increase of over 50 percent in consumer spending on health/fitness memberships (Figure 1-5).

As a result of both the under supply of health/fitness clubs and the growing financial performance of these commercial entities, the investment world began to look at the health/fitness club industry as a viable investment option. The movement of substantial equity into the industry from non-industry sources, such as equity groups, merchant banks, etc., represents one of the landmark

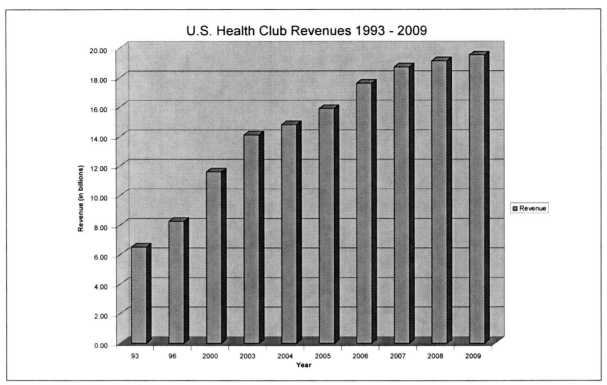

Figure 1-5. U.S. health club revenues

occurrences in the 1990s for the industry. In fact, this influx of investment was a precursor of many of the changes that would take place in the 21st century.

From a club and facility perspective, the 1990s brought several significant changes, including:

- Consolidation and the formation of larger multi-club operators on a local, regional, and national scale (e.g., Bally, 24 Hour Fitness, Town Sports International, Wellbridge, Sport & Health, Lifetime Fitness, Club One, etc.)
- The establishment of fitness centers (i.e., fitness- and exercise-only centers with no sports component)
- The development of large suburban multipurpose clubs that focused primarily on the family (e.g., Lifetime Fitness, Western Athletic Clubs, Leisure Sports, etc.)
- The creation of multiple-modality studios (e.g., aerobics, spinning, Yoga, etc.)
- The dawn of the club-based spa
- The creation of distinct club brands (e.g., Bally, Crunch, Equinox, 24 Hour Fitness, Lifetime Fitness, LA Fitness, etc.)
- The entry of hospital-based facilities into the industry, in large part driven by the aging population and the realization of the medical community that "prevention" should be an integral part of the medical business model
- The entry of expensive large-scale, community-owned and operated recreation centers, which would compete in the industry on a not-for-profit basis

From a club and facility perspective, the 1990s brought several significant changes, including the creation of distinct club brands such as Equinox.

- The expansion of the number of YMCAs and JCCs into a more competitive position in an attempt to serve the fitness market
- The development of apartment- and hotel-based fitness centers

The aforementioned changes in the types of health/fitness facilities and operations were driven by the evolving demographics, alterations in popular culture, additional research on the benefits of exercise, and the maturing of the industry from a purely business perspective. The 1990s also served as host to some of the most significant program and service trends to hit the industry since its earliest years. Among the more influential trends and program practices to arise during this period were the following:

- Spinning. Introduced by Johnny G in 1987, spinning became the rage during the early to mid-90s and has continued to be one of the industry's most sought-after group-exercise programs. Spinning served as the seed for a host of group-cycling programs that emerged on the market during this period (e.g., Schwinn, Keiser, Reebok, etc.); spinning involves group-based cycling that is done to music.
- Yoga and Pilates. As the average age of the club members continued to increase in the 1990s, classes in yoga and Pilates became mainstays of the industry. The trend was toward softer activity that emphasized stretching and movement, rather than aerobics. Yoga is an Eastern form of moving meditation that combines stretching with breathing. Pilates is a form of exercise that is based on principles that were developed by Joseph Pilates in the 1920s.

- Weight training. Research showing the beneficial effects of resistance training on bone health, weight control, and overall health led to an enormous increase in the popularity of weight training, particularly among women.
- Personal training. The public's perception of personal training changed dramatically in the 1990s. Once considered a fringe program that appealed to a very small audience of affluent members, personal training became the primary program thrust of the industry during this period, as even more individuals recognized the value of receiving personalized attention and instruction. By the end of decade, clubs operated by Equinox and Sports Club/LA were often generating personal training revenue in excess of $2 million annually.
- Packaged group exercise. In the 1990s, the focus on "aerobics" had generally been replaced in the industry with "group exercise," and with it, an emphasis on having more diversity in group-exercise programming. In the process, programs, such as STEP, Body Pump, Spinning, Precision Cycling, Body Rage, and Kickbox Fitness, among others, became household programs in the industry. By the late 1990s, Les Mills' packaged group-fitness programs (e.g., Body Pump, Body Rage, etc.) had become a dominant force in the health/fitness club industry.
- Kids' programming. By the end of the decade, most suburban clubs had come to realize that their ability to successfully attract a sufficient number of members would, in large part, be driven by their ability to offer a variety of youth-oriented programs.
- Seniors' programming. In the 1990s, the ever-increasing age level of the average club member, in part driven by the aging of the baby boomers, created a need for an entirely new focus of programming that was geared toward providing exercise alternatives for those individuals over the age of 50. For example, the development of Wellbridge was in response to this particular program trend.
- Day spas. By the end of the decade, the day-spa concept had taken hold in the industry, as many members perceived spa treatments to be an integral part of their overall approach to improving their level of well-being.

In 1996, possibly the most important landmark for the health and fitness industry ever to occur happened when the U.S. government released the *U.S. Surgeon General's Report on Physical Activity and Health*. In this report, the U.S. Surgeon General provided the American public with a clear, yet critical, message: Americans would benefit immensely from a regular program of physical activity. In essence, the message detailed the fact that engaging in physical activity on a regular basis contributes significantly to reductions in many health-related disorders. Furthermore, if specific activity guidelines were followed, individuals could improve their health and prolong the quality of their life. The full impact of this report has yet to be completely realized, since most Americans have not fully embraced the significance of the report. Nonetheless, the impact of this particular report on the industry was very significant.

The 1990s also served as a springboard for some of the most significant equipment innovations in the industry since the development of StairMaster,

In 1996, the U.S. government released the *U.S. Surgeon General's Report on Physical Activity and Health*.

Lifecycle, and Nautilus machines. Among the critically acclaimed equipment concepts that occurred during this period were the following:

- The elliptical trainer. Precor introduced the concept of elliptical training in 1995. Named the EFX, the Precor elliptical trainer had a major impact on equipment-based training. The elliptical trainer was designed to provide a low-impact, comfortable approach to training that would slowly lead to a significant decrease in the popularity of such activities as indoor cycling and mechanical stairclimbing.
- Spinning bike. The introduction of the spinning bike was a new twist on the bicycle ergometers of the 70s and 80s (for example, those that were manufactured by Body Guard and Monarch). The spinning bike allowed members to train in social groups, while simultaneously controlling the intensity level of their training.
- Plate-loaded resistance equipment. First introduced by Hammer in the late 1980s, but subsequently popularized in the 1990s, plate-loaded equipment combined the safety features of selectorized machines with the impact of free-weight training.
- Treadmills. While treadmills had been around for over 40 years, companies, such as Star Trac, Life Fitness, Quinton, and Precor brought new dynamics to this particular type of equipment in the 1990s. In the process, treadmills became one of the most popular pieces of equipment in the industry, as manufacturers included programming options, as well as audio and visual entertainment, as a basic feature on their products—all at a reasonable cost.
- Pilates-based equipment. While Pilates equipment has been around since the 1920s, it was essentially introduced to the club industry during the 1990s. By the end of the decade, Pilates equipment, continuing to grow in popularity, became one of the fastest growing trends, according to data released by IHRSA.
- Personal entertainment systems. The introduction of Cardio Theater in 1991 by Tony Deleede (and later Broadcast Vision) was a landmark occurrence in the industry. For many consumers, the introduction of Cardio Theater changed the way that they perceived their club experience.

> The introduction of the spinning bike was a new twist on the bicycle ergometers of the 70s and 80s.

The final noteworthy event that occurred in the 1990s was the change in direction taken by the International Health, Racquet & Sportsclub Association (IHRSA). From its inception and through the first half of the 1990s, IHRSA (formerly IRSA) had focused its efforts on being an association of quality clubs. This focus allowed it to develop resources to upgrade the professionalism of its membership. During the later half of the 1990s, however, IHRSA undertook a conscious shift in its strategy. In the process, IHRSA became an industry trade association, one that focused on public advocacy for the industry and one that expanded its role in the growing international market. This change in direction allowed IHRSA to partner with other organizations in an attempt to establish a more significant voice for the industry in public policy and industry promotion.

The Early 21st Century (2000-2010)

At the beginning of the new century, the United States had almost 16,000 health/fitness clubs that served approximately 33 million members. By the beginning of 2010, the number of U.S. clubs had grown to 29,750, with just over 45 million members (Figures 1-1 and 1-2). During this period, the percentage of Americans who were members of clubs increased from approximately 13 percent of the population in 2000 to 16 percent of the population by the beginning of 2010. In other words, in a decade, the number of clubs had increased by nearly 87 percent, while the number of club members had grown by slightly over 36 percent.

The aforementioned trend (the number of clubs growing faster than the member population) is the polar opposite of what occurred during the 1990s, when the growth in membership outpaced the growth in clubs, and demand exceeded supply. A review of industry data going as far back as 1987 shows that the average number of members per facility has dropped over the past 25 years from over 2,000 per club to approximately 1,500 per club.

The apparent reason for the aforementioned situation was an overdevelopment in the number of clubs, which, in turn, outpaced the growth in membership. In other words, the industry began to carve the pie into smaller pieces, rather than grow the size of the pie. Club growth had created saturation in several significant areas, such as New York, Los Angeles, and Chicago, as well as in other major metropolitan markets. In these areas, the number of clubs far surpassed the growth in market demand. Most of this shift in supply and demand was fueled by the influx of investment capital and the growth strategies of various regional and national club chains, including Bally's, 24 Hour Fitness, LA Fitness, Equinox, Sports Club/LA, Town Sports International, and Life Time Fitness, among others. The supply-and-demand equation has been further

In some areas, the number of clubs far surpassed the growth in market demand.

tilted by the fact that a significant portion of the club growth has occurred in what is commonly referred to as "fitness boxes"—club models that look and feel the same and that lack any real brand differentiation. Another contributor to this excess supply of clubs has been the rapid growth of small franchise operations since 2005 (e.g., Anytime Fitness with over 1,400 facilities, Curves with over 8,000 facilities, and Snap Fitness with over 1,200 facilities), and high-volume, low-priced clubs (e.g., Planet Fitness, Blink, etc.) brought additional operators to a relatively saturated market. On the other hand, all of the blame for this oversupply cannot be attributed purely to the growth in the number of commercial clubs, as there has also been a significant growth in not-for-profit facilities (e.g., community-based facilities, university-based facilities, and medical-based models) (see Figure 1-6).

Looking closer at industry research, as detailed in *IHRSA's 2010 Global Report,* it is apparent that during the first decade of the new century, the industry has had more success generating usage from its existing members, rather than attracting new members to the market. In 1990, average club members used their club 79 times a year, while by 2010, that usage figure had increased to approximately 102 visits a year. Furthermore, the number of core members (i.e., those individuals who utilized their club more than 100 times a year) had increased to over 19 million, or approximately 44 percent of the total membership base. In fact, the most active club members were those individuals who were over the age of 55. The available statistics indicate that by 2010, the industry had managed to elicit greater usage from its existing membership, to

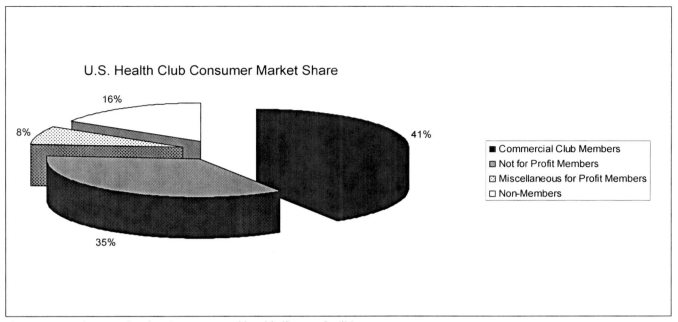

Figure 1-6. Industry mix of various types of health/fitness facilities

a greater degree than it had been able to drive additional nonmembers into the clubs. As a result of these trends, the industry currently faces three key challenges: an oversupply of clubs; an insufficient influx of new members; and a lack of product differentiation.

In 2010, statistics indicate that the demographic profile of a U.S. club member was shifting. By 2010, the U.S. health club consumer profile was as follows (refer to Figures 1-7, 1-8, and 1-9):

- Fifty-three percent of members were men and 47 percent were women, statistics that represent a radical shift from five years earlier when men composed 43 percent of members and women 57 percent of members. In essence, over the past five years, membership has swung from being heavily weighted toward women to now being more male oriented.

- The 55-and-over population was the fastest growing age segment during the first five years of the 21st century. Even by 2010, when the overall growth of this particular age grouping had slowed down somewhat, it still represented approximately 23 percent of the membership, up from under 10 percent in the mid-90s.

- The 35-to-54 age group encompasses the largest segment of club membership at 36 percent, having grown by over 140 percent over the last 20 years.

- While those individuals who are 18 to 34 years of age still entail 31 percent of the membership, this group had the least growth in the past two decades.

- The number of members under the age of 18 continued to grow, with approximately 10 percent of all members in 2010 being under the age of 18.

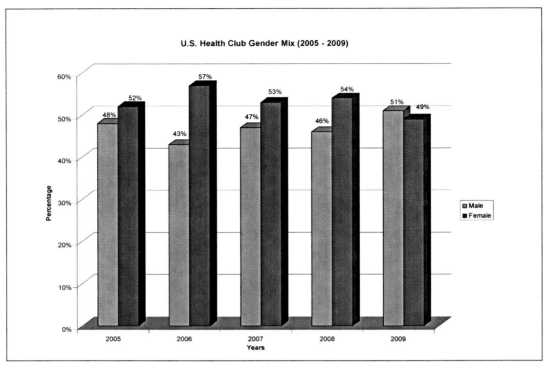

Figure 1-7. U.S. health club membership gender mix

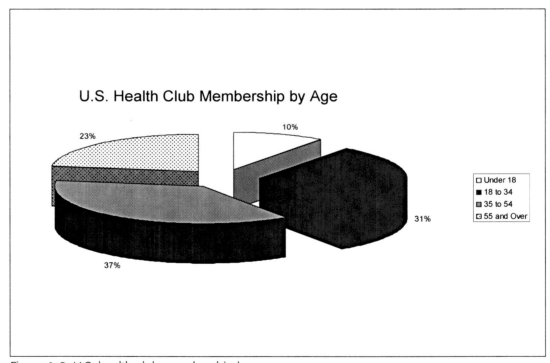

Figure 1-8. U.S. health club membership by age

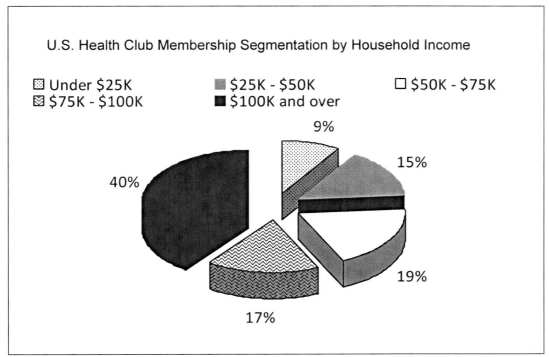

Figure 1-9. U.S. health club membership segmentation by household income

- Membership penetration is highest for women 35 to 44 and men 25 to 34.
- Thirty-six percent of all members have household incomes over $100,000 annually, while another 18 percent of members have household incomes between $75,000 and $100,000 annually. The industry continues to see its audience come from a higher income bracket than it did a decade earlier.
- Over half of all club members have a four-year college degree.

A Glimpse at Several Future Club Industry Trends

By 2010, a number of health/fitness club industry trends had shifted, as the facilities, equipment, and programs employed in the industry reflected the new demographics and psychographics of the American population. These trends represent the true state of the health/fitness club industry, as of 2010, and are precursors for what the industry can expect over the next one to two decades. Among the most significant trends that have evolved over the past few years are the following:

❑ Facilities
  - High-volume, low-priced clubs (HVLP). These are clubs that offer limited amenities, 24-hour access in most cases, an abundance of equipment, and relatively limited staffing all for under $20 a month. Examples of HVIP facilities include Planet Fitness and Blink.
  - Independent studios that are designed to appeal to niche markets (e.g., cycling studios, such as Soul Cycling, Pilates studios, yoga studios, personal training studios).

- Small franchise operations, for example, facilities that provide convenience and affordability (e.g., Anytime, Snap, etc.), or concerns, such as day spas and salons, that target women.

❑ Equipment
- Cardiovascular equipment that feature personal media centers that include a variety of attractions, such as LED touch screens, smart phone attachments, internet access, and cloud software applications.
- Functional fitness accessories, such as TRX, Bosu balls, kettlebells, Indian clubs, etc.

❑ Programs and services
- Boot camps and "extreme" training camps, such as mixed martial arts, and elite athlete training.
- Fusion fitness involving activities that blend diverse modalities, such as yoga and cycling, Pilates and weight training, yoga and Pilates, etc. This approach is designed to cater to consumers who want/need variety for motivational purposes.
- Core fitness classes that concentrate on working the core musculature.
- Packaged group-exercise programs, such as Les Mills and Zumba that offer predictable, entertaining, and effective exercise routines. These programs provide great efficiency for clubs, as well as compelling and constantly changing exercise routines for participants.
- Youth sports performance conditioning. The growing epidemic of childhood obesity and America's fascination with organized youth sports helps fuel this trend.
- Group training. As a result of the recession of 2008/2009, and an evolving consumer attitude toward materialism, group training offers members modified individualized attention in a small social setting at lower cost.
- Internet based training. As technology has evolved, and consumers have become more technology savvy and time-pressured, clubs have begun to offer a variety of Internet-based services, including personal training on the Internet.

The U.S. industry continues to face challenges brought on by an increasing demand from the public and government for professional accountability.

At the present time, the U.S. industry continues to face challenges brought on by an increasing demand from the public and government for professional accountability. As a consequence of IHRSA's and the industry's efforts to have the industry accepted as a mainstream entity and the maturation of the U.S. health/fitness club industry into a $20 billion undertaking, both the public and the government have begun to place ever greater demands on the level of accountability of both the industry and the professionals involved in the delivery of fitness services. Among the examples of some of the public and government expectations that have either occurred or are in the process of transpiring (as of the publication of this book) are the following:
- State-level legislation that mandates the placement of automated external defibrillators in every health club (as of 2010, 11 states have passed legislation requiring health clubs to have AEDs)

- State-level legislation that mandates the registration or licensure of personal trainers
- State-level legislation governing the operation of spa services
- Higher expectations by the public for business practices grounded in integrity from all health/fitness club operators
- Expectations from the financial world for greater accountability and standardization of accounting practices in health/fitness clubs
- Expectations from investors for quarterly earnings performances that are consistent with Wall Street expectations
- Expectations by the public that the franchising of health/fitness clubs will continue. In that regard, beginning in 2003 and continuing through 2010, the industry has witnessed a substantial growth in the level of franchising groups, such as Anytime Fitness, Gold's, Powerhouse, Curves, Snap, and Crunch, among others.

As of 2010, 11 states have passed legislation requiring health clubs to have AEDs.

2

The Physical Activity Beliefs and Behaviors of Americans and Their Implications for Health/ Fitness Clubs

Chapter Objectives

In order to gain a greater understanding of the physical activity practices of Americans and ultimately their potential suitability as health/fitness club members, it is important to understand the values and attitudes that Americans have toward physical activity. In that regard, research has shown that the values and attitudes held by individuals are the major determinants of their behavior. In other words, the core determinant of a person's actions is that individual's core values, which are at the heart of the attitudes they have. In fact, the success of the health and fitness club business is extremely dependent upon the physical activity beliefs and behaviors of Americans. This chapter provides an overview of the available research pertaining to both the attitudes of Americans toward physical activity and their actual physical activity behavior. The information in the chapter is designated to help club owners and operators better position their clubs for success by enabling them to more fully understand the beliefs and behaviors of those individuals that they potentially serve.

Core American Values Toward Physical Activity and Health

When Americans are asked to rank their core values and how those values align with their overall satisfaction with life, health and fitness are an integral part of their response. According to research conducted by Roper Starch for IHRSA in 2001, which was later updated in a report released in 2007 entitled Fitness American Style, Americans rank health as the third most important value behind family and spouse. Concurrently, they rank fitness seventh among

> The success of the health and fitness club business is extremely dependent upon the physical activity beliefs and behaviors of Americans.

their top eight values (family, spouse, health, friends, career, diet, fitness, and money). It is interesting to note that both health and fitness are rated as more important than money (refer to Figure 2-1).

On the other hand, when indicating the importance of each value to their overall level of satisfaction with life, health and fitness seem far less relevant to Americans than values, such as family, spouse, and money. Taken at face value, it is evident that when Americans prioritize their values, that health and fitness are important, but when measured as a contributor to their overall level of satisfaction with life, health and fitness fall lower on the scale.

When Americans are questioned in greater depth about their attitude toward the importance of health and fitness, they share the following:

- 97 percent of Americans say it is essential and/or important to maintain good health.
- 91 percent of Americans say it is essential and/or important to keep up their physical appearance.
- 83 percent of Americans say it is essential and/or important to get enough exercise.
- 81 percent of Americans say it is essential to become more physically fit.

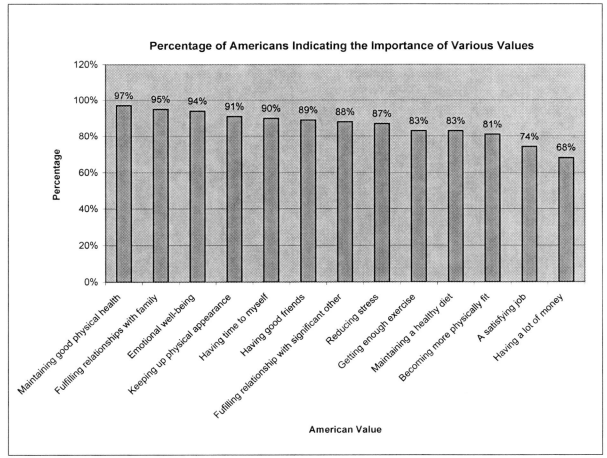

Figure 2-1. Percentage of Americans indicating the importance of various values

- Women are far more likely than men to say fitness is essential to good health (nearly 60 percent of women versus 50 percent for men). Women are also more likely (40 percent to 31 percent) than men to say fitness is important to appearance.
- 74 percent of Americans are satisfied with their physical health, while 73 percent are satisfied with their physical appearance. Only 49 percent are satisfied with the amount of physical activity they get.
- Younger men seem more satisfied than younger women with their health and appearance, but as both groups age, men become less satisfied and women more satisfied.

When this data and the supporting research are examined, the following conclusions can be drawn:

- Americans understand the importance of being healthy and fit, yet they don't see as much value in actually exercising to obtain the health and fitness that they say they value so much.
- Women, more than men, understand the importance of fitness to health and well-being.
- Americans as a rule, and men more than women, are generally satisfied with their health, appearance, and fitness. As a result, they already see themselves as having met the value equation when it comes to health and

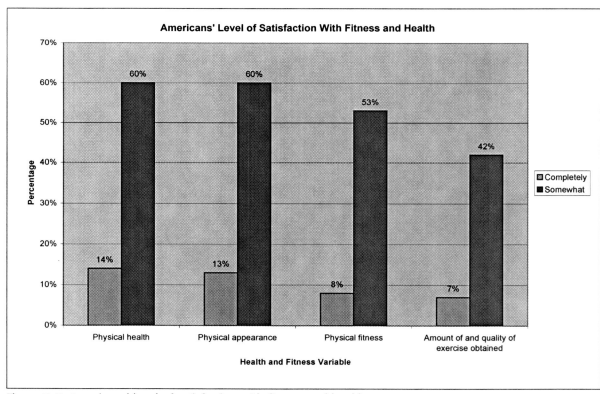

Figure 2-2. Americans' level of satisfaction with fitness and health

fitness and are less likely to see themselves as having a need to actually engage in an activity, such as exercise (refer to Figure 2-2).

What Active Americans Say Are the Reasons They Participate in Exercise and Sports

When men and women are asked for the reasons why they engage in physical activity (exercise and sports), their responses indicate that multiple variables influence their actual behavior. Figure 2-3, based on research conducted by Roper Starch on behalf of the International Health, Racquet & Sportsclub Association (IHRSA) in 2001, provides a concise overview of the multiplicity of reasons Americans give for exercising.

It is clear from looking at Figure 2-3 that men and women have different reasons for exercising. This information is important because understanding these gender-related differences can assist club owners/managers in developing club-based programs that can help attract and retain club members. For example, men are far more inclined than women to claim fun, enjoyment, personal challenge, and competition as driving forces for their exercise habits. Women, in turn, are far more inclined to see losing weight, staying fit, and helping prevent or assist with health-related conditions as their reason for exercising.

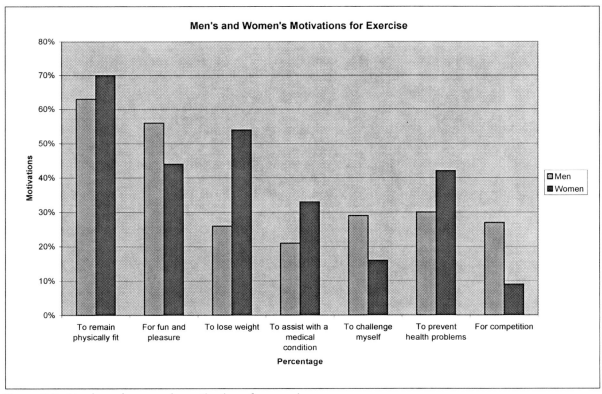

Figure 2-3. Men's and women's motivations for exercise

The Level of Fitness Consciousness Among Americans as a Predictor of Joining and Staying With Exercise

According to the research conducted by American Sports Data in 2003 and supported by the work of Dr. Rod Dishman, Americans can be classified in one of four categories of fitness consciousness: non-believers, indifferent, uninitiated believers, and hard-core participants. Understanding these categories and the accompanying traits and characteristics can assist clubs both in attracting new members and retaining existing ones. Figure 2-4 offers an overview of the traits associated with each basic category.

It is evident that those who are non-believers or indifferent are not good candidates for membership in a health/fitness club because the values and beliefs that they hold toward exercise would be very difficult to overcome when attempting to entice them to join a club. Even if they were sold a membership through "closing techniques," they would be unlikely to ever use their membership. The individuals who have hard-core, favorable attitudes toward fitness represent 16 percent of the population, a total which closely parallels the percentage of Americans who are currently health club members (16 percent). According to data presented in the *IHRSA Health Club Consumer Report*, published in 2010, the percentage of Americans who are enrolled as club members ranges from as low as 8.7 percent in Oklahoma to 23.7 percent in Massachusetts. These statistics suggest that the industry is close to extracting all of the low hanging fruit and needs to develop strategies that will attract the uninitiated segment (64 percent) of the population if it is to continue to grow the membership market.

Non-Believers 2% of the population)	**Indifferent** (16% of the population)	**Uninitiated Believers** (63% of the population)	**Hard-Core Participants** (17% of the population)
Do not embrace the fitness lifestyle	No real interest in fitness	Believe fitness has value	Embrace fitness
Don't believe exercise is important	Negative attitude toward fitness	25% are sedentary and 26% are very active	Doers and believers; apostles of exercise
Sedentary lifestyle	Likely to claim they are not healthy	70% claim to be overweight	Regard their health as excellent
Male dominated	Equally likely to be male or female	More likely to be a woman and younger	57% male
Least educated	Low income and education	37% are college educated	49% are college educated and 38% are making in excess of $75K

Figure 2-4. Traits attributed to each of the basic categories of fitness consciousness

What a Portrait of Those Who Exercise Can Mean to Clubs

In the work that Roper Starch conducted for IHRSA in 2001, exercisers and non-exercisers were identified by a set of personality or psychographic characteristics. Grasping the nuances of these classifications can help club operators better understand the dynamics of how to develop and deliver a personalized club experience that can help attract and retain members. According to Roper's research, there are a total of six classifications: balanced holistics, conscientious preventors, social competitors, abracadabras, woulda-shouldas, and sit-com skeptics. An overview of the key attributes that characterize each of these six different and important groups involves the following:

❑ *Balanced Holistics (13 percent)*. These individuals see exercise as important to both their emotional and physical health. They exercise regularly and focus on reaching a state of internal harmony. They are twice as likely to be club members in comparison to the average American. They define themselves as socially confident, goal-oriented, energetic, and intelligent. They are more likely to be female (58 percent), college educated (32 percent), have a higher household income (average of $42K), be married (69 percent), and younger (40) than the average American. Finally, this group is two-and-a-half times more likely to exercise "religiously" than the general public.

❑ *Conscientious Preventors (8 percent)*. This group takes a balanced approach to physical activity and sees exercise as an avenue for the prevention of health-related problems and as a means to manage existing conditions. They are twice as likely to be club members and describe themselves as health-conscious, family-oriented, religious, and perfectionists. They are more likely to be older women (60 percent female, average age of 55); college educated (32 percent), and have a higher income (average of $46K) than the average American.

❑ *Social Competitors (20 percent)*. These individuals prefer to spend their time in an environment that is social, engaging, and competitive. They are no more likely than other Americans to be club members. They describe themselves as professional, ambitious, risk-taking, and outgoing. They are also more likely to be male (62 percent) and single than the average American. They tend to fall within the average range when it comes to their level of college education and income, but are younger than the average American.

❑ *Abracadabras (14 percent)*. These individuals tend to be de-conditioned and have little desire to pursue exercise. They describe themselves as less socially skillful, health conscious, and energetic than the general population. This group is skewed toward married women with kids at home.

❑ *Woulda-Shouldas (12 percent)*. These are people who exercise, though not on a regular basis, and who tend to feel self conscious about themselves. They describe themselves as out of shape, emotional, shy, and undisciplined. They are most likely to be women (73 percent) and married (60 percent) who have average earnings and slightly less college education than the general public.

Grasping the nuances of personality characteristics can help club operators better understand the dynamics of how to develop and deliver a personalized club experience.

PART ONE   *Introduction to the Health/Fitness Club Industry*

❑ *Sit-Com Skeptics (12 percent)*. Members of this category see exercise as nothing more than a craze that is followed by self-absorbed individuals. They feel that a reasonable diet and clean living are the answer to good health. Generally speaking, they tend to be older married males (70 percent married and 56 percent male), with less education and less household income.

At first glance, a question might arise concerning what value exists in being aware of the aforementioned information. In essence, the answer is fairly straightforward. If club owners/managers were to create a profile questionnaire for their member prospects and existing members and then categorize these individuals into one of the four groups categorized by Roper, then they would have the capability of creating programs and services that would allow them to better tailor the club experience to each group's needs and interests.

What Americans Are Actually Doing When It Comes to Physical Activity

Up to this point, much of this chapter has addressed the beliefs and values that Americans have about exercise and sports. As was previously stated, understanding those values and beliefs will help club operators and/or fitness professionals better understand how they can exert greater influence on changing the exercise and sports behavior of the public and, as a consequence, grow their membership base. This section of the chapter presents an overview of the actual reported physical-activity behavior of Americans. The information is designed to provide further insight into the relationship between values, beliefs, and behavior when it comes to exercise.

In the 2002 American Sports Data (ASD) report on Trends in U.S. Physical Fitness Behavior, physical fitness activity was divided into three distinct categories: fitness, recreation, and outdoor activity. The fitness category included such activities as aerobics, aquatics, free weights, Pilates, yoga, etc. Recreation involved participating in such undertakings as basketball, football, ice-skating, tennis, racquet sports, volleyball, etc. Outdoor activity consisted of engaging in activities such as hiking, rock climbing, mountain biking, skiing, etc. According to Figure 2-5 (based on data compiled in the aforementioned 2002 American Sports Data Report), American involvement in physical-fitness activities on an active basis has increased from 42 million in 1987 to nearly 51 million in 2002 (it should be noted that "active" is defined as 100x in at least one activity annually).

	1987	1990	1993	1997	2000	2002
Millions	42.3	51.5	50	52.6	51.7	50.9
Percent of Total U.S. Population	19.7	23.2	21.8	21.8	20.8	19.8

Figure 2-5. Annual American involvement in physical fitness pursuits on an active basis

46

A review of Figures 2-5 and 2-6 indicates that the percentage of Americans who report being actively involved in physical fitness activity (fitness, sports, outdoor) has continued to drop since 1990, falling to a level of below 20 percent of the population in 2002. It is interesting to note that participation in fitness-only activities has increased from just over 27 billion participation days in 1987 to 30 billion participation days in 2002, although the number of individuals participating in sports activity and outdoor activity has remained relatively flat at 8.3 billion participation days and just under 1.4 billion participation days, respectively (refer to Figure 2-7). This data, along with other statistics provided by the ASD's research, indicate the following macro trends in physical-fitness behavior:

- The number of core or active participants in physical-fitness activity has continued to grow over the past 15 years, but as a percentage of the population, it has remained flat.
- Women are more likely than men to be core or active participants.
- Those 55+ are the largest segment of active individuals.
- 34 percent of those individuals with college degrees are active, while just 13 percent of those individuals who do not have a college education are active.
- Men are far more likely than women to be involved in outdoor activity.

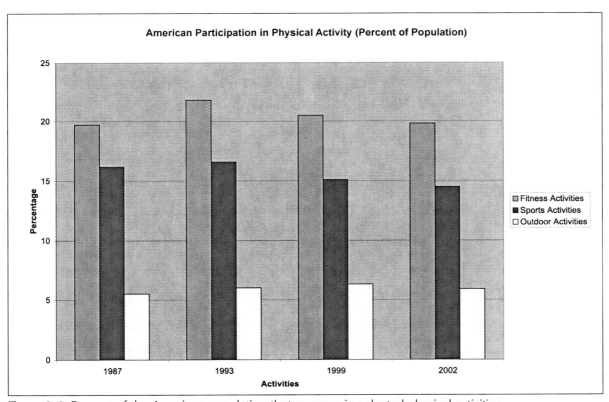

Figure 2-6. Percent of the American population that engages in selected physical activities

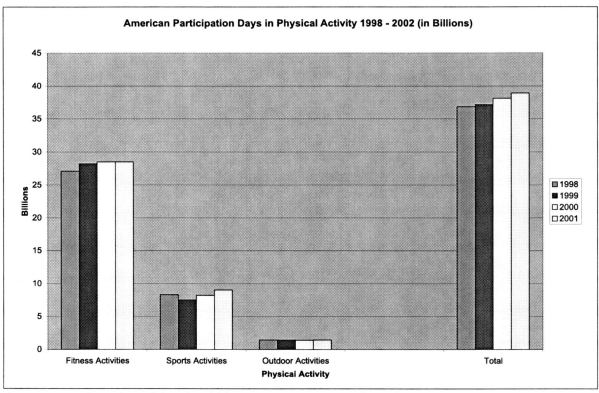

Figure 2-7. Total number of days in which Americans engage in physical activity

- Over the past 10 years, participation in club-based activities, such as high-impact aerobics (40 percent), step aerobics (30 percent), mechanical stairclimbing (10 percent), and stationary cycling (30 percent), have all declined.
- During the past 10 years, the following activities have shown continuous growth in participation: spinning (10 percent), elliptical training (100 percent), free weight training (50 percent), yoga (100 percent), and Pilates (150 percent).

Key Takeaways From Research on American Beliefs and Behavior With Regard to Physical Fitness Behavior

- Americans, in general, understand and acknowledge the fact that exercise and fitness are important to their health. Furthermore, they tend to view both factors as important values in their overall value hierarchy.
- While 80 percent of Americans claim that exercise is important, only 19 percent have adopted the appropriate behavior, in some fashion, that is consistent with this belief.
- While the fitness consciousness of Americans is higher than ever before (according to research and the media), actual fitness behavior is at one of its lowest points in 20 years. Obviously, a real disconnect exists between what the brain knows and the body does.

- Physical fitness behavior is slowly becoming the domain of an older, more educated, and more affluent segment of the American population. As such, exercise behavior seems to be tracking alongside the "baby boomer demographic."

- Health and leading a balanced life seem to be overtaking appearance as a prime factor in whether an individual engages in physical activity on a regular basis.

- One key to attracting people to exercise and fitness is to better understand the personality dynamics of individuals and have the club tailor its promotional and programming package to fit those dynamics. For example, if someone is an uninitiated social competitor, then the club's package must be different for them than it would be for an uninitiated balanced holistic. Likewise, if club operators are core users who could be classified as conscious preventors, they should not expect their target market to be attracted to those factors that attract them.

It is important to be aware of the difference in what motivates women and men and how an individual's age, education, and background can affect that person's behavior. This understanding can help club operators to adapt their efforts to attract and retain members accordingly.

One key to attracting people to exercise and fitness is to better understand the personality dynamics of individuals.

3

Consumer Attitudes Toward Health/Fitness Clubs That Affect Their Reasons for Joining and Staying

Chapter Objectives

The heart and soul of any successful health/fitness club is its membership. Without a thriving membership base, a health/fitness club will never reach its operating and financial potential. Membership, therefore, must be the top priority when it comes to building a successful club. The first step in building club membership is to understand what consumers perceive about the club experience and what triggers influence their decision to join a particular facility. This chapter initially focuses on providing an overview of consumer perceptions of health/fitness clubs and then details the reasons why consumers actually join a health/fitness club.

Consumer Attitudes About Health/Fitness Clubs

As discussed in the previous chapter, the attitudes and beliefs that consumers have about exercise are the primary drivers of their actual exercise behavior. This relationship also applies to consumer behavior with regard to actually joining a health/fitness club. What the consumers perceive about the health/fitness club experience has been shown to play a major role in their decision about whether to become a member. While more personally relevant needs and wants can alter the impact of consumer attitudes as they impact their decision whether to join a club, attitudes toward health/fitness clubs still play a very significant role in their decision whether to become a member of a and more importantly, which health/fitness club to join.

The heart and soul of any successful health/fitness club is its membership.

In 2001, Roper Starch, on behalf of IHRSA, studied the attitudes of both non-members, former club members, and existing club members to gain a more thorough grasp of the underlying attitudes about health/fitness clubs and why people join. This research was the first meaningful work in this arena since the 1985 study sponsored by IHRSA titled, "Why People Join." Among the key facts that Starch identified in his research are the following:

- 66 percent of consumers feel that the purchase of a health-club membership is worth the expense.
- 60 percent of consumers agree that health/fitness clubs offer more knowledge and expertise on fitness than consumers can obtain on their own.
- 56 percent of consumers believe that health/fitness clubs are fun.
- 48 percent of consumers believe that health/fitness clubs are only for those who are physically fit and not for those individuals who are just beginning a fitness program.
- 45 percent of consumers see health/fitness clubs as being for young people.
- 31 percent of consumers believe that health/fitness clubs are places to go to "pick up" others.
- 62 percent of non-members and 73 percent of members believe that health/fitness clubs are overcrowded.

One point that can be deduced from Starch's data is that consumers, in general, place a value on the health/fitness club experience, primarily in the ability of the club to provide an environment of expertise and enjoyment. Concurrently, a perception also exists among the public that health/fitness clubs are overcrowded, and are primarily entities for young people. In addition, a perception exists among nearly one-third of consumers that health/fitness clubs are particularly appropriate places to pick up dates. Obviously, these types of attitudes and beliefs present a challenge to any club that is attempting to attract prospects to its doors.

It should be kept in mind that the aforementioned highlighted findings are generalized across the three segments of the population that Starch studied— non-members, former club members, and current club members. When a closer look is taken at the attitudes by segment (refer to Figures 3-1 and 3-2), even greater understanding of the dynamics of consumer attitudes and their impact on health/fitness club membership can be gained.

Given the information presented in Figures 3-1 and 3-2, the health/fitness club operator could logically extrapolate the following concerning consumer attitudes about health/fitness clubs:

- The non-member is far less likely to see the value in a health/fitness club than either a member or a former member. From a club perspective, this determination means that clubs need to educate prospects better about the real value of the club experience.
- The non-member is far more likely to say a health/fitness club is not a fun place than either a former member or a member. From a club perspective, this conclusion suggests that clubs must do a better job of portraying to consumers the entertainment aspect of the health/fitness club experience.

The non-member is far less likely to see the value in a health/fitness club than either a member or a former member.

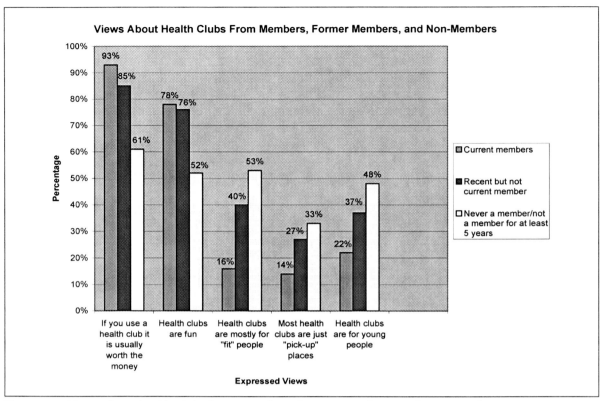

Figure 3-1. Views about health clubs from members, former members, and non-members

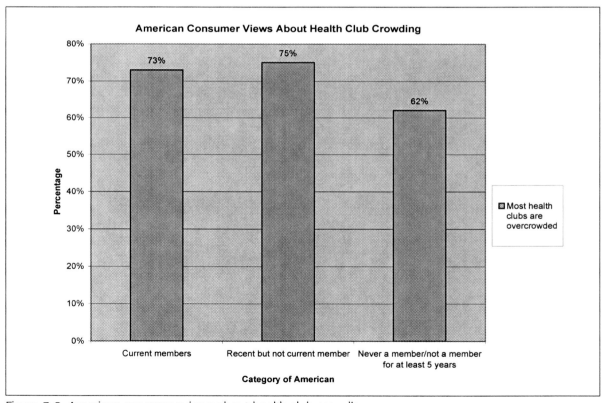

Figure 3-2. American consumer views about health club crowding

- The non-member overwhelmingly believes, in comparison to former members and current members, that health/fitness clubs are for the fit and young, as well as a place to "pick up" someone. In light of the research presented in the first chapter that concluded that the average age of club members is getting older, this perception is not in touch with the actual reality. The pertinent questions have to be, "What are club operators doing to perpetuate these beliefs among the public or what can they do to change them?"
- Non-members, former members, and members all hold a similar view that health/fitness clubs are overcrowded. From the club operator's perspective, this viewpoint is one of the most challenging and possibly damaging perspectives the industry could present. Research has shown that if consumers feel the clubs are too crowded, they will be far less likely to join a health/fitness club.

The Reasons Members Give for Joining a Health/Fitness Club

While the previous section examined the attitudes that consumers hold about health/fitness clubs, this section reviews the reasons club members give for actually joining a particular club. Since approximately 16 percent of the population in the U.S. are health/fitness club members at the present time, the reasons given for joining only reflect a small percentage of the total consumer population. It should be kept in mind that when reviewing this information, that while these reasons can play a critical role in how a club markets itself to the public, these reasons—by themselves—will not help a club overcome the public perceptions of the health/fitness industry. Understanding and then acting on both the attitudes that individuals have toward clubs and the reasons members give for joining a club will be most useful and helpful when developing and implementing a successful health/fitness club operation.

Consumers join health/fitness clubs for a variety of reasons. According to *Fitness American Style III,* prepared for IHRSA in 2007, the top three reasons that new members gave for joining their club were the following:

- Get in shape (64 percent of respondents)
- Convenience of a place to workout (54 percent)
- Stay in shape (49 percent)

An analysis of data from 2001, 2004, and 2007 IHRSA reports can lend clarity to whether the leading reasons for why individuals join a health/fitness club had changed over that period, or if the level of importance behind a specific factor had changed during that same time span. Figure 3-3 provides a graphic illustration of the trends from 2001, 2004, and 2007 concerning the reasons consumers give for joining a health/fitness club. Among the insights that can be gleaned from these trends are the following:

Getting in better shape remains the primary reason members join a club.

- Getting in better shape remains the primary reason members join a club. The percentage of consumers who give this response has dropped from nearly 80 percent of respondents in 2004 to 64 percent in 2007.

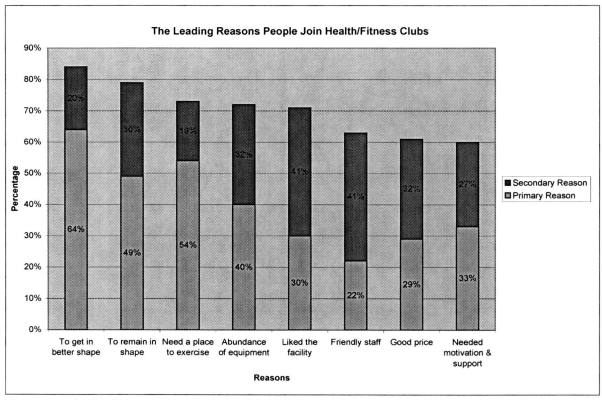

Figure 3-3. The leading reasons people join health/fitness clubs

- While needing a place to exercise was the third most frequently given reason for joining a club in 2007 (49 percent), it received a significantly lower response rate then in either 2004 or 2001, when nearly 60 percent of respondents indicated that this factor was why they joined a club.
- In 2001 and 2004, close to 60 percent of respondents indicated that they joined a club for the motivation, but in 2007, only 20 percent of respondents gave this reason for becoming a member.
- In 2001, consumers indicated that their number one reason for joining a club was because they liked the facility (70 percent), followed closely by the fact that the club was a great value (60 percent), and then by the fact that the club was a place to get in better shape. In 2007, liking the facility or indicating that membership in it was a good value took on less importance.

It appears that over the course of the first seven years of the 21st century, consumers moved from having an "extrinsic goods" perspective (placing their reason for joining a club in terms of how the facility looked or how much it cost) to more of an intrinsic reasoning, based on their personal goals.

In the IHRSA report, *Fitness American Style III*, researchers looked at the differences between why men and women join a health/fitness club. The differences are considerable and are reflected in Figures 3-4 and 3-5. Among the most salient points that can be derived from this gender-based comparison of why individuals join a health/fitness club are the following:

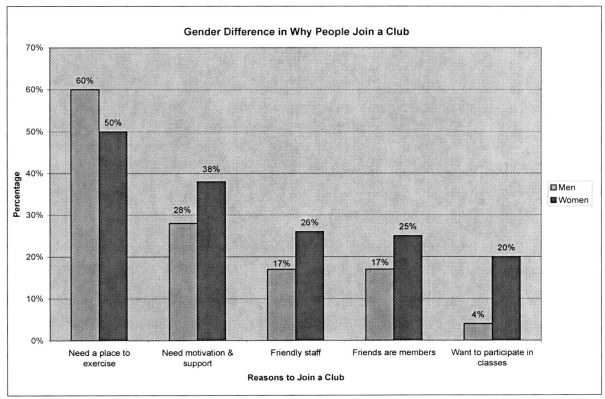

Figure 3-4. Gender difference in why people join a club

Men	Women
Location of the club to home or work (within 12 to 15 minutes)	Location of the club to home or work (within 12 to 15 minutes)
Convenience (easy to get in and out)	Convenience (easy to get in and out)
Quality of the facility and equipment	Cleanliness of the facility
The price—value equation. Is it a good deal?	Friends are members
Availability of equipment	Non-intimidating environment
Staff quality and service	Group-exercise programs and kids' services
Competitive environment	Staff quality and service delivery

Figure 3-5. Benchmark indicators concerning purchasing a club membership

- Men place the heaviest weight on having a place to exercise. Sixty percent of men list this factor as a reason for joining, while 50 percent of women indicate it is a reason for becoming a member.
- Women place a far greater emphasis on a motivating environment, educated and friendly staff, and friends who are members as reasons for joining a club. On each of the aforementioned factors, women think that it is more important than men do by a margin of at least 50 percent.

Approximately two years after *Fitness American Style III* was issued, a new report was released as part of the IHRSA's *2009 Profiles of Success*. In this updated report, members indicated that their leading reasons for joining a club included the following:

- Improving overall well-being (70 percent)
- Having access to a variety of equipment (49 percent)
- Working out, rather than socializing (46 percent)
- Having access to group-exercise classes (24 percent) and fitness programs (20 percent)
- Having friends and family as members (18 percent)
- Having access to the social aspects of the club (16 percent)

When the responses were segregated by gender, some important differences were identified, including the following primary significant differences:

- Women were far more likely to list looking better (70 percent for women versus 55 percent for men) and to feel better about self (70 percent of women compared to 63 percent of men).
- Men were far more likely to indicate building muscle (43 percent of men versus 34 percent of women) to maintain bodyweight (39 percent of men compared to 32 percent of women), and to address a specific medical concern (29 percent of men as opposed to 23 percent of women).

The 2009 report also looked at generational differences concerning why members join and use a club. The generations that the researchers investigated in this study included the Eisenhower generation (born before 1945; the baby boomers (born between 1946 and 1964); generation X (born between 1964 and 1981); and generation Y or the millennial generation (born after 1981). A summary of their key findings is shown in Figure 3-6. Among the most interesting insights from this research were:

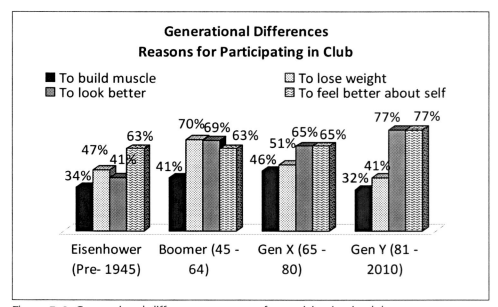

Figure 3-6. Generational differences re asons for participating in club

- Using a club to improve an individual's self-image and sense of self is much more important to those in generation Y (77 percent) than it is to any of the other generations (63 percent to 65 percent).
- Those individuals in generation Y also indicated that "looking better" was a significant factor for their joining and using a club, a response that was significantly higher than for the other generations (41 percent to 69 percent). Interestingly, the baby boomers were not far behind generation Y with regard to this factor.
- Baby boomers detailed losing weight (70 percent) and looking better (69 percent) as their leading rationales for joining and using a club.
- Generation X, similar to generation Y (although 12 percent lower than generation Y), considered self-image and looking better as their top reasons for joining and using a club.

Another interesting issue that the researchers addressed in their study involved what consumers perceived to be the barriers to joining a club. Perceived barriers are important to understanding joining behavior, because as they can represent a strong counterforce to the reasons behind joining a club. Because perceived barriers can often overwhelm good intentions, they can have an impact on the influence of rational reasons for joining and even remaining a member. Figure 3-7 provides a graphic representation of these barriers. According to research, the leading perceived barriers to joining a club were as follows:

- The club is too expensive, or I can not afford it (61 percent)
- I exercise elsewhere (30 percent)
- I feel out of place (18 percent)
- The club is not convenient (16 percent)
- The club is too crowded, and I don't know anyone at the club (12 percent apiece)

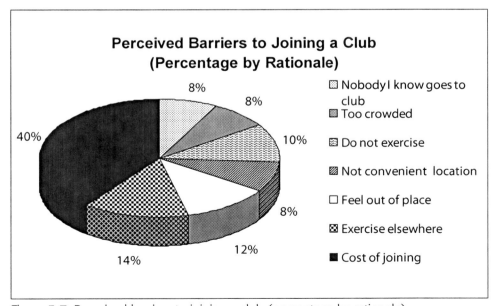

Figure 3-7. Perceived barriers to joining a club (percentage by rationale)

According to a report prepared by IHRSA in 2006 entitled *Why People Don't Join,* the top reasons given for not joining a club were the following:

- Lack of time
- Membership costs too much.
- The club was intimidating.
- Lack of a social support network

Interestingly, these reasons for not joining a club in 2006 are not too dissimilar from the barriers that consumers expressed in the aforementioned 2009 report. Among the general takeaways with regard to consumer attitudes toward clubs and the beliefs that drive them to join or not join a health/fitness club are the following:

❑ Many consumers believe that health/fitness clubs offer a "fun" environment, a perception that is different than the opinions expressed about exercise itself.

❑ Consumers still retain some negative perceptions about health/fitness clubs. In particular, they perceive clubs as being overcrowded (a strong influencer of member retention), a place for young and fit people, and a pick-up place. What is most interesting is that some of these perceptions have been around for decades, and yet the industry has not been able to change them. The perception of overcrowding may be the most damaging factor, especially since club members and former club members have a stronger perception of this aspect than non-members.

The primary reasons for joining a club are related to getting in shape, staying in shape, or enhancing self-image.

❑ Regardless of whether an individual is a man or woman, the primary reasons for joining a club are related to getting in shape, staying in shape, or enhancing self-image. All factors considered, women tend to look more closely at feeling better and looking better, while men are more inclined to focus in on the availability of the facility and the possibility of gaining muscle. Each of these variables that impact the decision to join a club also plays a role in why members remain a member of a club, a topic that will be discussed in the next chapter.

❑ Women place much greater emphasis on the quality of the club's staff, whether friends or family are members, and if the club has a socially engaging environment. While not one of their leading reasons, the cleanliness of the facility is also a critical factor for many women.

❑ Men who are thinking about joining a club tend to evaluate the amenities offered by the facility more than the anticipated experience. For example, men want a club to have a variety of equipment, be convenient, and have a competitive environment. Men also seem to be more inclined to look at a club for health reasons, which is counter to what they express when asked about their feelings about exercise.

❑ Generation Y seems to be very concerned with the club's ability to assist them in looking better and feeling better about themselves, which is much different than the reasons expressed by the other large generation—the baby boomers. As such, baby boomers tend to focus on whether the opportunity to lose weight and look better exists in a club.

Reasons Why Members Either Stay in or Quit Clubs

Once a consumer decides to join a health/fitness club, the process of keeping that member involved begins. This process is referred to as membership retention. Similar to the factors attendant to the joining process, members have specific reasons that they give for quitting a club and/or remaining a member. This section reviews the reasons that members offer for leaving or staying with a health/fitness club that they have joined.

In IHRSA's 1998 publication entitled, *Why People Quit*, researchers identified six key drivers that members cite for resigning from their club (Figure 3-8). The three leading reasons were the cost of the club (23 percent), overcrowding (20 percent), and not having enough time to use the club (19 percent).

If the aforementioned reasons for leaving a club are compared to those reasons that individuals point out for their joining a club, two responses stand out when the consumer perceptions of the "club experience" are considered. The first factor is overcrowding, which existing members indicated was a barrier to their overall satisfaction with the club experience. Overcrowding was also listed as a leading negative perception that consumers have about clubs.

All factors considered, it would appear that not only are the perceptions of consumers genuine, worse yet, the industry has been unable to overcome an important negative influencer of member satisfaction and membership retention. In reality, when the reasons for resigning are separated into intrinsic motives (e.g., reasons driven by members' perceptions of their own experience, operational reasons, or reasons that reflect management's approach to the members), several valuable insights can be discerned.

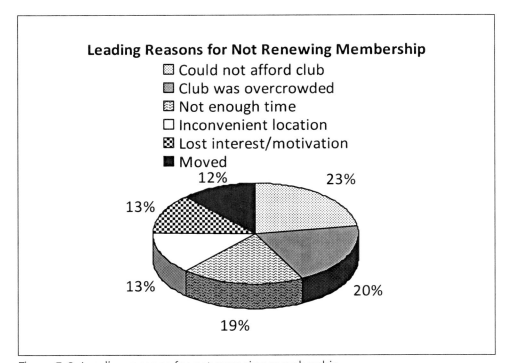

Leading Reasons for Not Renewing Membership
- ▨ Could not afford club
- ▩ Club was overcrowded
- ▨ Not enough time
- ☐ Inconvenient location
- ⊠ Lost interest/motivation
- ■ Moved

Figure 3-8. Leading reasons for not renewing membership

When detailing the intrinsic factors that members give for resigning their membership (Figure 3-9) the top three reasons are: the level of club usage, the lack of motivation, and not having an exercise partner. Obviously, because members who don't use the club frequently enough tend to see less value in their membership, they identify it as a reason for their leaving (a connection that has been documented in numerous studies).

The other two intrinsic reasons that consumers provide for resigning from their club can also have a critical impact on member retention levels—a lack of motivation and a lack of an exercise partner. Given that each of these reasons is a key driver of member usage, it is logical to assume that members expect clubs to provide them with an environment that is motivating and supportive. In addition, these factors may be an indication that clubs may have a responsibility to help members connect with other members, particularly if member retention is an important aspect of their business model. In reality, when members share their reasons for joining a club, neither motivation nor having an exercise partner are identified as primary factors, although for women, having friends and family as members of the club is viewed as important.

It is important to understand the discrepancy that exists between the reasons that impact the joining behavior of individuals and those reasons that influence a member's decision to resign. As such, it appears that either members' expectations change once they join a club, or individuals don't realize how important certain beliefs are until they actually join a facility.

When researchers looked at the extrinsic reasons (Figure 3-10) that people provided for choosing to resign, or, as was discussed previously, the reasons that were affected by management's approach to the facility's customer and

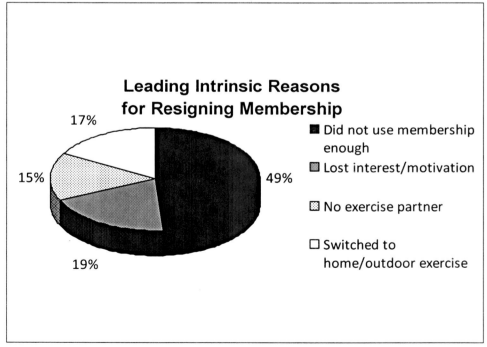

Figure 3-9. Leading intrinsic reasons for resigning membership

business model, several alarming issues arose. The first issue was the fact that overcrowding of the club is the leading reason given (41 percent) by members for resigning. As has been noted, not only do consumers have a negative perception of clubs with regard to this factor, existing club members also indicate it is a key driver of their level of satisfaction. Frankly, while the issue of overcrowding is one that can be easily managed, the industry's apparent lust for overselling memberships (i.e., selling more memberships than a club can actually accommodate) is in large part to blame for this particular driver of membership terminations.

Possibly more important than overcrowding for why individuals drop their club membership are three reasons directly linked to management:

❑ *Dissatisfied with staff.* This factor indicates that the members are either dissatisfied with the qualifications of staff, the level of staffing, or the manner in which staff treats members.

❑ *Lack of attention from staff.* This aspect is relatively simple to interpret. Members feel that the club's staff do not focus their efforts on providing members with assistance and guidance. This particular problem tends to be exasperated by the industry's current love affair with paid personal training, which has resulted in many clubs forgoing any type of service to members who are otherwise unwilling to pay for hands-on guidance. In research conducted in the United Kingdom by Dr. Paul Bedford who interviewed over 24,000 club members, the issue of attention from club staff also arose. It seems that in many cases, members had not been approached by staff since they joined their club, which in numerous instances had been over one year.

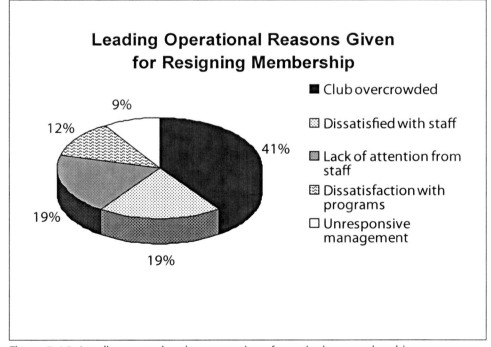

Figure 3-10. Leading operational reasons given for resigning membership

❑ *Unresponsive management.* This measure references the inability of management to resolve member issues in a timely and satisfactory manner. Both directly and indirectly, it is related to the level of communication and transparency between management and the members.

In another study commissioned by IHRSA in the early part of the 21st century, members were asked why they resigned from a club, and whether those reasons would also have an effect on their decision to rejoin the facility instead of quitting. In response, they indicated reasons (Figure 3-11) that were very similar to the intrinsic and operational reasons that were previously mentioned:

• No exercise partner
• Lost interest
• Did not fit in
• Favorite staff left

These responses, similar to the others that have been detailed in this chapter, indicate that members expect clubs to provide staff, programs, and a social environment that motivates them to continue their membership.

Variables Associated With Remaining a Member

When individuals are asked what factors impact their decision whether to remain a club member, their answers are very similar to those that individuals give for quitting a club, only the opposite. Among the primary reasons given by individuals for remaining a member of a health/fitness club are the following:

• Their relationship with the staff. The better the relationship, the more likely they are to remain with the club.
• Positive first impressions with the staff and the facility
• Their initial connection with the club, both with meeting other members and meeting staff
• Achieving their expressed fitness and health goals

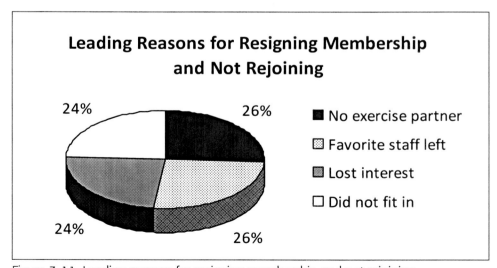

Figure 3-11. Leading reasons for resigning membership and not rejoining

What Should Clubs Learn From the Research on Consumer Attitudes Toward Clubs

As has been discussed previously, multiple, mitigating reasons exist concerning why people join a club, many of which are different in nature from their actual perceptions of what a club is. In order to bring consumers into the club, operators must focus on overcoming any negative attitudes that prospects may initially hold toward the club. Even when these negative attitudes are reversed, the club must be able to offer an experience that is consistent with the reasons that consumers give for joining a particular facility. Finally, having brought new members into the club, club operators should try to better understand the basis for the reasons that members give for leaving and staying and how they can impact those reasons in a meaningful fashion. In this regard, it is interesting to note the disconnect between consumer attitudes about the health/fitness club business, their reasons for joining a club, and finally their reasons for leaving (refer to Figure 3-12).

Figure 3-12 shows that the perceptions that consumers have about the health/fitness industry are mostly related to beliefs around the "people" in the business, such as the quality of the staff, the type of members using the club, and whether individuals believe that they will have fun if they become members of the club. When it comes time to join a club, the attitudes that consumers have regarding people-related issues impact their decision. On the other hand, their decisions concerning whether to purchase a club membership seem to be more driven by facility and program-related factors (women are an exception given that they have certain social expectations). Finally, when a member makes the decision to stay in or leave a club, their reasons are primarily relationship and connection driven, with the obvious exception of whether they achieved their personal fitness goals.

Consumer Perceptions of Health/Fitness Clubs	Reasons Given for Joining Health/Fitness Clubs	Reasons Given for Relinquishing Membership in a Health/Fitness Club
Clubs are worth the money.	Good price	Didn't use the club enough to warrant the cost
Clubs are fun.	Group exercise programs	Poor programming
Club staff is knowledgeable.	Staff quality	Lack of attention from the staff
Clubs are for the young.	Friends are members.	No partner
Clubs are overcrowded.	Non-intimidating environment	Overcrowded
Clubs are for those individuals who are already fit.	Get in shape or stay in shape	Didn't achieve fitness goals

Figure 3-12. Dichotomy between consumer perceptions, attitudes, and behaviors

Given the aforementioned, it is logical to conclude that if a health/fitness club wants to create the most favorable environment for attracting and retaining members, they need to focus on the following factors:

- Target their message to their market. A successful club should not create a generic marketing message, especially if it features young, fit people as role models. Rather, it should try to develop a message that speaks to a non-intimidating environment, where everyone is welcome and comfortable.

- Align the price with the experience. Clubs should try to avoid falling into the pricing game. Potential members see value as being a balance between the experience they have in a club and the price that the club charges for membership. In reality, if a club can deliver great service, provide an enriching social ambiance, and offer educated fitness professionals who can assist members in achieving their goals, then the facility can charge an appropriate price for becoming a member without having to discount it.

- Send a message that their club is clean.

- Make sure their club is seen as having staff who are not only credible and professional, but also warm and service-driven. Remember, members say they want to be acknowledged.

- Build programs that are entertaining, diverse, and motivating.

- Encourage staff to engage members immediately and make sure that the staff introduces these individuals to other members. To the degree possible (and appropriate), the focus of staff should be on partnering.

- Have their employee team engage each new member; focus on helping them establish relationships at some level with every member.

- Find out exactly what prospects and new members want to achieve physically and emotionally, and then make sure that the club's professional staff is there to help guide, motivate, and support the achievement of each member's goals.

- Create activities in the club that are member-driven and in which members can take ownership.

- Recognize the achievements of the club's members.

- Make sure that the club has more equipment than the number of members expected to be in the facility at any given time.

- Make the club convenient; remove any barriers that might otherwise prevent the relatively easy use of the facility and don't make the members sacrifice their time or needs to use the club.

- Create a system so members can communicate with management about club-related issues that they perceive to be important and what their experiences are in the club.

- Make parts of the club non-intimidating, especially if attracting women is important to the club's business model.

Club operators should not sell their club on "closing techniques" and price. Instead, they should align the benefits that their club offers with the needs of the customer and create value for the members.

Clubs should try to avoid falling into the pricing game.

MEMBERSHIP IN THE HEALTH/FITNESS CLUB INDUSTRY

Jupiterimages

- Chapter 4: Membership in the Health/Fitness Club Industry
- Chapter 5: Branding and Marketing of Health/Fitness Clubs
- Chapter 6: Selling Club Memberships

Part Two

4

Membership in the Health/Fitness Club Industry

Chapter Objectives

To a great degree, the financial success of the health/fitness club industry is dependent upon its ability to offer an experience that attracts and retains members. According to the report, 2010 IHRSA Profiles of Success, approximately 74 percent of all health/fitness club revenues come from membership dues, making sustained membership growth the top priority of club operators. This chapter reviews the types of membership offerings currently offered by operators in the health/fitness club industry, and then discusses membership pricing and membership structures. Finally, the chapter examines what these membership policies and procedures mean to the club operator.

Defining the Differences Between a Member and a Customer

The health/fitness club industry is unique in that to a great degree, its success depends upon selling and retaining memberships, whereas in most other hospitality and retail industries, success depends upon customer volume. With regard to the impact of membership on the level of success that a health/fitness club achieves, it is important to note that some very important differences exist between customers and members. In order for a health/fitness club to perform well financially, it must clearly understand that difference and create an experience that drives membership, not customer traffic. While the differences between a member and a customer are often subtle, they are nonetheless, very important.

A customer can be defined as an individual who uses a service, such as a health/fitness club visit, for a fee. A customer asks for no other privilege other than the right to use the service that they have paid for and understands that the fee is based upon the level of service provided or used. Customers are people who gain access based on a fee and have no commitment to the business they are accessing. In essence, a customer is involved in a transactional experience, in which success is measured by the direct outcome of the actual transaction.

To a great degree, the financial success of the health/fitness club industry is dependent upon its ability to offer an experience that attracts and retains members.

A member, on the other hand, is someone who pays for the privilege and right to use a health/fitness club, as well as the privilege to associate with others of similar interests and backgrounds. Members establish an agreement with the business that they intend to honor. Members take a sense of ownership in the organization they join, connecting not to a service or facility, but to other people who are members of the same organization. A member expects certain privileges, which in most cases, extend far beyond just access to a service. Members pay not just for access, but for the unfettered privilege (schedule-wise) to access, with no restrictions placed on them when they access the service.

Types of Memberships in the Health/Fitness Club Industry

During the modern era of the health/fitness club industry, the membership offerings of clubs have varied, ranging from a customer-driven model of daily access for a fee to a model that is based on the payment of annual dues for the privilege of open-ended access year around. At the present time, the industry has three relatively standard types of membership offerings:

❑ *Membership Contract.* The membership contract was first introduced back in the 1940s by Vic Tanny, and based on *IHRSA's 2007 Profiles of Success*, represents approximately 47 percent of the industry's accounts. Membership contracts are an agreement between the club operator and the member, which commits the member to a specified membership time period, usually one year to three years, for a specified amount of dues. In essence, the member is agreeing to pay the club operator a set fee (usually discounted) for the privilege of a long-term membership, whether they actually use the club or not.

> In the past, many clubs offered lifetime contracts, but more recently, the length of a contract has been determined by laws that exist in most states. At the present time, most states limit a club membership contract to three years, and in many states, that limitation is set at one year in duration. These membership contacts can also include certain discretionary provisions, for example, renewal periods of equal length or an option to convert to a month-to-month plan at the completion of the contractual period. According to data from 2007, approximately 5 percent of all membership accounts are contracts of greater than one year in duration, while 18 percent are one-year contracts, with a 12-month renewal. Twenty-nine percent are one-year contracts, with a month-to-month plan at the completion of the initial contract period. A member perceives a value in the contract based on the opportunity to gain privileges for a reduced fee (a price-driven decision), while the operator sees value in the agreement arising out of the fact the club has received an agreed-upon amount of dues (resulting in a higher retention level of dues), that might otherwise not be available if a member chooses to leave before the year is out.

> Many consumers who are looking to join a health/fitness club view membership contracts as legal agreements that require them to commit to a set length of membership and financial commitment, even though they are not sure that they will either want or need to use the club for the time commitment set forth in the contract. Membership contracts tend to be

The membership contract was first introduced back in the 1940s by Vic Tanny.

used most frequently by clubs that offer high-volume membership sales at lower price points, while also experiencing a high volume of member turnover (attrition).

❏ *Month-to-Month Membership*. This type of membership offering has been around the industry for years. Month-by-month memberships provide a member with club privileges for a period of one month, for which, in turn, the member commits to paying one month's dues in advance. This type of membership package, based on data from 2007, is offered by 85 percent of all clubs and is selected by 49 percent of all health/fitness club members, making it the most popular offering in the industry. Many members and prospective members believe that the month-by-month membership is their more attractive option because it does not require them to make a commitment beyond a month's period of time. At the same time, owners tend to find this type of membership offering desirable because it presents less of an up-front barrier to joining their club based on price.

Month-by-month memberships are the most popular offering in the industry.

On the other hand, this type of membership offering also has some downsides for both the member and owner. For the member, a month-by-month membership is easier to terminate and requires less of a commitment to using the club. For the club, a month-by-month membership tends to be associated with higher turnover than with a membership contract, and as a result, also offers slightly less financial security to the owner and operator of a club.

Month-by-month memberships tend to be used frequently by clubs that are focused on providing a higher degree of member service, as well as serving a more affluent population of members. These clubs tend to focus less on the volume of membership and more on the quality of the membership.

❏ *First-Year Membership Contract, With Monthly Membership*. This type of membership agreement is the most recent contractual offering of the industry. Years ago, the industry discovered that by offering a blended membership package, they were able to provide an offering that appealed to prospective members more than the standard contract. A blended package also gives a club more financial protection than a month-by-month membership.

A driving force behind the development of this type of membership offering was research showing that if a member was engaged for a full year, they would be far more likely to stay active in the club going forward. Owners believe that a blended-membership package presents a viable strategy to reduce the first-year attrition of a month-by-month membership, yet offer the member the ability to stay or leave as they choose after the first year.

This type of membership package is offered by approximately 49 percent of the industry. This particular membership offering is the second most popular among members, given that 29 percent of members select this package when joining a club. This membership offering is equally popular among the high-volume and low-dollar health/fitness clubs as it is among the lower-volume, higher-dollar health/fitness clubs.

Membership Categories Typically Offered in the Health/Fitness Club Industry

As was previously detailed in this chapter, health/fitness clubs have developed three basic types of membership offerings. To help differentiate these offerings, the industry has gone one step further and created special membership categories that allow the industry to further personalize their membership offerings to their prospects. In this regard, the categories most frequently offered by clubs include the following:

- *Individual Membership*. This type of membership bestows the privileges of membership on one designated individual for a specified dues rate. The most frequently selected type of membership, this particular membership category is most popular in urban settings.

- *Couples Membership*. This type of membership bestows membership privileges to two individuals for a specified membership dues rate. In some cases, clubs refer to couples as two people from the same family (e.g., a married couple, a parent and child, etc.), while in other markets a couple might be defined as two individuals who live or work together. This basic category is most often employed in large metropolitan markets.

- *Family Membership*. This type of membership provides membership privileges to an entire family, usually defined as two adults and their offspring who are under the age of 21, for a specified membership dues rate. This particular category is popular in the suburban market. The greatest challenge with this category comes when a club has a large family using the membership, which can result in a club losing potential dues revenue that might otherwise be derived from selling separate memberships to several members of the same family. In recent years, many club operators have begun to limit the number of offspring allowed on a family membership (most frequently, two to three) before charging an additional monthly fee for offspring who exceed the predetermined limit.

- *Individual Membership With Family Add-on*. This type of membership offering grants membership privileges to an individual for a designated dues rate, but then allows that individual to add on additional individuals at lower price points. This category is designed to permit an individual to determine who else in the family should receive membership privileges, whether it is a spouse, offspring, or a combination of the two. This type of membership can also be used by someone who joined the club as an individual and later has someone else who wants to become a member of the club with that person. This category of membership has become popular in both suburban and urban markets and provides the club operator and member greater flexibility and value. For members availing themselves of this type of membership, they only have to pay dues for those individuals who have privileges, which might not be the case with a family membership structure. For club operators offering this type of membership, they gain benefit by collecting membership dues from every family member with access to their facility. It should be noted that in today's marketplace, a family might be a married household with kids or an unmarried household with kids.

In recent years, many club operators have begun to limit the number of offspring allowed on a family membership.

While the four previously mentioned categories dominate the industry, clubs employ some less frequently offered membership categories to target specific niche markets. The following categories provide a sampling of the growing trend in the industry to branch out to less typical membership offerings:

- *Singles Membership.* This category does not involve an individual membership, which could be purchased by a single or married person, rather it is a membership offered only to someone who is single. This category is popular in urban markets that have a large population of single professionals.

- *Junior Membership.* First offered in the country-club industry, junior memberships provide membership privileges to younger individuals who might not yet have the earning potential and expendable income to purchase a standard full-privilege membership. This type of membership usually has an upper age limit for eligibility, such as being under the age of 21 or under 30. The Cambridge Group of Clubs in Canada, for example, offers two membership categories that could be classified as junior-style memberships—intermediate executive (ages 31 to 34) and young executive (under age 30), each of which enables an individual to join the facility at a price reduction.

- *Seniors Membership.* This category of membership is offered in markets that have a high concentration of seniors (usually defined in the industry as individuals who are over the age of 55). This category allows senior adults to have full club privileges at a reduced cost.

- *Corporate Membership.* This category is very popular among clubs that are located in settings surrounded by a high concentration of businesses. A corporate membership usually allows groups of individuals from a specific company to join a club at a reduced rate.

- *Off-peak Membership.* In many urban markets, club operators offer customized off-peak or non-prime time memberships that restrict the hours that a member can access the club in return for a lower dues payment. For example, a club might create an off-peak membership that limits an individual's access to the facility to between the hours of 9 a.m. and 5 p.m. on weekdays, and after 11 a.m. on weekends at a dues price-point that is 10 percent to 20 percent less. The rationale for establishing this category of membership is two-fold. For one, they target consumers who might not otherwise be drawn to the club, and for another, they provide an attractive price-point for consumers who have flexible time schedules.

- *Executive Membership.* Sometimes referred to as a VIP membership, this category of membership is relatively new to the industry and is based on packaging special benefits with the membership, such that a member will pay additional dues for the perceived extra benefits included in the category. Among the examples of special benefits often that are packaged into this type of membership are complimentary locker rental, access to a special locker room with custom features, discounts on club services, a specified number of complimentary services each month, etc.

- *Multiple Club Membership.* With the expansion of club chains, many club operators have found value in offering a membership option that gives members access to more than one club in a chain. Most of the regional club

With the expansion of club chains, many club operators have found value in offering a membership option that gives members access to more than one club in a chain.

chains (e.g., Multiplex in Chicago, Healthworks in Boston, New York Sports Clubs, in New York, Equinox in multiple demographic markets, Western Athleltic Clubs in California, etc.) currently offer multiple-site memberships. Many national chains offer both regionally based and nationally based multiple-club memberships as well (e.g., Equinox, 24 hour Fitness). This type of membership offering has gained popularity with members because of the convenience factor, especially for those members who commute within a city or for those individuals who travel a lot around the country or world. For the club operator, this category provides an avenue for up-selling and adding incremental dues dollars at minimal cost.

Packaging Membership Category Offerings

Up to this point, this chapter has reviewed how clubs package their memberships from the perspective of a particular category and contractually. In most cases, the industry sees differentiation of a membership being based on the length of the contract, category of membership, and the associated pricing. In essence, the industry, as a whole, has created multiple membership offerings, using a commodity and goods approach, where the difference in the offerings is based mostly on how the product is priced and wrapped.

In recent years, several of the leading health/fitness club operators have created differentiation in their membership offerings not just on the basis of category and price, but also on what additional benefits they ultimately roll into the offering. This approach to membership differentiation follows a service or experience model, allows clubs to create greater separation from their competitors, and generates improved margins on their membership offerings. Examples of how clubs package their various membership offerings (categories and contracts) include the following:

- Package a specified number of complimentary personal training sessions with the membership
- Incorporate certain discounts to various club services, such as child care, dining, massage, etc.
- Include special privileges to certain areas of the club, such as executive locker rooms, Pilates room, private training area, etc.
- Include affiliated services with other service providers, such as restaurants, dry cleaning, car washes, etc.
- Incorporate charging privileges at the club

In recent years, several innovative club operators have been looking at offering outcome-driven memberships (weight loss, anti-aging, sports achievement, healthy back, etc.), which, instead of providing specific privileges for a monthly fee, promise a specific outcome, bundled with specific services. This approach is less about providing access and more about tailoring the membership to the specific needs of the prospective customer base.

Pricing Strategies for Memberships

The health/fitness club industry has developed a replicable model for the pricing of its membership packages and categories. This pricing model is based

In recent years, several of the leading health/fitness club operators have created differentiation in their membership offerings not just on the basis of category and price, but also on what additional benefits they ultimately roll into the offering.

on a fee associated with entry or access to the membership privileges and then another fee associated with the actual usage of that privilege. In that regard, the two types of club charges are initiation fees and dues:

❑   *Initiation Fee.* The initiation fee is the up-front fee a prospective member pays to a club for the privilege of becoming a member and associating with the individuals who belong to that club. The initiation fee is often used as a differentiating factor for clubs, with those clubs that charge a higher upfront fee often being seen as more exclusive and less crowded. Research conducted both by IHRSA in the United States and by the Fitness Industry Association (FIA) in England shows that members who pay a higher initiation fee tend to remain members for a longer period of time. As a result of this research, the initiation fee is also seen as a pricing strategy related to gaining a greater level of commitment from members and therefore enhancing the retention level of members.

Research conducted both by IHRSA in the United States and by the Fitness Industry Association (FIA) in England shows that members who pay a higher initiation fee tend to remain members for a longer period of time.

Initiation fees range from a low of $0 to as high as $24,000 in the health/fitness club industry, with the average initiation fee equaling 2x to 4x the average monthly dues. According to the published report, the *IHRSA 2010 Profiles of Success*, the average initiation fee paid to clubs in 2010 was $95, down from over $150 at the beginning of the 21st century, figures that represent a decline of nearly 100 percent in net present dollars over the past decade. The initiation fee often is classified under other names, such as enrollment fee, administrative fee, processing fee, induction fee, etc. The tendency in the industry is for clubs that sell higher volumes of membership at lower dues points to refer to their initiation fees as administrative or processing fees, as a way of getting fees despite the fact that they proclaim that they have no initiation fees. Initiation fees are more common in clubs that sell month-to-month memberships. Clubs that sell membership contracts rarely charge initiation fees, instead offering low upfront processing fees.

In most cases, initiation fees are collected by the club at the time the new member enrolls for membership. The initiation fees are normally collected via a check or credit card. Since 2000, a new approach has arisen with regard to the pricing and collection of initiation fees. Taking the lead from the car industry, many clubs are now offering installment initiation fees, which allow a member to put down a percentage of the initiation fee upfront, and then over a period of time, pay off the balance of the initiation fee. In most cases, the initiation fee balance is included with the monthly billing of dues. In some cases, clubs are promoting initiation fees similar to car leases, in which they show the initiation fee as a monthly payment to be made over a designated time period. This strategy allows clubs to charge a higher initiation fee, but also enables the customer to have more flexibility to complete the payment.

In recent years, a number of clubs have moved away from straight enrollment fees and have emigrated toward charging two fees—a processing fee (described as the actual administrative costs of setting up a membership) and a one-time initiation fee. This approach enables many clubs to reduce their initiation fee to zero to attract customers and to still collect an administrative fee.

❑ *Dues.* Dues are the fees charged to members for the ongoing privilege of being a member. Dues allow the member freedom to access the various privileges of the club, per the terms of the membership they have purchased. Dues, as previously presented in this chapter, are billed either on a monthly basis, on an annual basis, or some combination of both. Clubs bill dues using various methods, including monthly statements from the club, billing through a designated charge card, or an electronic funds transfer, also known as EFT. The most popular form of billing dues is through EFT, with the second most popular being credit card billing. A few clubs exist, however, that have members pay their dues monthly, using a coupon that they forward in with their check. EFT is very popular because members are automatically charged their dues, and the club receives its dues income with limited liability for uncollected dues income. Dues for health/fitness club memberships range from a low of around $10 a month for an individual to as high as $500 a month for some family memberships. The average monthly dues, according to the most recent edition of the *IRHSA Profiles of Success*, was $60 a month. In fact, from 2000 to 2009, the average monthly dues collected by clubs remained relatively flat, a situation that actually involves a decline in relative revenues, when accounting for the net present value of the dollar.

By combining initiation fees with dues, clubs have the ability to differentiate their product offering and create multiple price points for the various markets they are attempting to target. Figures 4-1 and 4-2, based on data compiled in the *IHRSA 2010 Profiles of Success*, show some of the variability that exists in the market when it comes to the pricing of both initiation fees and dues.

While the data in Figures 4-1 and 4-2 reflects industry averages when it comes to initiation and dues pricing, the industry has increasingly moved toward a dues-pricing strategy as a point of brand differentiation (e.g., a commodity- or goods-differentiation model). Among the various dues-pricing strategies that are employed in the industry are the following:

• *Under $20 a month.* Clubs that offer memberships that are priced at this level are referred to as "high volume-low priced" facilities in the U.S. and as budget clubs in Europe. This strategy has grown in popularity over the past five years and is exemplified by several U.S. club operators, such as Planet Fitness in the Northeast (monthly dues range from $9.95 to $19.95 a month), Blink in New York (monthly dues range from $15 to $20 a month), Crunch franchise clubs in California ($9.95 to $19.95 a month), and Cardinal Fitness (now Charter Fitness) in the Midwest, as well as a number of European club companies, such as McFit in Germany (under $18 Euros a month) and the Gym Group in the United Kingdom (under 20 pounds a month). Clubs that take this approach to pricing tend to focus on delivering a "fitness box" that provides a workout facility that has abundant equipment, offers no amenities (e.g., no towels, no locker room facilities, etc.), provides no programming, and has limited staff, other than sales people. In recent years, in an effort to enhance the efficiency and profitability of these low-priced clubs their operators have moved to an online method of membership sales and sign-up. As part of their business

> By combining initiation fees with dues, clubs have the ability to differentiate their product offering and create multiple price points for the various markets they are attempting to target.

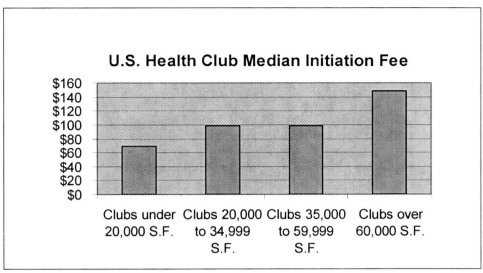

Figure 4-1. U.S. health club median initiation fee

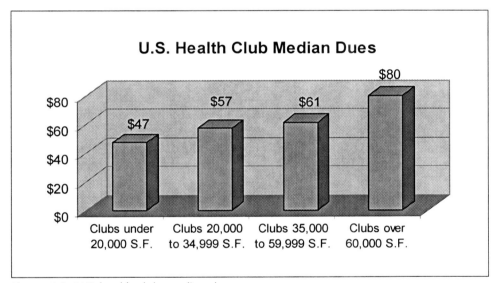

Figure 4-2. U.S. health club median dues

model, these clubs target high-volume membership sales in order to generate the revenue that they need to be profitable. On average, most of these facilities have over 7,000 members per club.

- *$20 to $49 a month*. Based on a premise that is often referred to as premium economy or affordable fitness, this pricing strategy seems to be the most popular approach to membership pricing in the market, especially among the major domestic multiple-club operators that are located in numerous geographic locations (e.g., LA Fitness, 24 Hour Fitness, Gold's, Bally's, etc.), as well as several regional players, such as X-Sport Fitness in Chicago and Urban Active in the Midwest. Clubs such as Fitness First in the UK and Germany also subscribe to this model. Clubs that adopt this approach focus on providing a medium-to-large "fitness box" that is very well-equipped and offers the basic amenities. For example, 24 Hour Fitness and Bally currently design their clubs at 45,000 square feet. This type of club provides basic programming opportunities for members, especially in the area of group exercise. Due to their low pricing, these facilities focus more on their equipment offering and convenience, than on service. In most instances, these clubs have limited staffing and programming. Similar to the facilities that subscribe to the affordable fitness pricing strategy, these clubs also target high-volume membership sales in order to generate the revenue that they need to be profitable. As a rule, the average club in this membership-pricing category has between 6,000 and 10,000 members per facility.

- *$50 to $74 a month.* This pricing strategy has grown in popularity over the past 10 years. It is the strategy most often taken by independent clubs in smaller markets and local/regionally based multiple-club operators (e.g., Wisconsin Athletic Clubs, New York Sports Clubs, Lifestyle Family Fitness in Florida). Clubs that take this pricing approach are focused on delivering a service-driven experience for their members and provide a balance of more-than-adequate facilities, plentiful equipment, amenities, program options, and reasonable levels of staffing. These are the clubs that have shifted their focus from mostly on sales to achieving a balance of membership sales and member service. These clubs, depending upon their size, will normally have membership levels ranging from 2,000 to 5,000 members, with the exception of the clubs in smaller geographic areas.

- *$75 to $99 a month.* This pricing strategy reflects what is frequently defined as the premium market segment, i.e., the high-service area of the club industry. This strategy is found among many regional club operators (e.g., Spectrum Clubs, Sport and Health in the Washington, DC area, and Club One in California), as well as in larger independent club operators in small- and medium-sized markets (e.g., the Maryland Athletic Club in Timonium, Maryland). Clubs that take this approach primarily focus on the goal of delivering high levels of member service. Facilities in this category normally commit to having a greater level of finish-out for their facilities (i.e., the level of interior finish, such as type of tile, lighting, etc.), as well as providing a relatively wide variety of equipment. These clubs offer considerable programming options, especially in the area of group exercise. These clubs also are focused on providing a reasonably high level of staff-to-members ratio. These clubs, depending upon their size, will normally have between 1,500 and 4,000 memberships.

- *$100 a month or more.* This pricing strategy is often referred to as the upper premium and luxury segment of the industry. This differentiation strategy is employed by operators who are targeting the affluent segment of the market. Facilities in this strategic pricing category focus on delivering a high-end service experience that resembles a resort-type experience. This approach has been undertaken by several well-known independent club operators, including the Houstonian, Houston, and the East Bank Club, Chicago, as well as some regional and national club operators, such as Western Athletic Clubs, Sports Club/LA, and Equinox. These clubs provide luxurious physical environments that are supported by well-trained staff as well as innovative and extensive programming.

The "$50 to $74 a month" pricing strategy is the strategy most often taken by independent clubs in smaller markets and local/regionally based multiple-club operators.

Over the past 10 years, the average initiation fee charged by U.S. clubs has declined, while the average monthly dues have remained relatively flat. In fact, in terms of real dollars (current revenues compared to a decade earlier) club dues have actually declined. Figure 4-3 provides a graphic depiction of this trend.

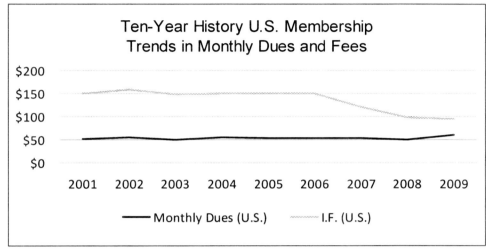

Figure 4-3. Ten-year history U.S. membership trends in monthly dues and fees

Key Points to Consider

Without question, decisions concerning membership pricing, procedures, and policies are some of the most important issues with which club operators will ever have to deal. In that regard, this chapter has addressed the following key points:

- Membership is the heart of the health/fitness club industry, contributing over 70 percent of a club's overall revenue in most cases.
- Membership is about privileges and benefits, not just about access. Membership is about connecting with the club's people.
- Clubs have many options for packaging their membership offering. They can offer membership categories that are grouped by such factors as age, size of group, family status, level of privileges, access to multiple sites, etc.
- Clubs can offer their membership packages on a month-by-month basis or through contracts of specified periods of time.
- When pricing memberships, clubs can consider both initiation fees and dues as a means to differentiate themselves from their competitors. Research shows that higher fees usually lead to greater membership retention. In reality, membership pricing (fees and dues) has either declined or remained flat over the past decade, a situation that is a reflection of the industry's inability to differentiate itself, other than on pricing. All factors considered, over the long run, predatory pricing practices can cause immeasurable damage to the industry.
- Clubs should not fall prey to pricing as the main differentiation of their club membership offering from their competitors. Rather, they should consider the benefits and privileges that they bundle into the membership offering as a means to differentiate themselves.

5

Branding and Marketing of Health/Fitness Clubs

Chapter Objectives

As was discussed in the previous chapter, the health/fitness club industry has a unique product offering—membership. While the membership offerings of clubs can vary widely, a basic question arises concerning what is it that allows some clubs to achieve success with their membership offerings while others do not? With regard to that issue, one fundamental factor is how clubs market and sell their membership offerings. As such, this chapter focuses on how clubs brand and market their membership offerings. Branding and marketing are the processes by which a club develops a distinct position of the club's membership offerings in the public's mind and makes the public aware of its membership offerings, thus creating an enhanced opportunity to uncover leads and prospects for membership.

Branding in the Health/Fitness Club Industry

Branding involves the efforts of a club to create a distinct perception of what its membership offering is in the mind of its audience. A club's brand is its membership promise; it is what a club is able to get its prospective members and the public at large to believe is the membership experience that the club has to offer. When a brand is developed for a club, the effort involves creating an image that the public and the facility's members will associate with the experience that will be delivered by the club.

Branding is particularly important when the goal of a club is to differentiate its membership experience in the mind of the public. The clubs that are successful at branding are those that the public and members talk about and that individuals associate with a specific message. Great brands have several common characteristics that allow them to be easily identifiable in the mind of the consumer, including the following:

- They engage the emotions of the consumer by creating an emotional bond between the consumer and the actual or perceived experience that the

> Branding and marketing are the processes by which a club develops a distinct position of the club's membership offerings in the public's mind and makes the public aware of its membership offerings, thus creating an enhanced opportunity to uncover leads and prospects for membership.

consumer has with the brand. A great example of this attribute is Apple, a brand that elicits a substantial degree of fanatical loyalty and allegiance from its customers. Another company that creates an emotional bond with its customers is Facebook. In the health/fitness club industry, McFit in Germany has established a brand that evokes an extraordinary level of emotional engagement from its audience, as witnessed by the incredible "buzz" it receives on various social media sites (e.g., Facebook, YouTube).

- They define the aspirations of their customer and provide a means for those aspirations to be achieved. An excellent example of a brand that achieves this objective is BMW, which features a slogan ("the ultimate driving machine") that targets a compelling customer-based aspiration. BMW, through is slogan and advertising, as well as through the experience its customers have when they're driving a BMW, communicates and fulfills a promise that speaks to the ultimate driving experience.

- They anchor customers around something familiar, something important. The brand creates a sense of emotional community. Several brands accomplish such a goal, for example, Apple, Blackberry, and the UFC (Ultimate Fighting Championships). Two notable examples in the health/fitness industry of clubs that exemplify this particular characteristic of a successful branding strategy are the Eastbank Club in Chicago and the New York Athletic Club in New York.

McFit in Germany has established a brand that evokes an extraordinary level of emotional engagement from its audience.

In general, a business tends to establish a brand promise that falls into one of four broad categories, driven by the audience it is targeting and the promise it wishes to foster:

- *Being brands*. These are brands that say directly or indirectly to the customer that they have arrived, and confirm for the customer that they are important, not just to themselves, but to the world. Examples of "being brands" include Armani, Rolex, Porsche, and the Mandarin Oriental. In the health/fitness club business, a few of the most recognized "being brands" in their respective markets include Eastbank Club, Chicago; Houstonian, Houston; and the Harbour Club, London.

- *Aspiration brands*. These are brands that speak to what the customer aspires to be. They elicit an emotional response akin to, "This is what I want to be even if I am not that now." Examples of aspiration brands include Apple, Prius, and Nike. In the health/fitness club industry, examples of aspiration brands might include Equinox, U.S.; Exhale, U.S.; and body + soul, Germany.

- *Doing brands*. These are brands that communicate to their audience that "we empower you to accomplish a goal; we provide a means for you to achieve your goals." Examples of "doing brands" include Amazon, Blackberry, Google, and Honda. In the health/fitness club industry, examples of "doing brands" might include 24 Hour Fitness, U.S.; Fitness First, Europe and Asia; and Lifetime Fitness, U.S.

- *Belonging brands*. These are brands that communicate to their audience that they are part of a group with similar needs and interests. Belonging brands elicit a sense of community. Examples of "belonging brands" include Facebook, Starbucks, and YouTube. In the health/fitness club industry, examples of "belonging brands" include Ecofit, Brazil; McFit, Germany; and Healthworks, Boston.

Branding does not happen by accident, but rather through disciplined business practices. While many factors influence the ability of a health/fitness club to create and sustain a strong brand, several business practices are critical to the branding process, including the following:

Branding does not happen by accident, but rather through disciplined business practices.

- *Create a brand promise*. A brand promise is the experience that a health/fitness facility promises to deliver to its customers. It is the experience that members perceive they receive when they use the club. A brand promise must be customer-centric, not product-centric. It must also be emotionally engaging, so that the customer or member establishes an emotional memory of the experience. For example, Rolex is referred to as a "being" brand, since it emotionally confirms that the owner of a Rolex has arrived, that the person wearing a Rolex is important, etc. In the health/fitness club industry, organizations such as the Houstonian in Houston, Texas and the Harbour Club in London, England have established themselves as recognizable "being" brands in their respective markets.

- *Deliver on the brand promise*. Too often, businesses think that if they communicate their brand promise, that is all that is required. To effectively establish a brand, clubs must ensure that everything they do aligns with their promise. In other words, the colors used in the club, the behaviors of the employees, the type of programming, etc. must all consistently support the brand message. In the health/fitness club industry, McFit in Germany is a good example of a company that consistently delivers on its promise of inexpensive, self-directed, high-tech, and socially connected fitness. McFit's ability to consistently deliver on its promise has allowed it to grow to an organization of over 120 clubs throughout Europe, with most of that growth occurring during the past decade.

- *Narrow the focus.* Great brands know who they are and focus all their energy on delivering on the brand promise. In this situation, a narrow focus refers to the fact that a club selects a targeted audience and then applies all of its energies toward fulfilling a promise that is targeted at that particular audience. Narrowing the focus is the opposite of trying to be everything to everybody. In the health/fitness club industry, Curves is an example of having a narrow focus. Curves focuses on older women, who typically are intimidated by the "normal" club environment, and delivers a very social and non-intimidating fitness experience.

- *Be authentic.* Authenticity means being real, being trusted, and delivering an experience that is credible. A strong brand will be authentic when consumers put their trust in the brand promise and the resulting experience. Authentic brands are not copycats; they don't deliver a karaoke-style product. For example, consumers look at Apple as authentic because their products are unique, innovative, and, most importantly, inspire trust from their customers. In the health/fitness club industry, facilities such as Gainesville Health and Fitness in Gainesville, Florida and Red's in Lafayette, Louisiana have great authenticity, because their members believe that they embody the fundamental attributes of being authentic.

- *Tell the story.* Great brands make sure to tell their story. Telling the story involves spreading the organization's brand message through authentic and credible means. A facility's best method of telling stories about its brand is by having members share their experiences about the club with others, People see friends and associates as the most trusted source of information about a brand. In the current marketplace, social media sites, such as Facebook and YouTube, have proven to be one of the most effective avenues for friends and associates to share messages that are perceived by others as authentic. Another credible and important storytelling mechanism is the media. Stories that originate in the media are typically perceived as credible, because they come from a trusted source.

The following companies have some of the more successful brands in the global health/fitness club industry:

❑ *Gold's Gym.* The Gold's brand is widely considered as one of the top national brands in the health/fitness club industry. When the public sees the Gold's name and logo, the image of a facility catering to weightlifters and bodybuilders comes to mind. If average citizens were asked what they initially think about when they hear someone refer to Gold's Gym, most individuals would probably respond that it's a club for serious fitness people. This brand image is built partially by being one of the first gyms to receive substantial publicity (e.g., from the movie Pumping Iron), by extensively

Great brands know who they are and focus all their energy on delivering on the brand promise.

When the public sees the 24 Hour Fitness brand, they tend to think about a facility that is characterized by such attributes as convenience, all-day access, plenty of equipment, and affordability.

merchandising its logo, and by the visibility offered of its first spokesperson, Arnold Schwarzenegger. It is interesting to note that the Gold's Gym name, through its franchising efforts, has come to be much more than what its brand is perceived to be.

❏ *24 Hour Fitness.* The 24 Hour Fitness brand is one of the more visible brands in the United States. When the public sees the 24 Hour Fitness brand, they tend to think about a facility that is characterized by such attributes as convenience, all-day access, plenty of equipment, and affordability. 24 Hour Fitness has built its brand image through a combination of mass-media promotions, building and locating clubs in large numbers in major markets, and keeping its clubs open 24 hours a day. Recently, 24 Hour Fitness has aligned themselves with several celebrity sports stars (e.g., Andre Agassi, Magic Johnson, Lance Armstrong, Jackie Chan, etc.) in an attempt to create an even more recognizable brand.

❏ *Healthworks.* Healthworks is a women's-only group of clubs in the Boston area that is one of the most familiar regional brands in the Northeast market. Healthworks has built its brand recognition by being the first quality women's-only club to market, by delivering an experience women respect and enjoy, and by marketing that image in the community. Healthwork's marketing, in large part, has been developed through its community involvement and charitable work for women and families in need, both of which play a significant role in the strength of its brand.

❏ *McFit, Germany.* McFit was originally established in 1997. Over the past five to eight years, it has become a phenomenon in Germany. McFit promises its customers a convenient (24-hour access), inexpensive (under 18 Euros a month), high-tech (nearly all operational and membership services conducted over the Internet) and communal experience (McFit has an incredible fan and friend base on both YouTube and Facebook). The success of its brand is the result of it consistently delivering on its promise in every location in which it operates.

❏ *Companhia Athletica, Brazil.* Companhia Athletica opened its first club in Sao Paolo, Brazil in the early 1980s. The company built its brand promise around delivering an entertaining, family-friendly, high-quality service experience for the affluent residents of San Paolo. Recently, the company celebrated 25 years of excellence. In the process, it has grown from one club to over a dozen clubs, with revenues exceeding $30 million U.S. annually.

❏ *East Bank Club.* The East Bank Club is a 450,000 square-foot club that is located along the river in Chicago. It could be argued that everyone in Chicago knows of the East Bank Club. East Bank's reputation as a premier club, providing every imaginable service to its members, has been built through each of the three key steps to branding. East Bank was the first mega high-end club to market, it continues to deliver an extraordinary service with incredible facilities, and its members seem to willingly serve as promoters of the club's numerous positive features. Over the past 25 years, many high-end mega clubs have been built in Chicago, but every one of them finds itself measured against East Bank as the top brand in the market.

❏ *Red's*. Red's is located in Lafayette, Louisiana. Red's was founded in the early 1960s as a small 3,000 square-foot club and has expanded over the years to become a 180,000 square-foot facility. As of 2004, Red's club had approximately 15 percent of the total city population as members, even though it had over a dozen competitors, including a Planet Fitness only a few blocks away. A local landmark, Red's is an exceptional brand. Not only was it first to market, more importantly, it has built a strong reputation as a result of having a great product and being extensively involved in the community.

A number of other brands exist on an international, regional, and local level that are excellent examples of well-established brands, including the New York Sports Clubs (regional), Sports Club/LA (regional), Houstonian (local), Cooper Activity Center (local), Curves (national and international), and Lifetime Fitness (national).

Marketing in the Health/Fitness Club Industry

As was discussed in the previous section, marketing is one of the critical steps in branding. Marketing, however, involves much more than just establishing a brand image. Not only does marketing help create awareness of the club in the mind of the public and help establish a reason for the public to visit the club, in essence, it also assists in bringing leads to the club. Marketing is not selling, however, since marketing never closes a membership sale. Instead, marketing enables a club to instill an image in the public's mind and then provides a compelling reason for the public to consider the club to pursue their exercise and recreation needs. Too many individuals in the health/fitness club industry, however, equate marketing with engaging in advertising and placing lead boxes in the community. In reality, marketing can take many forms, each with the ability to create an image and provide the public with a compelling reason to visit the club.

> **Not only does marketing help create awareness of the club in the mind of the public and help establish a reason for the public to visit the club, in essence, it also assists in bringing leads to the club.**

Proven Marketing Approaches in the Health/Fitness Club Industry

❏ *Advertising*. Advertising represents a very broad-stroke approach to marketing in the health/fitness club industry. As a rule, advertising is not a targeted approach to marketing, but rather a method for hitting a larger, less-targeted audience. Advertising can take many forms, including:

• *Print media*. Print media advertising includes placing advertisements in such venues as newspapers, magazines, company newsletters, etc. Print media varies in its effectiveness. If a club is in a small market with a relatively small local paper, then print advertising can be an effective approach. On the other hand, if a club is located in a large market, such as New York, print advertising's success is highly dependent on the audience to which it is speaking, the demographic radius from which it will be pulling, and the scalability of its business. For example, New York Sports, with over 90 clubs in the New York metropolitan region, has had considerable success with print advertising. At the least, print advertising can be very expensive. Not only must a club pay for the expenses involved in the production of the advertisement, it is also responsible for the cost of its placement as well. In some cases, the cost of producing a quality print media ad can run thousands of dollars, while the cost to place it can run over $25,000 for a full-page advertisement in several large papers, and even more in some of the most well-read magazines. Clubs that chose to use print media may want to consider using other print media, such as local community circulars, or flyers, which are less expensive and can be more easily targeted to their audience. Two club companies, in particular, that have set themselves apart with their print advertising are Companhia Athletica, with corporate offices in Sao Paulo, Brazil and Equinox Fitness, with its corporate offices based in New York, New York. At Companhia Athletica, three of their most successful print marketing campaigns (each subsequently won awards) were the "Body Fat Imprisonment" campaign in 2007, the "Flowers" campaign in 2009, and the "Switch Your Routine" campaign in 2010. Equinox, which many in the marketing community consider the leader in print marketing, received acclaim for both its 2008 "Happily Ever" campaign, which generated considerable positive press and social media commentary, and its 2010 "My Body. My Biography" campaign.

> **Most radio stations will agree to broadcast live from a club, which can really add some visibility to the facility's marketing efforts.**

- *Radio.* Advertisements on radio can be placed on stations that have a demographic audience similar to demographics the club wishes to target. In fact, every radio station has detailed information on the demographics of its audience, which can help a club determine with which stations it should place its advertising dollars. Furthermore, most radio stations, for an extra cost, will also agree to broadcast live from a club, which can really add some visibility to the facility's marketing efforts. Radio advertising is not inexpensive, but if a club is relatively selective in how and where it advertises, such an approach can be effective.

- *Local and regional cable television.* Using cable television to communicate the club's desired message can be a very effective approach to advertising, especially if a club does it on a regional or local level. On the other hand, it is important for a club to keep the cost of production and placement of an ad on cable television in mind when deciding whether this approach is an appropriate way for it to advertise.

- *Billboards and banners.* Billboard advertising is an excellent alternative for advertising, especially in large, urban markets, such as Dallas, Houston, and Los Angeles, where people spend considerable time in their cars. Billboards and banners, if placed along the proper thoroughfare, can bring considerable attention to the club. For example, in Moscow, Russia, the number-one source of leads for the top operators is generated by banners that are hung over the streets (drivers in Moscow typically spend a few hours each day in traffic). Like most advertising efforts, billboard advertising involves both production and placement costs. With billboard advertising, similar to the other media, the club can pay for the space it chooses to use for a given period of time.

- *Internet advertisements.* Over the last few years, Internet advertising has become extremely popular. The most common form of Internet advertising has been the use of banner and pop-up advertisements. Club operators, however, should be aware of the fact that Internet advertising does not always work as intended. For example, with the increase in software that stops pop-ups, the value of Internet advertising to a club might not be as high as the other available forms of advertising.

- *Yellow Pages.* The *Yellow Pages* are still a good source of information for much of the public. Accordingly, given a choice of the various types of advertising media, club operators should seriously consider utilizing the *Yellow Pages*.

When contemplating the use of advertising, club operators should be aware that two basic types of advertising exist—image advertising and call-to-action advertising. With image advertising, a club is sending a message about the image of its brand. Image advertising involves efforts by a club to create awareness of its brand and establish exposure of its business in the marketplace. Call-to-action advertising, on the other hand, focuses on providing a compelling reason for the club's audience to take action (e.g., join the club, sign up for a product or service, etc.). Call-to-action advertisements typically offer some inducement for the public to visit the club, such as discounts, a free week's membership, a raffle for a free membership, etc.

❑ *Social Media Marketing.* Employing social media has become the hottest trend in marketing over the past few years. Social media has the advantage of being able to reach millions of consumers in a matter of seconds. Furthermore, among today's tech-savvy public, social media sites have become extremely popular destinations for potential consumers of a club's product offering. The leading forms of social media marketing include:

- *Social media sites.* The newest favorite delivery-platforms of the promotional world, social media sites, offer a host of alternatives for exposing a club's offering to the public. Social networking sites, such as Facebook and YouTube, allow clubs to create large fan bases, as well as attract numerous unique visitors to their sites. For example, YouTube has become the go-to-social media site for clubs that deliver video messages. Equinox Fitness, a New York-based operator of premium clubs throughout the U.S., has been very successful at leveraging YouTube to promote its brand. Its video campaigns, such as "Happily Ever After," the Allen Enlow video segment, or the recent video clip entitled "Behind the Scenes with Equinox," have been highly successful at generating publicity, as well as steering traffic to its website. Another company that has successfully leveraged YouTube to enhance its brand message and attract new customers is Companhia Athletica of Sao Paulo, Brazil. Companhia Athletica's "Get in Shape" series of video clips on YouTube have attracted a relatively large following of fans and in the process, enabled the organization to sign up countless new members. Other club companies that have done an excellent job of leveraging the social and mass market appeal of YouTube include McFit of Germany (member-generated video clips), Leo Sports Club of Germany (its "Nut Cracker" clip was one of the most watched on the Internet), Fitness First of the United Kingdom, and 24 Hour Fitness of the U.S.

Social networking sites, such as Facebook and YouTube, allow clubs to create large fan bases, as well as attract numerous unique visitors to their sites.

Facebook is often the other social media outlet that clubs around the globe utilize to connect with members and reach out to the public. Tech-savvy clubs employ their Facebook page as a portal into their website, thereby creating a simple one-stop site for members, prospective members, and the public to experience their brand. In fact, several renowned club companies, such as Equinox, U.S., Club One, California, 24 Hour Fitness, U.S., and McFit, Germany, leverage Facebook to attract fans and friends. In addition to Facebook and YouTube, Twitter has become another popular social site for clubs. Twitter, although it only allows short messages (less than 140 words), has become a "hot" messaging tool for many clubs, enabling these facilities to send relatively brief, focused messages to both member groups and prospects.

• *Social buying sites.* Over the past few years, social buying sites, such as Groupon, Living Social, and Tippr, have become extremely popular sites for businesses to promote their product offering. As such, these social buying sites are virtual group-purchasing platforms that enable a business to promote its products and services through special one-time offers and coupons. These sites provide consumers with the opportunity to leverage the purchasing power of a group. In essence, they provide a virtual form of collective bargaining that can help ensure that a consumer can acquire a particular "product" at the lowest possible price. Social buying sites benefit a club by exposing its product offering (i.e., programs and services) to a relatively large audience in its respective market (most social buying sites have a very large audience of fans in their respective markets). Typically, when a club puts together a special promotion that will appear on one of the social buying sites, the price associated with that offer is triggered when the critical mass of purchasers within that particular market is reached. For every customer who purchases the club's offer (e.g., a one-month membership, massage package, etc.), that facility not only earns money, it also obtains a valuable lead. Club One, based in California, has found that Groupon, the current granddaddy of all social buying sites, is very effective in generating both leads and prospects, as well as simultaneously producing incremental revenue that far offsets the cost of delivering the offer.

❑ *Buzz Marketing.* Buzz marketing is often referred to as word-of-mouth (WOM) marketing or viral marketing. The premise behind "buzz" marketing is that a club creates a message that is then shared with others through the personalized sharing of information, based on trust between the source and target. Buzz marketing works like a virus by having the message spread from one source to multiple targets. Each of those targets then becomes a source that spreads the message to multiple other targets. Another factor critical to the success of buzz marketing is that it allows the source to have unfettered access to the mind of the targeted audience. In other words, the intended message is communicated with minimal or no external interference. In the health/fitness club industry, member-referral programs are an example of buzz marketing. In the current marketplace, social media sites, such as Facebook, Twitter, and YouTube, have become great vehicles for implementing a buzz-marketing campaign. Social media sites allow

In the health/ fitness club industry, member-referral programs are an example of buzz marketing.

sources to rapidly spread the message to many like-minded targets. Two keys to a successful buzz-marketing campaign include:

- *Authenticity*. The target of the message must see the source as credible. Member referrals, testimonials, and messages passed through social network sites are often considered credible by the public. Ruth Berstein, executive strategic director of Yard Advertising in New York, was quoted in an article that appeared in 2010 in the *New York Times* about Equinox's "My Body, My Biography" campaign. Her statement that "the campaign was designed to be more authentic and emotional" is a reflection of how important authenticity can be when targeting a promotional message.

- *Stand out*. The message must be different and unique. In essence, it must stand out among all of the other messages that the intended target receives. Standing out can take any number of forms, such as being taboo, outrageous, funny, remarkable, or even secretive. All factors considered, Equinox's "Happily Ever" campaign was perceived as taboo and racy, while Companhia Athletica's "Flower" campaign was viewed as being remarkable and different.

❑ *Direct Mail Marketing and Email Blasts*. Direct mail marketing provides a more targeted approach to attracting audience eyeballs than standard print advertising or promotions distributed over social media sites. Direct mail allows a club to select its audience based on key demographic characteristics. The effort can be as small or as large as the club likes. On average, most print direct-mail efforts will generate a response rate that varies from .5 percent to three percent. Email direct mail promotions, on the other hand, have been found to garner a somewhat larger percentage response, occasionally reaching levels as high as 10 percent. The more targeted a club's initial audience, the higher its percentage of responses will be. Direct mail can be accomplished either through actual mailings, email, or most recently, through SMS or text messaging. In the area of email direct marketing, Equinox, a premium club operator based in New York, does a particularly outstanding job. Equinox's email blasts typically incorporate print advertisements that originally were generated as part of its print promotional and social website campaigns. While text messaging has just recently become popular in the U.S., it has been used extensively in Europe and Russia for several years. Text messages tend to generate a larger response than either print direct mail or email-delivered direct mail. Recently, a U.S.-based company, Fit Messenger, has begun offering text or mobile marketing services to the health/fitness club industry. Among the ways that clubs can enhance their direct-mail marketing efforts are the following:

- *Keep the message simple*. A direct-mail message needs to be direct and simple, otherwise consumers will not spend much time reading it. Simplicity is what makes text message blasts so successful.

- *Make the message different and appealing*. Because consumers get hit all the time, if a direct-mail piece does not "knock their socks off" at first glance, it is quite likely that the level of attention of the recipient of the message has probably been lost. Some of the best direct-mail pieces feature unique pictures, special offers, and a look and feel that

Direct mail marketing provides a more targeted approach to attracting audience eyeballs than standard print advertising or promotions distributed over social media sites.

is different. The best examples of these pieces are what are termed 3D direct-mail. A 3D piece could be a box that when opened has a barbell paperweight or it could be a tennis-ball container that when opened has a ball with a gift certificate attached to it. Clubs that are using email to forward their direct mail messages should consider either attaching a link to their website or employing a podcast to significantly boost the appeal of their message.

*   *Personalize the mailing.* If a club employs pre-printed labels in its direct mailings, they don't separate themselves from the crowd. Research has shown that handwritten cards and envelopes get far more attention when they arrive in the mail. When it comes to email and texting, the message should come from someone the targeted consumer either has met or with whom is familiar.

*   *Make an offer.* A direct-mail piece needs to provide a reason for the consumer to visit a club. For example, the piece could include/feature an eye-catching enticement, such as a guest pass, a gift certificate, a complimentary month's membership, or a discount coupon.

*   *Obtain good contact lists.* The club's best source for names to contact is names provided by its members. As a rule, the next best avenue for securing names is from a direct mail house that provides mailing lists (for a fee). At the present time, a number of firms, for a fee, provide mailing lists, email lists, and even cell phone lists (used for text messaging). These lists can be sorted (organized) by a number of critical factors, including zip code, age, gender, household income, phone number, email address, etc. The better job a club does in identifying the desired parameters, the better its mailing list will be.

Reputation management can be one of the most powerful marketing avenues a club can employ.

❑ *Reputation Management.* Reputation management is another way of expressing involvement in community and public relations. Reputation management is about a club creating and sustaining its brand image through relationships in the community. Reputation management can be one of the most powerful marketing avenues a club can employ. Examples of reputation management include:

*   *Serving on community boards and committees.* A club can have members of its staff get involved in the community by serving on local boards or groups, such as the chamber of commerce, rotary, local hospital board, school board, PTA, or other locally active organization serving the public.

*   *Sponsoring community activities.* A club can get involved with community activities by serving as a sponsor for a local community event, such as a rotary function, school PTA function, special charity event, etc. If a club is particularly sensitive to the value of such an approach, it will go one step further and actually agree to host community events and meetings. For example, a club could host the parent meetings of the local Little League.

*   *Creating a press kit and sending out press releases.* Every club should create an attractive and compelling press kit. Such a press kit should include a background statement about the club, a fact sheet, some

biographies of key staff, etc. The press kit should then be forwarded to the local media, along with a human-interest story. The club should consider inviting the press to special events conducted at the club (e.g., grand opening, special activities, community-interest events, etc.) and get the media actively involved in promoting the occasion. Finally, the club should make sure to send stories to its media contacts on a regular basis. The press is almost always looking for great human-interest stories, and almost every club has members or employees who have compelling stories.

- *Becoming a health and fitness resource for the community.* A club could contact the local press and see if it can write a question-and-answer column for the paper. A club could also take this approach with a local radio or television station. For example, in Dallas, Texas, Larry North, owner of the Larry North Fitness clubs, is frequently featured as an expert on health and fitness matters on local radio.

- *Developing a charity event or foundation.* A number of clubs in the United States have created actual charity foundations that involve their members and staff in providing support and funds to a specified charity. The charitable activities of Healthworks in the Boston area are a perfect example of a club taking this approach.

❏ *Club Marketing Materials and Literature.* Clubs need to develop marketing materials that they can provide to leads and prospects that will articulate the "story" of their club. These marketing materials can be used as handouts, both when they're utilized outside the club, and when potential leads are visiting at the club. Examples of some of the most effective marketing literature and media used by clubs include:

Clubs need to develop marketing materials that they can provide to leads and prospects that will articulate the "story" of their club.

- *Print brochures.* Every club should have a print brochure. The brochure should represent the image of the club and tell the story of the club. An effective brochure, in this instance, should feature a number of items, including pictures, testimonies by members, bullet points on the attributes and benefits of the club, a map with the location of the club, and information on how to contact the club (including email and website addresses). Sample brochures are included in the appendices of this book. Cost-wise, a wide variety of print options are typically available. It is money well-spent, however. A quality color brochure might run as high as one to two dollars a brochure when the club prints 500 or more at a time.

- *CD/DVD brochure.* One of the most recently developed tools that a club uses to market and promote itself is an actual CD or DVD brochure. At a minimum, the DVD/CD should contain a virtual tour of the club, clips of member testimonies, information about the club in story format, and a direct link to the club's website. CDs and DVDs are a relatively inexpensive item to produce (generally ranging from 50 cents to one dollar to replicate). It should be noted that this cost is the same or less than for a printed brochure. Clubs, such as The Athletic and Swim Club in New York, ACAC in Charlottesville, Virginia, and LeClub in Wisconsin, are excellent examples of facilities that have successfully employed this approach.

- *Website brochure or smart-phone application.* No club should be without a web-based brochure. Such a tool can enable a club to use streaming video, photos, samples of club schedules, and other relevant information from the facility. Furthermore, a club can link its site to the web-based *Yellow Pages* and to IHRSA's healthclubs.com. The Equinox Clubs, based out of New York City, have done an incredible job with this approach. In the last few years, a number of companies, such as Crunch, Equinox, Planet Fitness, and others, have released smart-phone applications. These applications are another means for clubs to provide current information about themselves.

❑ *Strategic Alliances.* Another effective marketing approach that can benefit a club is to develop strategic alliances or cross-marketing relationships. A strategic alliance or cross-marketing relationship involves a situation where a club establishes a working relationship with another organization that allows each of the respective organizations to benefit from the relationship, for example, in attracting new customers. Among the types of strategic alliances that a health/fitness club might consider are the following:

- *Alliance with local restaurants.* Clubs can approach restaurants whose clientele have the same demographics and establish a relationship in which both organizations are marketing the others to its clients. This approach can be as simple as employing table-top advertising, or could involve special coupons that members and customers receive when they use the club or restaurant.
- *Alliance with local healthcare organizations.* By establishing an informal relationship with other healthcare organizations, a club could gain valuable leads.
- *Alliance with local homeowner associations.* A club could establish a relationship in which new homeowners obtain, as part of their homeowner membership, a coupon that enables them to join the club at a discounted price or even a one-month, complimentary membership.
- *Alliance with local realtors.* Clubs can work with local realtors to create special welcome gifts. These gifts could be included with all new home purchases or could be positioned as a special-benefit package if individuals satisfy some set of predetermined criteria set by the local realtor. In an urban market, a club might want to work with local apartment/condominium landlords to create the same type of package.

❑ *Community and Corporate Health Fairs.* Clubs can build their reputation as a member of the healthcare network by sponsoring local health fairs. If the club is in an urban market or an area heavily populated by corporations, the club should contact the various companies and offer to sponsor a health fair for the company. These health fairs can include both club-related services and demonstrations, but also involve bringing in outside healthcare providers, such as physical therapists, opticians, etc. In some urban settings, building landlords are often receptive to activities such as these to offer as a benefit to their tenants. If a club is in a suburban or residential market, contact should be made with local city leaders or local associations to gage their possible interest in having the club sponsor a community-based health fair.

> A strategic alliance or cross-marketing relationship involves a situation where a club establishes a working relationship with another organization that allows each of the respective organizations to benefit from the relationship, for example, in attracting new customers.

❑ *Member Referral and Sponsor Programs*. Research has shown that the single best source of new members is the club's existing members. Clubs who understand the value of leveraging existing member involvement in their club as a marketing tool usually achieve the greatest success. Every club should have an ongoing member referral program that provides a process and incentive for existing members to share the club's story with friends and associates. Over the years, club companies, such as ClubCorp in Dallas and Western Athletic Clubs based in California, have done an excellent job with their referral programs. Among the factors that referral programs focus on are the following:

- *Providing a means for members to submit and refer the names of friends and associates.* This process could be as simple as having referral cards and a box, a special web address, or encouraging members to contact the membership sales department.

- *Providing recognition for the members who provide referrals*. This policy can vary from providing special awards for club services to special grand prizes.

- *Resisting the tendency to overextend the welcome.* A good member referral program is not promoted too blatantly; rather, it is incorporated into the overall fabric of the club's membership and marketing process.

❑ *Lead Boxes.* Lead boxes were among the first marketing tools employed by health/fitness clubs. Lead boxes involve placing a special box, accompanied by a promotional offer and a special information card, at specific locations throughout a particular market. As a rule, a club will place the lead boxes in various retail locations, where the demographics of the retail customers match the profile of the club's membership. A lead box is normally accompanied by a flyer or poster that extends to the public a chance to win a membership or other service just by filling out a card and placing it in the box. Clubs subsequently check their lead boxes on a regular basis and collect the names of those individuals who want a chance to win whatever prize has been promoted. A prize is always awarded. At the same time, however, the club has also collected the names of people who are potential prospects and future members.

Key Points to Consider

Branding and marketing are critical undertakings for clubs that are interested in building and sustaining a vibrant membership. Branding helps establish the image and the story of the club in the mind of both the public and the members. Such an image can help create a greater level of awareness of the club in the market and help attract the public to its front door. Marketing involves the steps undertaken to help build the brand image of the business and generate interest in the club's membership offering. Marketing is critical to generating both membership leads and membership prospects. Membership sales staff cannot sell memberships if they do not have a sufficient number of leads and prospects. Accordingly, marketing should be a significant part of the prospecting strategy utilized by a club's membership sales staff.

> **Research has shown that the single best source of new members is the club's existing members.**

6

Selling Club Memberships

Chapter Objectives

In the previous two chapters, the principles of membership and the art of marketing were reviewed. This chapter logically extends that line of discussion by examining the process of selling memberships. To many individuals in the health/fitness club industry, the word "sales" elicits negative perceptions. In reality, however, sales essentially involves nothing more than providing a worthwhile product for which a market exists, a needed service, or an exceptional experience that fulfills a prospect's wishes. This chapter initially presents an overview of the sales process, and then discusses several actual practices, such as the club tour, corporate sales, and sales management, which can assist club operators in driving their membership sales. This chapter concludes with a short presentation on the newest form of membership sales, on-line sales without sales staff.

Understanding the Mathematics of Selling Memberships

As was discussed previously, a thriving membership is at the heart of every successful club. The challenge of sales is to make sure that the club's membership level continues to grow, thus ensuring the overall profitability and vitality of the club. According to the published report, the *IHRSA 2010 Profiles of Success*, a profile of the health/fitness club industry, IHRSA health/fitness clubs had net membership growth of negative .5 percent in 2009, which was in sharp contrast to 2008 and 2007 results, when participating clubs experienced positive net membership growth of 4.2 percent and 1.9 percent respectfully in the two previous years. The negative growth in 2009 can be attributed in large part to a decrease in new membership sales, rather than to any increase in the loss of existing members. Based on data from 2010, as reflected in Figure 6-1, most clubs have to sell between 300 and 1,000 new memberships on an annual basis to maintain their existing membership levels. In fact, some of the larger club "big box" operators have to sell as many

> The challenge of sales is to make sure that the club's membership level continues to grow, thus ensuring the overall profitability and vitality of the club.

as 5,000 new memberships annually to maintain a stable membership base. IHRSA tracks a metric entitled, "account replacement ratio," which reflects the ratio of new sales made to the number of existing memberships terminated. A ratio of 100 percent would mean that for every 100 memberships sold, 100 memberships also terminated. In 2009, the account replacement ratio was 1.02, which means that in 2009, clubs sold 102 memberships for every 100 memberships terminated. This metric was the lowest replacement ratio the industry had seen in the past several years.

What is most evident from the aforementioned figure is the fact that most clubs, whether small or large, are generating new sales on an annual basis at a rate ranging from 25 percent to 50 percent of their base membership. The point is that when it comes to membership sales, health/fitness clubs have established a historical pattern requiring a high rate of membership sales. If, for example, in 2009, the median number of total sales for clubs over 60,000 S.F., which is 1,021 memberships, is used as a basis for identifying the extent of the need to sell club memberships and that number is converted to a weekly sales rate, a club ends up having to sell 20 memberships a week. If the 2009 annual sales ranges indicated in Figure 6-1 are examined, the average sales required on a weekly basis for the majority of clubs would range from a low of six sales a week to a high of 20 sales a week. It is interesting to note that some of the clubs operated by big box players, such as Lifetime Fitness, LA Fitness, 24 Hour Fitness, and Bally's, often have to sell an average of 50 to 100 memberships a week. It is important to understand that a high performing sales person will, on average, make approximately 10 membership sales a week. In other words, most clubs will need to have at least two full-time membership sales people. In fact, high sales volume clubs, such as Lifetime Fitness or LA Fitness, will often need as many as 10 to 15 membership sales people. Obviously, sales are most definitely a numbers game.

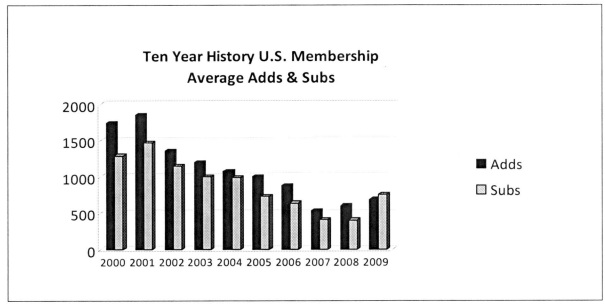

Figure 6-1. Ten year history U.S. membership average adds and subs

Understanding the Membership Sales Continuum

Membership sales involve three distinct stages: identifying leads, qualifying prospects, and closing the sale. Each of the sales stages is like a filtering screen, with the number of people at each stage being screened until it becomes a smaller population with better qualifications for membership. As Figure 6-2 indicates, the sales process can begin with 100 leads that then develop into 30 prospects, and finally result in 15 sales.

Using the aforementioned example as a reference, a club that requires 20 new memberships a week would need to generate a total of 40 prospects and 130 leads weekly. When examined in this perspective, the sales process requires a club to create a large reservoir of leads in order to produce the required level of membership sales. While the percentages tend to vary from market to market and club to club, the average club can expect to convert 20 percent to 50 percent of its leads to prospects and 20 percent to 80 percent of its prospects to actual members.

Figure 6-2. Membership sales continuum

Membership Sales Stages Up Close and Personal

❑ *Identify Leads.* A lead is defined as an individual whose demographics (personal characteristics and behaviors) align with the demographics of a club's membership and whom has given an indication that they might be interested in a club's membership offering. Examples of leads include individuals who complete a lead card, individuals who respond (i.e., called or possibly walked in) to an advertisement, and individuals who respond to an email blast, text message, or social media promotion. Leads are just that, individuals who, when exposed to the features and benefits of the club, may become more interested and eventually decide to join the club.

The process of generating leads should be considered the top priority of a membership sales team and the marketing department. By generating a sufficient reservoir of leads, a club can be assured of generating a sufficient number of membership sales. The lead generation process involves two distinct phases. The first phase is marketing, which is designed to generate consumer interest and awareness of the club, while the second phase is lead tracking or database mining, which enables a club to place a name with a lead. Because marketing was reviewed in the previous chapter, this chapter does not reexamine this aspect of lead generation. Instead, this section details some of the key aspects of database mining (name recording), including the following:

- Every time a club gets a phone call or inquiry, an effort should be made to get the caller's address, phone number, and email address.
- Clubs should make sure that their lead cards provide space for the name, address, phone number, and email address. An incentive should be offered to the lead to provide this information.
- For any marketing piece that gives an individual an opportunity to respond to the marketing offer, the response form should require the lead to provide the appropriate contact information.
- If a club is engaged in a health fair or community event, contact information should be collected on every individual with whom the club comes into contact.
- A club should make it a habit for its sales staff to collect the required contact information on every individual with whom they come in contact.
- If a club utilizes guest passes as a marketing strategy, the guest pass should include space for the contact information.

If the club extends complimentary guest passes or trial visits using its website or Facebook page, then as part of the process of obtaining the guest pass, the inquiring individual should have to provide that person's contact information. An example of this approach is Club One Fitness. On Club One's website, shoppers are offered an opportunity to apply for either a trial visit or a complimentary three-day guest pass. As part of the process, the site captures the necessary contact information, data that then allows the club's sales staff to conduct the proper follow-up.

As the aforementioned points indicate, generating leads is a full-scale effort that ties marketing to information collection.

> Generating leads is a full-scale effort that ties marketing to information collection.

❏ *Qualifying Prospects*. A prospect is a lead who has expressed a need for or an interest in the club. A prospect differs from a lead in that that person has been identified as having a desire, need, or want that can be filled by the services offered by the club. Accordingly, a prospect is more likely to become a member than someone who is a lead. Turning leads into prospects and qualifying people as prospects occur in many ways. The most critical factor in qualifying prospects is to talk with the lead/individual and identify that person's desires, needs, and wants and then get that individual to express it to the sales person. Several core marketing strategies exist that are relatively likely to be successful at generating prospects, including member referrals, guest visits from distributed guest passes and trial memberships, and referrals from corporate accounts. In the end, to turn a lead into a prospect requires that a conversation take place between the membership sales person and the individual who is a prospective club member, during which the membership sales person picks up an indication that qualifies the lead as a prospect. Among the more common indications that a lead is now a prospect are the following:

- An individual indicates verbally or non-verbally that the club offers them an opportunity to fulfill a specific need.
- The individual has been a member of another health/fitness facility in the past.
- The individual has a history of being physically active and is looking to resume exercising.
- The individual is looking for a way to achieve a personal fitness or weight-loss goal.
- The individual contacted the club, based on the recommendation of a current club member.
- The individual has taken a tour of the club or has utilized a guest pass they received and has actually used the club.

> When a sales person determines that a lead has become a prospect, it is that person's responsibility to move forward with the final process of closing the sale.

When a sales person determines that a lead has become a prospect, it is that person's responsibility to move forward with the final process of closing the sale.

❑ *Closing the Sale.* The process of closing a sale refers to the process of moving a prospect to the point where that person decides to become a member of the club. The process of moving a prospect to membership usually takes place in one of two ways. The first way is what is referred to as relationship selling, where prospects choose to become members because the club has demonstrated to them that the club can fulfill an expressed need. The second method is often referred to as "high-pressure sales," a practice in which the membership sales representative, using certain "closing" techniques, applies pressure on the prospect to join. Relationship selling is likely to generate the highest closing percentage (i.e., the percentage of prospects who become members) and the highest quality member. "High-pressure" closing techniques (i.e., high volume sales), on the other hand, usually produce lower closing percentages and low-quality or often unqualified members. The primary differences between the two basic methods of closing are highlighted in the following points:

- *Relationship selling.* This approach to selling is preferred by those clubs that are interested in bringing in members who will remain members. A technique that is most frequently practiced in premium and luxury clubs, this approach to turning a prospect into a member involves an in-depth process of uncovering a prospect's needs and then connecting the club's services to the expressed needs of the prospect. The process involves creating a series of benefit statements that enable the prospect to see how the club can fulfill their expressed needs. This process does not intimidate the prospect, and it does not employ discounting or other rehearsed processes to move the prospect to membership. The relationship sale involves the following simple steps:
  - ✓ Asking questions of the prospect so that that individual's needs can be determined. Normally, at least two expressed needs must be identified. The questions usually start as open-ended probes (no definitive answer) and then move into closed probes (yes- or no-type questions).

✓ When a need is uncovered, the sales person will reiterate what has been said and then create a benefit statement that connects a particular service to the expressed need of the prospect.

✓ When a prospect confirms (verbally or non-verbally) that the benefit exists, then the membership sales person will confirm the benefit.

✓ After confirming the benefit agreed to by the prospect, the membership sales person will repeat the process to inject yet a second confirmed benefit into the process.

✓ Once the prospect has confirmed that the club benefits them in at least two ways, the membership sales person will ask for the sale in a non-intimidating way.

Relationship selling is far more effective in generating quality membership sales than high-pressure selling and typically will lead to a very high closing ratio. The primary challenge with relationship selling is the time it can take to close the sale. While "high-pressure" sales tactics are geared to close a prospect immediately, it is not uncommon for a prospect exposed to relationship selling to take a day, or even longer, to make the final purchase commitment.

Relationship selling is far more effective in generating quality membership sales than high-pressure selling and typically will lead to a very high closing ratio.

• *High-pressure closing.* Clubs and membership sales people who use this process start by asking questions that uncover a prospect's needs and vulnerabilities. While uncovering the prospect's needs is an important facet of this process, what is more important is identifying the prospect's vulnerabilities, such as time, cost, support of a significant other, self-confidence, etc. When the membership sales person identifies the vulnerability, the next step involves having the sales person use rehearsed closing lines that have a proven record of intimidating and pressuring the prospect, based on that individual's specific vulnerability, to sign up for membership. Vic Tanny clubs, which initially opened in 1947, were the first facilities in the health/fitness club industry to leverage this approach to sales. The Vic Tanny organization later introduced the high-pressure methodology to a host of other clubs and club companies, including Health and Tennis Corporation (now called Bally Total Fitness). In an article that appeared in *Time* magazine in 1961, the leadership of Vic Tanny was quoted as saying, "If you fail to get an appointment, then take a gun out of your desk and shoot yourself." This quote exemplifies the intensity and ethics that underlie clubs that rely on "high-pressure" selling.

The following case study can help illustrate the process. For example, a membership sales person has uncovered the fact that the prospect has low self-esteem and does not perceive that he has sufficient funds to join the club. A possible high-pressure closing technique that this membership sales person might use is to say, "You don't want to continue feeling so bad about yourself, so why don't you join now and get started with changing your image! I know you don't think you have the necessary funds for joining, so the club is prepared to offer you a $0 initiation fee and reduced membership dues of $19 a month if you sign up for a two-year contract."

Membership sales representatives who use this approach to attempt to turn a prospect into a member tend to discount the price of the memberships that they are selling and present multiple closing lines, before allowing the prospect to leave. In many cases, the membership sales representative will tag team with another membership representative to further intimidate the prospect. While this approach to closing is considered inappropriate by much of the industry, consumers are likely to face such strategies from clubs who depend on high-volume sales.

Staging the Membership Tour

The club tour is the strategy that has been shown to produce the highest percentage of prospects from leads and also the highest percentage of memberships from prospects.

Earlier in this chapter, the various strategies for moving a lead to a prospect and then turning that prospect into a member were discussed. Among the many approaches employed in the health/fitness club industry in this regard, the club tour is the strategy that has been shown to produce the highest percentage of prospects from leads and also the highest percentage of memberships from prospects. A membership sales person who has mastered the art of the club tour can be assured of generating quality prospects and membership sales. Staging the winning club tour involves the following steps:

❑ *Begin the Tour With a Relaxed Q-and-A Session.* When sales people first meet prospects, they should sit down in an open, non-intimidating setting. The sales person should offer the prospect a beverage or water and then proceed to uncover the following key pieces of information:

- Are they currently a member of a sports or health club, and if so, what activities do they currently pursue?
- If they are currently a health/fitness club member, why are they considering another club?
- Do they currently exercise? If yes, what kind of exercise do they currently perform? If not, what factors do they feel will help them be more likely to engage in a regular exercise program?
- What is it they would like to accomplish as the result of joining the club? Do they have any specific goals that they have established?
- Are there any activities that are of particular interest to them, such as group exercise, yoga, running, weights, etc.?
- Do they have a friend or associate who currently uses the club?
- Do they prefer a competitive or social atmosphere or are they more inclined to prefer a relaxed, private atmosphere?
- How much time do they have available at the moment to learn about the club and the benefits it can offer?

The aforementioned inquires are the most critical questions that should be asked. Obtaining answers to these questions will not only increase the chances of the membership sale being closed, but the information can prove invaluable in setting up for the prospect's first visit to the club. This information can also be used by a club's fitness department to help identify those members who may be at a heightened risk for attrition. The information obtained by this process can also help the entire club to focus on improving membership growth and retention.

❑ *Start the Tour at the Prospect's Hot Spot.* It is critical that the club tour begins in the area the prospect indicates as having the highest importance to them. It is important to keep in mind that the "club shoppers" of today are very knowledgeable about clubs and to give them a "canned" tour is one of the worst things a club can do. It can turn them off and detract from the club staff's level of professionalism. The tour should be personalized for each prospect, based upon the areas that the prospects indicated were their priorities in the Q-and-A session. A sales person should not waste time taking the prospect through the entire club, unless the sales person asks the prospect first.

❑ *Introduce the Prospect to the Experts.* It is critical during the tour that the sales person introduces the prospect to the club's experts in the prospect's indicated areas of interest. If the tour has been scheduled, arrangements should be made for the experts to be present. For example, if the prospect is interested in group exercise, then the group-exercise coordinator or an instructor should be made available. If the prospect is interested in free weights, then the fitness director or a personal trainer should be present to answer the prospect's questions. If the tour is unscheduled and an expert is not available, an effort should be made to get the fitness director or an assistant to show the prospect around the fitness area.

   A sales person should never lead off a tour of the fitness area by saying, "this is our cardiovascular room," or "we have Nautilus equipment." These statements are obvious, and to the club shopper, who has probably been a member of other clubs, these statements indicate a lack of professionalism and understanding of the prospect's specific needs by the individual leading the tour. The sales person should focus on what sets the club apart from all the other clubs. The sales person should address what the key differences mean to the prospect and why the individual should join the club. At this time, the sales person should focus on the staff, service, members, programming, etc.—not the equipment.

❑ *Extend the Invitation to Try the Club That Day.* The sales person should make sure that the prospect is given the opportunity to use the club that day if the prospect desires. Better yet, the prospect should be connected with another member or a staff person who can provide any needed assistance.

❑ *Introduce the Prospect to a Member.* From a sales perspective, nothing is stronger than the testimony of a member in showing a prospect the value of a club. The introduction between a prospect and a member should be short and brief. The club should always keep in mind that a satisfied member can be their best sales person.

> From a sales perspective, nothing is stronger than the testimony of a member in showing a prospect the value of a club.

❑ *Provide a Brochure/Club Information Package.* Every prospect should be provided with the club's brochure, which will enable certain parts of the information presented in the brochure to be referenced during the tour.

❑ *Use the Club's Program/Events Calendar.* The tour should include a brief review of the club's program and/or events calendar. It is important that the prospect gets a feel for the various activities that the club sponsors, along with a sense of the traditions of the club. This situation also represents a great opportunity to allow prospects to ask any questions that they may have and it gives the sales person an excellent chance to elaborate on the level of activity in the club.

❏ *Ask for the Sale.* After the tour is completed, the sales person should sit down with the prospect in a non-intimidating setting and ask if the prospect has any further questions. After answering the prospect's questions, the sales person should ask for the sale. If the tour went as planned, the sale will be made. If the sale doesn't occur, the sales person should make sure that the prospect is given a guest pass and then follow-up with the prospect at a later date to see how the individual's visit to the club went.

The Corporate Membership Sale

In urban markets and suburban markets with a high concentration of businesses, corporate membership sales present an unparalleled opportunity for clubs to develop large reservoirs of leads and prospects, which often result in high closing rates.

The corporate membership sale involves a unique process and situation in the health/fitness club industry. In urban markets and suburban markets with a high concentration of businesses, corporate membership sales present an unparalleled opportunity for clubs to develop large reservoirs of leads and prospects, which often result in high closing rates. For many health/fitness clubs, the corporate market represents a majority of their membership growth opportunity. According to the published report, the *IHRSA 2007 Profiles of Success*, clubs, on average, generated 15.6 percent of all sales from corporate memberships, a number that declined during the 2008 to 2010 economic downturn. Since the process of generating corporate leads and prospects, along with the process of closing those leads, is different than the typical sales process, this section of the chapter reviews the most effective approaches for selling to the corporate market.

❏ *Learn and Understand the Corporate Mindset Toward Club Memberships.* The club's first step should be to learn about the corporate fitness arena and what corporations are seeking when they purchase corporate memberships. In this regard, the University of Michigan's Health Management Research Center produces an annual report detailing the current research on the benefits and costs associated with worksite wellness. This report offers a useful overview of the cost benefit data that corporations typically consider when they evaluate the need for a corporate membership program. Another excellent resource is the 1998 IHRSA publication, *The Corporate Market: How to Capture and Keep Corporate Memberships.* In general, most corporations purchase corporate memberships for one of the following reasons:

• Use it as a tool for recruiting high-caliber talent. Many corporations indicate that fitness memberships are a benefit frequently sought by new employees.

• See it as a means to help improve employee morale and productivity.

• See it as a means to reduce healthcare-related costs for the company (current research validates the fact that low-risk employees cost companies less).

• See it as means of improving the image of the company.

- See it as a means to reduce worker's compensation costs, absenteeism, and work-related disability.

  While most companies pursue a fitness membership program for their employees based on one or more of the aforementioned factors, they also evaluate a corporate fitness membership program based on a club being able to provide one or more of the following services:

- Corporations look for health/fitness programs that include fitness, nutrition, health education, health screening, and behavioral change.
- Corporations look for membership packages that offer more than just memberships, but also allow access to specific programs, such as back care, weight loss, stress management, health fairs, health-risk screening, etc.
- Corporations look for clubs to provide them with reports on employee usage of both the club in general and particular programs specifically. These reports should provide the corporation with detailed insight into how much use their employees are getting out of the membership.
- Corporations prefer a situation where clubs offer a variety of options for billing, including the options of dues sharing with employees, payroll deduction, discounted fees, etc.

❑ *Identify the Club's Corporate Market.* Once a club gains an understanding of the corporate market, its next step should be to develop a list of the most appropriate corporations to pursue. Among the most effective means for accomplishing this task are the following:

> Corporations prefer a situation where clubs offer a variety of options for billing, including the options of dues sharing with employees, payroll deduction, discounted fees, etc.

- *Identify which corporations are represented by the club's current membership.* This step can be done by doing a search of the club's membership roster and identifying the corporations listed on the membership applications. If the club has a good relationship with its members, it might also consider having discussions with those members of the club who are known to be affiliated with local companies. Clubs should always keep in mind that its members are the best source of information in this arena.
- *Compile a list of companies that fall within the club's market area.* While not as effective as utilizing the club's membership roster, this strategy is a good alternative. Clubs should focus primarily on those companies that are located within a few miles of the club.
- *Find out who the decision-makers are at the corporations.* In most cases, either the human resources department or the medical department is involved in the process of deciding whether to purchase health/fitness club memberships for their company's employees. In smaller companies, it might be the manager or president of the company. Of course, if a club has a good relationship with its members, it may be able to find out from them who the key decision-makers are at the companies at which they work.
- *Learn about the company's values and needs.* As part of the process, clubs should make an effort to learn as much about a company as it can. The club can start the effort by searching the company's website.

Most companies, both small and large, expect the sales process to feature professionally presented materials.

The best approach in this regard, however, is for a club to talk to its members who are employed by the company. The club should learn as much as it can from these discussions with its employees.

❏ *Develop a Corporate-Presentation Package.* Most companies, both small and large, expect the sales process to feature professionally presented materials. As a result, a club needs to prepare a professional presentation about the club and the value of corporate memberships. Among the key elements that such a presentation package might include are the following:

- *Develop a PowerPoint or DVD presentation.* A PowerPoint or DVD presentation should be put together that not only tells the story of the club, but also integrates information on the benefits of fitness and wellness for the corporation.

- *Make the presentation company relevant.* The materials should be customized to the respective company with which the club is dealing.

- *Have a printed presentation package or DVD/CD package.* The club should leave a professionally done package with the company after its presentation is completed. In this regard, the most recent trend is for a club to use CDs or DVDs that also link to the club's website.

- *Get away from a standard corporate discount package.* The club should avoid making its presentation a discount presentation. The club's primary goal during a presentation should be to increase the perceived value of what it has to offer the company.

❏ *Get an Audience at the Corporation.* This step is often the most challenging aspect of corporate sales. Similar to the typical membership sale, when converting a lead into a prospect can be a demanding task, getting an opportunity to meet with the corporation can be a long tedious process. Clubs experienced in corporate sales have found the following approaches to be effective in getting the club's foot in the door:

- *Arrange for a member referral.* The best approach for getting an audience at a corporation is for a club to have one of its existing members introduce a designated person from the club to the company decision-maker by setting up an appointment for them. If members cannot set up an appointment for that person, then the member should be asked to at least provide an introduction for the sales person.

- *Build relationships in the community.* If possible, appropriate staff members from the club should join the local chamber or business-networking group. They should establish relationships that they can later use to help get them an audience at the targeted company.

- *Forward a personalized invitation.* If the company contact is known, the club should forward an invitation inviting them to the club for a special presentation. The invitation should be compelling and eye-catching. The more professional and out-of-the-ordinary it is, the more likely it is to get the company's attention.

- *Always confirm an appointment with a follow-up call.* Whether the club's appointment is obtained by an invitation or a personal introduction, the club should be sure to follow-up by phone and/or email to confirm the appointment.

❑ *Make the First Appointment a Learning Experience.* In corporate sales, the first appointment is not designed to close the sale, but rather as a means to learn about the company's needs and wants (sound familiar?) and to present general information on the benefits the club can offer. At this meeting, typically more time is spent learning about the company than presenting information on the club. The basic goal of this first meeting should be to have the company agree to have the club forward a proposal specific to the company.

❑ *Forward a Customized Presentation.* Upon completion of the initial meeting, the club should prepare a customized proposal on membership for the company. The proposal should be relevant to what the club has learned about the company. The proposal might include an invitation for the contact to use the club or possibly an invitation that allows the company to send its employees to the club for a week's complimentary usage. Some clubs have developed special activities at the club, such as featured evenings for the targeted companies. In any event, the club should make sure to follow-up its proposal with a call to confirm that its proposal has been received. The call should include an inquiry about when a good time to follow-up might be.

❑ *Maintain Contact.* Once its proposal has been forwarded to the company, the club should be vigilant with following up. The club will often find that it may take a few months between the time it forwarded its initial proposal and the next meeting it has with the company.

❑ *Be Prepared for Additional Meetings and Counterproposals.* When pursuing corporate sales, the club needs to be prepared for the fact that it will typically have to deal with additional meetings and revised proposals. It is a rare event that a club's first proposal becomes the one the company accepts.

❑ *When Closing the Sale, the Club Should Throw a Party for the Company.* Once the company agrees to the club's proposal, then a special function should be held at the club in honor of the company, welcoming the company to the club.

❑ *Make Sure to Assign a Corporate Representative.* Over the years, clubs have found that it is essential for them to assign a staff person to represent the account and maintain an ongoing contact with the company representative once the contract has been signed. More often than not, corporations need hand holding. Accordingly, clubs should make sure that they have a staff person meet with the designated corporate representative on a regular basis. These meetings should include providing information about the usage of the club by company employees and other relevant data to the company representative. Maintaining regular contact with the company can help assure ongoing support from the corporation.

Corporate membership sales are a high-reward and high-risk approach to membership sales.

It is important to understand that corporate membership sales are a high-reward and high-risk approach to membership sales. While corporate sales can lead to a relatively large number of sales, they can also often lead to high level of turnover.

Sales Management: Creating a Culture of Sales Success

The clubs who constantly achieve membership sales success are fully aware of the fact that membership sales must become part of the club culture. The most critical part of creating a sales culture is to establish disciplined sales-management practices. In the health/fitness club industry, a disciplined sales management approach would encompass several activities, including the following:

❑ *Identify and Appoint a Sales Manager.* It is extremely important that a staff person be accountable for the club's overall sales performance. The sales manager should be the individual who helps set sales goals, leads sales meetings, provides coaching and instruction for the sales staff, and otherwise supports the efforts of the sales staff.

❑ *Establish Sales Goals for the Team and Individuals.* The sales manager, working with ownership, needs to establish annual, monthly, weekly, and even daily sales goals for the team and individual sales staff. Many clubs set goals based on the number of membership units sold, but the wise sales manager focuses on sales goals founded in dollar volume. The individual and team sales goals that are established should be somewhat of a stretch, so that if they're achieved, the club exceeds its baseline membership parameters for being successful.

❑ *Monitor and Track Sales Performance.* The sales manager should implement a system that allows the club's sales-performance level to be tracked on a daily, weekly, monthly, and annual basis. The system should enable the sales manager and sales staff to identify positive and negative sales trends.

❑ *Conduct Weekly Team and Individual Sales Meetings.* The sales manager needs to have weekly sales meetings with the team that focus on results, challenges, and solutions. Concurrently, the sales manager needs to meet individually with their sales team members to provide support, coaching, and education.

❑ *Create Special Incentives.* Sales are filled with highs and lows. Sales managers need to create incentives that reward exceptional performance and also help drive performance during down times. While these incentives can be ongoing, in many cases, they should be designed to be employed during specific time periods.

❑ *Recognize Success.* Sales managers need to realize how important recognition is to sales people. Accordingly, a means to recognize individuals who perform well should be designed and implemented. Such an undertaking can produce very positive results.

❑ *Compensate the Sales Staff, Based on Performance.* Sales people need to be compensated, based on how well they achieve their individual and team sales goals.

❑ *Integrate the Sales Team With the Operations Team.* Club managers and sales managers both need to realize that the greatest level of membership

> The individual and team sales goals that are established should be somewhat of a stretch, so that if they're achieved, the club exceeds its baseline membership parameters for being successful.

sales success comes when the sales team and the operations team work together. Unfortunately, some clubs forget this precept and create organizational slots (individual pockets of focus), in which membership sales are not connected to the other areas of the club. An effective sales manager will realize that the entire club staff can have a positive impact on the success of the sales department and will do whatever is feasible to integrate the two.

❏ *Hold the Sales Team Collectively Accountable.* The club manager needs to hold the sales manager accountable for the club's level of sales performance against the predetermined sales plan. By the same token, the sales manager should hold the sales staff accountable for their individual and team performance.

A New Approach to Sales: Online Prospecting and Sales

Over the past few years, a new approach involving membership sales has occurred in the health/fitness club industry—online prospecting and sales. This trend not only has removed sales staff and sales systems from the process, it has experienced an ever-increasing level of acceptance and success. Beginning with the advent of "budget clubs" in Europe and "high-volume, low-price clubs" in the United States, membership sales have moved out of the club and out of the hands of a trained sales staff into the realm of the "cloud." This new approach to membership sales relies on the following three critical factors:

❏ *Attracting Prospects With a Very Low Price.* Industry practice over the last few years has shown that if a club is able to effectively market itself through an attractive pricing offer (typically under 20 Euro or $20 a month), then it does not need to have sales staff involved in such tasks as generating leads, providing tours, and conducting sales sessions. All factors considered, it appears that when the price is low enough, a club can generate a plentiful quantity of leads, without the involvement of a sales team.

❏ *Demonstrating the Club Value Proposition Over the Internet.* With the advent of 3D technology and interactive modeling, clubs are able to provide prospects with virtual tours of the club online. In addition, websites can go beyond just providing virtual 3D tours. They can also provide member testimonials, class schedules, staff qualifications, etc. In essence, with the proper technology, everything that was once done in person in the club can now be done online.

❏ *Allowing a Prospective Member to Apply and Pay Online.* With the advancements in technology and online payment systems, clubs are able to have their entire membership application and dues-collection process to be conducted and completed over the Internet. This approach involves having the member actually complete an online application for membership, including providing the necessary payment information. After the membership application is completed and the payment method is approved, members receive their initial new-member information online. Shortly thereafter, they also receive their membership card and related materials in the mail.

An effective sales manager will realize that the entire club staff can have a positive impact on the success of the sales department and will do whatever is feasible to integrate the two.

Two examples of clubs that successfully leverage this approach to membership sales are the Gym Group, a leading budget club operator in the U.K., and McFit, the leading budget club operator in both Germany and Europe. In both instances they:

- Offer memberships at less than 20 Euro a month.
- Perform extensive Internet and social media-based marketing, an effort that promotes their price and the great value proposition.
- Have elaborate websites that allow a prospect to tour their clubs, view their offerings, and obtain any information that might otherwise be critical to the decision to purchase a membership. Prospects can see the club, view member testimonials, and even see parts of the club life.
- Have an online membership application and payment process.

Neither of the aforementioned clubs have a sales staff. Each of these companies generates, on average, between 5,000 and 7,500 members per club, and in many instances more.

Membership sales are a by-product of very disciplined business practices that require a detailed system of checks and balances.

Key Points to Consider

As illustrated by the information in this chapter, membership sales are a continuation of a club's membership and marketing efforts. More importantly, membership sales are a by-product of very disciplined business practices that require a detailed system of checks and balances.

MEMBERSHIP RETENTION IN THE HEALTH/FITNESS CLUB INDUSTRY

Ingram Publishing/Thinkstock

Part Three

7

Member Retention and the Value of a Member

Chapter Objectives

Members are the heart of every club. Without them, health/fitness clubs would cease to exist. It is a widely held belief in the industry that membership is all about sales. In reality, however, membership is a balance between the process of selling and retaining memberships. Membership retention is about engaging members in the club experience so that they continue to stay a member. The more members stay, the fewer the number of memberships a club has to sell. In other words, membership retention involves the process of keeping members after the sale. This chapter begins by providing an overview of membership-retention data in the health/fitness club industry. The chapter then features a clarification of what retention and attrition are and how they are measured. Next, the chapter discusses the value of a member. Finally, the chapter details several of the variables known to influence a club's membership retention level and some of the steps that clubs can take to affect those retention variables.

The Industry's Recent Experiences With Membership Retention

According to the published report, the *IHRSA 2010 Profiles of Success*, the average retention rate for U.S. clubs in 2009 was 71 percent. Ten years earlier, the U.S. club industry's retention rate was 65 percent, which indicates that over the past decade the industry has made strides in its ability to retain members (Figure 7-1). Most of that gain was achieved over the first five years of the 21st century, going from 65 percent in 2000 to 71 percent in 2005, and then remaining at 71 percent, on average, for the next five years. The key takeaway from these statistics is that the industry was able to improve its overall retention level of performance during the first half of the decade, and over the last half of the decade, was able to sustain that achievement. From a retention perspective, that is good news. Interestingly, some of the largest players in the industry have been unable to duplicate these industry-wide retention levels.

> It is a widely held belief in the industry that membership is all about sales. In reality, however, membership is a balance between the process of selling and retaining memberships.

According to Lifetime Fitness's public filings, its retention rates from 2006 to 2010 have floated between 58 percent and 65 percent. Equinox, one of the premier operators of quality clubs in the industry, has indicated, off the record, that its retention rates tend to fluctuate around 65 percent.

According to IHRSA's survey data, the average number of membership terminations a club experiences has declined steadily over the past decade, going from an average of 1,300 in 2000 to an average of 750 in 2009. On an absolute basis, this situation is a significant improvement in the average club's ability to retain members. Over the past five years, the average number of member resignations in a particular club has remained relatively flat at around 725 to 750 annually, with only two aberrations, one occurring in 2007 and the other in 2008.

According to the aforementioned data concerning the average number of new memberships sold and the average number of memberships cancelled, the average club in 2009 experienced more membership terminations than sales. This instance is the first time in the 10-year history that these statistics have been kept that membership terminations have been greater than new member sales, resulting in a negative level of net membership growth (Figure 7-2). As before, the data would seem to reflect that the U.S. health/fitness club industry was able to make inroads into member attrition during the first part of the decade, and since then has been able to maintain those achievements. Unfortunately, as clubs continue to experience logging new member sales, retention efforts will need to intensify, if indeed the industry wants to grow over the next decade.

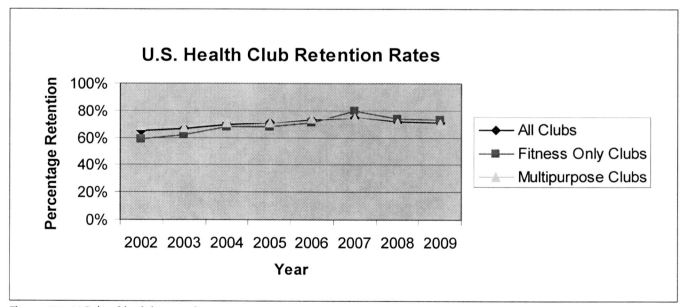

Figure 7-1. U.S. health club retention rates

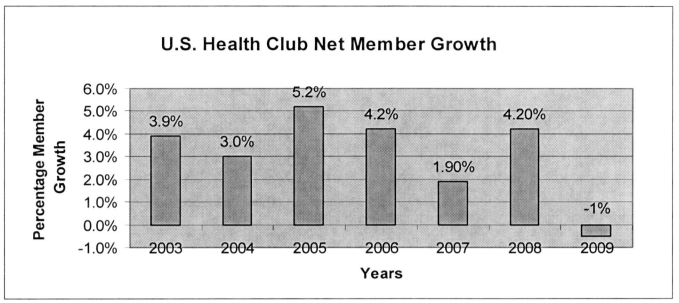

Figure 7-2. U.S. health club net member growth

The retention data presented in Figure 7-1 is a reflection of the sample of U.S. clubs that were surveyed by IHRSA. In a study conducted by researchers in the United Kingdom in the early part of the 21st century, U.K. clubs that were surveyed had retention levels that ranged from as low as 39 percent to as high as 89 percent. In reality, some clubs in the U.S. industry report retention rates closer to 50 percent, while others report retention rates that are as high as 90 percent to 95 percent. According to IHRSA's research, the larger clubs (over 60,000 S.F.) and those clubs generating over five million dollars in annual revenues have retention percentages that approach 80 percent. In fact, a number of clubs, such as the Houstonian in Houston, the Cooper Activity Center in Dallas, the Pacific Athletic Club in Redwood City, California, and the East Bank Club in Chicago, report that they are able to keep their retention rate at 80 percent or more on an annual basis.

Common Industry Definition of Member Retention

Membership retention describes the business outcome of a club holding on to (keeping) its members after the initial membership sale, and subsequent enrollment of the new members. As in any successful business, the objective is to retain the highest possible number of clients for the longest possible period of time. In the health/fitness club business, retaining members is as important, or even more so, than retaining clients can be for other businesses, given that members represent the "lifeblood" of clubs. The health/fitness club business represents a form of "closed economic model," one in which clubs are dependent on their ability to drive ongoing business from a restricted or limited market of clients (e.g., members). As a result, retention becomes a key driver of long-term profitability. The majority of health/fitness clubs measure retention on an annual basis.

An Alternate Definition of Member Retention

In their groundbreaking research on membership retention in the United Kingdom, Paul Bedford, Ph.D. and Melvyn Hillsdon, Ph.D. defined retention as the proportion of members who remain a member for a predetermined period of time (e.g., 3 months, 6 months, 12 months, 18 months, etc.). This definition takes into account the variable of a member's tenure. The rationale for tying membership tenure into the retention equation lies in the understanding that the longer a member remains with a club, the more likely it is that person will spend money in the club.

Common Industry Definition of Member Attrition

Attrition of clients, like death and taxes, is inevitable for any business, but like the other two factors, most clubs would prefer to minimize and delay it as long as possible.

Membership attrition is the opposite of retention, and represents the departure of clients and members from a club. Attrition of clients, like death and taxes, is inevitable for any business, but like the other two factors, most clubs would prefer to minimize and delay it as long as possible. In the case of the health/fitness club industry, delaying and, if possible, preventing the attrition of members can have a very positive impact on a club's financial performance. Each time a member leaves a club, that facility loses a valuable source of income. Furthermore, the expenses involved in replacing that member costs far more than it does to provide an environment that might otherwise help that member decide to remain with the club.

While the majority of clubs measure attrition on an annual basis, health/fitness facilities monitor this factor on a monthly basis. These operators believe that monitoring monthly attrition provides an additional perspective with regard to the seasonality of the health/fitness club business. For example, publicly held companies, such as Lifetime Fitness and Town Sports International, often report their monthly attrition figures as part of their monthly calls with investors.

An Alternate Definition of Member Attrition

In their aforementioned groundbreaking research in the United Kingdom, Dr. Paul Bedford and Dr. Melvyn Hillsdon defined member attrition (as opposed to their description of member retention) as the rate of member churn or turnover per 1,000 members. The authors believe that attrition is best measured not as a percentage of the total membership, but instead as a turnover rate, based on an objective and comparable metric. Such a methodology enables a club to objectively measure its attrition at any point in time.

Calculating Membership Retention: Two Approaches

The IHRSA Methodology for Calculating Attrition and Retention

- Begin by calculating the number of members at the end of each month.
- Take the number of members at the end of each month, and then add them together and divide by 12 (e.g., the number of months in the year). This calculation gives a facility its average member count for the year.
- Calculate the total number of members who resigned during the year.

- Divide the average member count by the total number of members who terminated their membership during the year, which will yield a club's annual attrition rate.
- Subtract the annual attrition percentage from the integer "one," which will provide the club's annual retention rate.

Figure 7-3 illustrates an example of using IHRSA's recommended approach to calculate a club's annual attrition and retention levels.

Month	Members at the end of the month	Resigned members	Monthly/annual attrition
January	3,200	60	1.8 percent
February	3,250	80	2.5 percent
March	3,300	90	2.7 percent
April	3,350	85	2.5 percent
May	3,350	90	2.7 percent
June	3,325	100	3.0 percent
July	3,275	105	3.2 percent
August	3,250	120	3.7 percent
September	3,275	95	2.9 percent
October	3,350	85	2.5 percent
November	3,350	90	2.7 percent
December	3,300	100	3.0 percent
Year-end average	3,298	1,100	33.3 percent attrition 66.7 percent retention

Figure 7-3. An example of employing IHRSA's recommended methodology for calculating membership attrition and retention levels

Retention and Attrition Measurement Approach Recommended by Bedford and Hillsdon

As part of their research efforts, Dr. Paul Bedford and Dr. Melvyn Hillsdon proposed using a form of "survival analysis" for accurately measuring a club's retention level. Their approach takes into account the time between events, as well as the proportion of members who remain at specific points in time. It is postulated that this approach provides a more accurate reflection of member retention, since it takes into account both the proportion of involvement and the tenure of the relationship. As shown in Figure 7-4, the two clubs (A & B) have identical retention rates after 14 months. On the other hand, with the exception of a few months, club A has been able to sustain a much higher level of retention at key periods of time, which may help to explain why it is able to retain its members for a longer period of time.

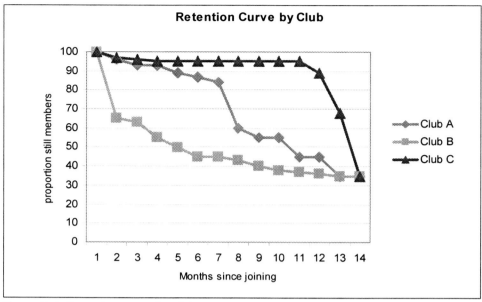

Figure 7-4. Retention curve by club

The Value of a Membership and the Value of Retention

With regard to member retention level, two key issues arise: what is the real value of driving retention to both a club and the industry, and why is it so important? An answer to both inquiries is provided by Dun & Bradstreet, a renowned financial research firm that states that the primary reason most businesses fail is that they either lack sales and/or fail to retain their existing customers. In the health/fitness club business, the value of retaining a customer (i.e., member) is even more significant than in many other businesses, because of the fact that a limitless supply of new customers for their business offerings does not exist. A better idea of the "real dollar" value of a typical club member can be obtained by looking at statistics on member pricing, member spending, and membership retention that appear in the book the *IHRSA 2010 Profiles of Success* (Figure 7-5).

Average initiation/enrollment fee for an individual:	$95
Average monthly dues for an individual:	$60
Average annual dues:	$720
Average percentage of revenue from non-dues:	30 percent
Average annual non-dues revenue:	$308
Total annual revenue per member:	$1,028
Average attrition rate:	29 percent
Average lifespan of a member:	3.3 years (based on attrition)

Figure 7-5. Typical club member pricing, member spending, and membership retention level (based on the average of club statistics)

In the case of the "average club member," according to the statistics detailed in Figure 7-5, the average club member spends $1,123 in that person's first year of membership. Furthermore, if the net present value of the dollar is not factored in, that member will, on average, be worth approximately $1,028 annually for the duration of that individual's membership. In turn, if the tenure of an average member is 3.3 years, then the total dollar value of an average club member over the membership period is approximately $3,487.

Given the 2010 IHRSA statistics that indicate that the average health/fitness club lost 601 members in 2009, it would mean that the average club lost over $2,095,000 in revenues in the course of that 12-month period. As such, if a club could decrease its attrition level by just five percent, thereby retaining an additional 30 members, the average club would save approximately $104,600 annually.

It should be noted the aforementioned example does not factor in the potential impact of member referrals or consider the value those referrals might bring to the bottom line. It also does not account for the fact that the longer an individual remains a member, the more incremental spending takes place. As such, it is obvious that when a member leaves a club, especially the earlier a member leaves a facility, the club's profitability will be negatively impacted.

All factors considered, the value of retaining a club member becomes even more important during periods of economic volatility, such as during recessionary periods or times when the economy is experiencing financial bubbles. Not surprisingly, when people are less secure about their financial position, they are less likely to spend money on a new purchase (e.g., a club membership). On the other hand, they are also more likely to stay with existing investments. Given the experiences that occurred during the economic turmoil of 2008/2009, existing members who had already invested in a club membership tended to use their club more frequently. As a consequence, they were less likely to surrender their membership. On the flip side, during the most recent recessionary period, new sales in clubs experienced a significant downturn. As a result, when the economic environment is less than ideal, retention becomes an even more critical factor to the profitability of a club.

> The value of retaining a club member becomes even more important during periods of economic volatility.

Variables Known to Influence Attrition and Retention

In 1998 and more recently in 2007, IHRSA funded research into uncovering the reasons why members leave clubs, with the intent of gaining a greater understanding of what factors might influence the individuals to stay. In 2000, IHRSA sponsored additional research that looked at these factors that correlated to individuals remaining as a member of a club, in an attempt to identify which of those variables might be alterable. Finally, in 2001, the Fitness Industry Association of England undertook research into membership retention. Cumulatively, the results of those three separate research endeavors provide considerable insight into why individuals forego their memberships in health/fitness clubs.

The decision a member makes to remain a club member or leave the club is impacted to a significant degree by personal and relationship factors.

The decision a member makes to remain a club member or leave the club is impacted to a significant degree by personal and relationship factors. It seems that such a decision is most often influenced by not having an exercise partner, not fitting in, losing motivation, lack of attention from the staff, and dissatisfaction with the programs and activities of the club. Each of these variables involves an individual's social connection to the club, to the club's staff, the other members, and the activities of the club. These factors are also affected by how well the club gets each new member "engaged" with their new purchase.

In addition to the aforementioned data, research has also identified the following factors as critical determinants influencing membership retention:

• Members who feel the staff helped them to achieve their personal fitness goals were far more likely to remain a member.

• Members who felt that the staff was professional and took a personal interest in them were far more likely to remain a member.

• Members who made friends quickly and developed a sense of belonging or fitting in were far more likely to remain a member.

• Members who used the club most frequently during their first month reported they had a better relationship with the staff.

• Members who rated their satisfaction with the club as the highest were also the most likely to have a great relationship with the staff and were the most likely to remain a member.

• The percentage of members who remain in a club falls proportionally over the first 12 months. According to the FIA research, at 12 weeks, retention is around 93 percent. It then drops to 78 percent by 24 weeks, just less than 70 percent by 36 weeks, and around 60 percent by 52 weeks.

• Older adults have a higher retention rate than younger adults, with those over 45 having the highest retention percentage of any age group.

• Those members who pay a higher initiation fee have a higher retention rate. According to FIA research, the retention rate for those paying an initiation fee is 21 percent greater than for those who don't pay a fee.

• Members who pay annually have higher retention rates than those who pay on a month-by-month basis. After one year, the difference between the two retention rates is negligible.

• A dose-response rate exists between use of the club and membership retention. In other words, the more engaged a member is in using the club, the more likely that person is to remain a member.

• The first month is the most critical period for the retention rate process. Those individuals who use the club less than four times in the first month have a significantly higher attrition rate.

• Those new members with a higher level of education and a higher level of income are more likely to remain members.

• Smokers and those individuals who are overweight are more likely to drop their membership.

As can be seen, a host of reasons exist why people decide to either remain a member or chose to leave. The aforementioned factors are similar in many respects to the data presented in the earlier figures. These factors lend further support to the contention that club members need to be engaged and connected with their clubs as soon as possible in order for them to continue with their membership. This step entails facilitating a connection between the individual member and both the staff and the other members. This undertaking also involves helping members achieve their personal goals and providing an entertaining and motivating environment for club members. Accordingly, club operators, with regard to membership retention, need to identify and focus on those factors that can have the greatest impact on their club's retention level and its bottom line.

Proven Strategies for Improving Retention

The process of retaining members ultimately revolves around the club's ability to deliver experiences that are personally relevant and are facilitated by exceptional service. This section reviews several proven approaches for not only increasing the level of member connection, but also driving member retention. In the next two chapters, some of the key elements involved in creating positive experiences and establishing a service culture and a service-oriented level of programming will be addressed. Among research-based strategies for enhancing the membership-retention level are the following:

> The process of retaining members ultimately revolves around the club's ability to deliver experiences that are personally relevant and are facilitated by exceptional service.

- *Don't sell the club membership short.* Retention begins at the time of joining. Research shows that members who pay an enrollment fee stay longer than those who don't. Furthermore, the higher the initial fee, the higher the retention level. The key point is that the club operator should assign a real value to the club's membership experience. If membership is given away, all factors being equal, members will feel their membership is not worth very much. One exception seems to exist to this rule, involving budget clubs, where the dues payment is under 20 Euro or $20 a month. It appears that at this low-price point, membership retention may actually increase slightly.
- *Identify the members' fitness needs and focus on getting them to the goal.* The data is clear that with regard to membership retention, it is crucial that members achieve their fitness goals. This process not only involves identifying what those goals are, but also developing a program that provides a realistic avenue for them to be achieved. Finally, all clubs should provide monitoring, support, and encouragement to their members so their members' goals can be achieved.
- *Connect the new member to other members.* Most members express a strong desire to have a partner or to feel a sense of belonging. Satisfying this desire requires getting the members to meet other members and establish friendships. Clubs can accomplish this goal by having the staff introduce new members to other members. They can also achieve this objective by organizing and implementing such undertakings as welcoming parties, new member/existing member activities, member chat spaces, partner programs, etc.
- *Staff and members need to connect.* Clubs need to establish a service culture that is passionate about caring for the members. The staff should

be encouraged to meet with members, learn about them, and respond to their needs and feedback. Responsive and friendly are two key attributes of a caring-oriented staff.

- *Get the members active.* The research is very clear about the "use-it-or-lose-it" aspect of membership. Members who are more active, especially in the initial stages of their membership, are far more likely to remain members (IHRSA and FIA data both reflect this phenomena). Clubs need to establish systems that introduce new members to club-based activities in a non-intimidating way and then track their activity-involvement levels so they can monitor and help reinforce each member's efforts to be physically active. Clubs might even consider offering incentive programs tied to activity during an individual's first three months of membership.

- *Be attentive to the members' comments and interests.* Club management needs to establish a system for maintaining an open dialogue with its members. This process should involve the use of such factors as a feedback system, service recovery system, focus groups, surveys, and even member committees. The members need to perceive management as being interested in and responsive to their experiences.

- *Keep the club clean and well-maintained.* While not a primary reason given by members for quitting, research shows that whether the club was kept clean and whether the club kept its equipment and facilities updated had an impact on the desire of individuals to maintain their club membership. Members want to feel that the dues they are paying are going back into the club. Clubs need to keep this factor in mind and let members know when the club is doing something to upgrade its facilities or equipment.

- *Make retention a part of everyone's job description.* All employees, from the membership sales staff to the manager to the housecleaning staff, must view the process of helping retain members as an integral part of their job. Sales people help retention by not selling the club short and by helping connect members at the time of joining. The fitness staff drives retention by helping members achieve their fitness goals and helping connect the members to other members. The front desk staff can have a positive impact on retention by making members feel welcome and responding to member comments. The house maintenance staff affects retention in a positive manner by keeping the club clean and by looking for ways to respond to member needs.

All employees, from the membership sales staff to the manager to the housecleaning staff, must view the process of helping retain members as an integral part of their job.

As club operators attempt to identify strategies that can help them retain members, they should remember that retention begins with a culture within the club that focuses on connecting people, creates memorable experiences, and always puts the member first. The next two chapters take a more in-depth look at member satisfaction and the need for a club to create exceptional experiences and service-oriented programs that will satisfy the needs and expectations of its members.

8

Creating Memorable Member Experiences

Chapter Objectives

In the previous chapter, the value of a membership and the importance of retaining members in driving the profitability and vibrancy of a club were addressed. As research indicates, members either stay in or leave a club based on whether their experience at the club meets or does not meet their expectations and needs. Research also shows that in the majority of instances, the situations in which member expectations were not met revolved around the connection of members to members, members to the staff, and members to the club's activities. This chapter explores the importance of the fact that clubs should create a culture that drives memorable experiences that meet and exceed the expectations of their members. The chapter examines how individuals who belong to clubs respond to experiences that they encounter as members of a club and the impact that these experiences have on their level of retention. The chapter then reviews the importance of creating memorable experiences. Finally, the chapter details the process of creating the experiences that drive member retention.

How Members Respond to the Service Delivery and the Experience Provided by the Club

When individuals decide to become members of a club, they join with certain preconceptions and expectations. For some, those factors may involve achieving a certain fitness goal, while the objective of other individuals may be to meet other people within the club setting. Regardless of whether one or more of these factors is the primary reason driving their joining a club, each of these variables affects whether they remain a member. In this regard, these factors may include such diverse matters as personal attention from staff, recognition from the club, facility cleanliness, program variety, program convenience, meeting other members, and a host of other reasons. In reality, because club operators cannot always identify these expectations, they must be prepared to create and deliver experiences that can meet or exceed expectations of which they may not even be aware.

Members either stay in or leave a club based on whether their experience at the club meets or does not meet their expectations and needs.

Research conducted on how individuals respond to their experiences indicates that four basic responses exist—one of which is good, one of which is outstanding, and all of which can be used to drive a club's ability to retain members.

A club's first indication of how members have accepted or perceived the delivery of the club experience is by the response they make (both verbally and non-verbally). Collectively, the members' responses then become an important factor in how club operators and their staff adjust the services and experiences they provide.

Research conducted on how individuals respond to their experiences indicates that four basic responses exist—one of which is good, one of which is outstanding, and all of which can be used to drive a club's ability to retain members. The impact of these responses on a club varies from factor to factor:

❑ *Outrage.* Outrage is an emotional response that members have when their experience has fallen well short of their expectations. Members who exhibit outrage feel great emotional displeasure and a sense of betrayal. When clubs do not deal immediately with member outrage, they are contributing to the formation of what can be called, "business terrorists," people who go out of their way to harm the business. Many of the individuals in the health/fitness club business are familiar with this response. Most clubs tend to ignore members who respond with outrage, not realizing that they are creating terrorists.

Over the past decade with the evolution of the Internet, outraged customers have used the social media to voice their unhappiness. Some outraged consumers search for vengeance by posting complaints on company Facebook pages and websites, while others take a more aggressive stance and create "complaint sites" or "gripe sites." As such, several of America's leading companies, including one of the leading health/fitness club operators in the United States, have been the target of dedicated gripe sites. Because these sites can damage reputations and profitability, finding ways to avoid creating customer outrage should be a priority for every business. When a club or business is able to actually overcome the outrage (not an easy thing to do), it is building a strong bridge to retaining that customer and/or member.

❑ *Dissatisfaction.* Dissatisfaction is an unemotional response that members have when they do not receive the service or experience they expect. This response often occurs when a club makes its members "sacrifice" something of importance, the absence of which then becomes an inconvenience. Dissatisfied members normally don't tell the club about their sense of dissatisfaction. In one large global fitness club company's semi-annual survey of its members, it was determined that over 50 percent of the members who experienced an inconvenience never filed a complaint. This statistic is a great example of what happens with members who are dissatisfied with the club experience; they may have a problem, but they don't voice it. Rather, they might grumble to other members of the club or show up less often at the club. An example of a circumstance that could result in a degree of member dissatisfaction could be something as simple and basic as a trainer arriving five minutes late for an appointment with the member or the sauna not working. Eventually, dissatisfied members will leave the club if they are not identified. On the other hand, they are easily taken care of if the source of their dissatisfaction is addressed by the club.

❑ *Satisfaction.* To many individuals in the health/fitness club business, member satisfaction is considered the end point, the response of choice. A satisfied individual means that the club has been able to meet the member's expectations. A satisfied member is not necessarily a happy member, rather an individual who, for now, will continue as a member. Satisfied members are often the first to leave when a new club opens elsewhere, because although they are satisfied, they have not developed a sufficient sense of loyalty to the club. Far too often, satisfied members are relatively unknown to the club, because they haven't expressed their true feelings to the club.

❑ *Delight.* Delight occurs when the club exceeds a member's expectations. In other words, the club has provided an experience that was both memorable and beyond the member's perceptions or expectations. Delight is an indication of an emotional buy-in or personal ownership. Delighted members are often referred to as "business apostles"—individuals who "tell and sell" the club's story to others. Typically, club operators know who these individuals are, because they are often the most active, outgoing, and loyal members of the club.

Delight occurs when the club exceeds a member's expectations. In other words, the club has provided an experience that was both memorable and beyond the member's perceptions or expectations.

In the late 1990s and early 2000s, ClubCorp sponsored research that was designed to identify how the various aforementioned member responses impacted retention and profitability. In particular, ClubCorp wanted to better understand how these responses affected the members' desire to remain a member and their willingness to refer others for membership. This research found that delighted members were twice as likely to remain a member over the next 12 months as a satisfied member and one tenth as likely to leave. Furthermore, a delighted member was nearly 10 times as likely as a satisfied member to refer someone for membership. The conclusion, which paralleled research results in other customer-service environments, was that a delighted member is the most valuable member a club has. These findings support the contention that a club should create a service and experience culture that is focused on driving member delight. Figures 8-1 and 8-2 illustrate the findings of the ClubCorp investigations. When the membership retention and membership sales implications of these figures are considered, it is very clear that clubs can benefit by creating a culture that is focused on delivering the service necessary to create experiences that drive a member's sense of delight, which collectively enhances member loyalty.

The Value Equation Behind Member Satisfaction and Loyalty

One key issue concerning creating memorable member experiences that often arises is how does a club first achieve member satisfaction, and then move beyond it to establish member delight and loyalty? It begins with understanding the underlying elements of how a customer, or in the case of the club business, a member, perceives value and how that value creates either satisfaction or emotional delight and loyalty. In that regard, a members' perception of value can be calculated using the following formula:

$$Value = \frac{Facility\ Quality + Product\ Quality + Service\ Quality + Emotional\ Quality}{Price + Time}$$

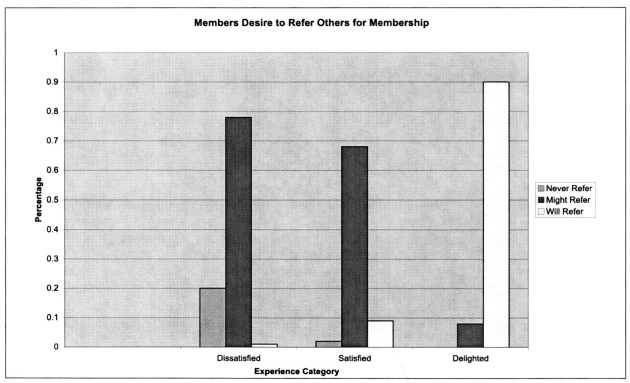

Figure 8-1. The members' desire to refer others for membership

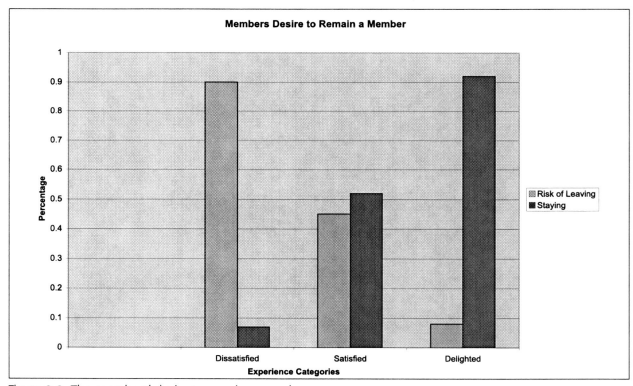

Figure 8-2. The members' desire to remain a member

❑ *Numerator*
   • Facility quality is defined by the overall quality of the facility and includes several elements, such as cleanliness, amount of equipment, accessibility of equipment, condition of the facility, etc.
   • Product quality is defined as the overall quality of the club's products offerings, based on the expectations the member has, including a variety of elements, such as class schedule, special events, training programs, etc.
   • Service quality is defined as the level of service the club provides, based on the member's expectations, and includes elements, such as smiles, greeting members by name, fast and courteous attention, service recovery, etc.
   • Emotional quality is defined as the level of emotional attachment that is created for the member by the club experience and is affected by several elements, such as relationships with staff, relationships with other members, sense of pride in the club, etc.

❑ *Denominator*
   • Price reflects the actual cash price an individual pays to use the club, encompassing such expenses as enrollment fees, dues, and possibly fees for extra services. It may also involve whether the payment is made monthly or annually.
   • Time reflects the time that the member must spend to achieve the perceived/expected benefits offered by the club, for example, factors such as visits per week, time spent each visit, and any time necessary to get to and from the club each visit.

Member satisfaction occurs when the numerator is higher than the denominator. Loyalty, on the other hand, can only occur when the emotional quality in the numerator is very high (delighted members). For example, Apple has created incredible customer loyalty because all of the elements in the numerator are powerful, but in particular the emotional quality. Obviously, Apple products are not inexpensive (typically, they're considerably more expensive than comparable products). The point, however, in Apple's case, is that Apple's numerator contributors, when combined together, are far more valuable and powerful than the costs reflected in Apple's denominator.

As a result, in order for clubs to establish a high value, they must deliver the facility, products, and services, along with emotional engagement at a level far greater than the actual cost and time required for a member to use the club.

Measuring Member Satisfaction and Loyalty

The standard approach for measuring satisfaction and loyalty is to survey the membership on a regular basis, asking a series of questions or proposing specific statements to which members can then respond, using a simple numerical scale (e.g., the five-point Likert scale—an instrument commonly employed in most surveys). The Likert scale (in its simplest, most common format, the simple scale has five points, more advanced scales can have as many as seven

> In order for clubs to establish a high value, they must deliver the facility, products, and services, along with emotional engagement at a level far greater than the actual cost and time required for a member to use the club.

or nine points) is a standardized psychometric scale that allows researchers to easily assess respondent answers. The basic five-point scale involves the following classifications:

5 = strongly agree (delighted)

4 = agree or somewhat agree (satisfied)

3 = not sure or neither agree or disagree (partially satisfied)

2 = disagree (dissatisfaction)

1 = strongly disagree (outrage)

By employing this scale, researchers are able to accurately measure the degree of delight, satisfaction, and dissatisfaction that may exist around a specific situation, a series of situations, or an entire experience.

The most frequently used and quoted metric or indicator of member loyalty is called the *"Net Promoter® Score,"* a measure that was introduced in 2003 by Harvard University professor Fred Reicheld. The term *Net Promoter Score* is actually a trademarked title of Reichheld, Bain & Company. The purpose of the *Net Promoter Score* is to clearly identify those customers and/or members who are actual promoters of a business (loyal members, raving fans, etc.). Typically, while Net Promoters are determined using a 10-point scale, they can also be identified by using a simple five-point scale, like the aforementioned Likert scale. A *Net Promoter*, or loyal and delighted member (raving fan), is a member or customer who rates a club as either a 9 or 10 on a 10-point scale or a 5 on a five-point scale.

A facility's *Net Promoter Score* is determined by taking the percentage of members who rate the club experience as excellent (e.g., "5" on a five-point scale) and then subtracting that number from the percentage of members who rate the club experience as less than satisfactory (e.g., "3" or less on a five-point scale). The resulting number is a club's *Net Promoter Score*. A score of zero or better is considered good, while a score greater than +50 is considered excellent.

Many businesses focus on one simple question to determine their overall *Net Promoter Score*, which is, *"How likely are you to refer a friend or colleague?"* On the other hand, many researchers feel that this single question and the resultant *Net Promoter Score* are not a true indicator of customer loyalty. Rather, it is merely a score that indicates how likely a member is to refer another member. The underlying premise of these detractors is that the *Net Promoter Score* should be determined by using the responses to a series of questions. In the health/fitness club industry, one leading market researcher suggests calculating the *Net Promoter Score*, using members' responses to the following four questions:

- How likely are you to remain a member over the next 12 months?
- How likely are you to refer someone for membership over the next 12 months?
- How would you rate your overall experience with the club?
- How much do you love the club?

> The most frequently used and quoted metric or indicator of member loyalty is called the *"Net Promoter Score."*

In reality, taking the responses to these four questions and calculating the percentage of responses that fall into each of the three response categories (promoter, passive, detractor), totaling them up, and then subtracting detractors from promoters provides a far more accurate portrayal of a club's *Net Promoter Score*.

Using their *Net Promoter Score* enables clubs to more easily identify the general level of member delight and loyalty that exists within their membership. On the other hand, even though they may have their *Net Promoter Score* in hand, health/fitness clubs need to realize how important it is for them to get a reading on other important issues that can affect how their members perceive the experiences that they are having in the facilities, and most importantly, to understand the specific variables that can contribute to driving their *Net Promoter Score* upward.

Defining a Positive Club Experience

As the previous sections discussed, if a club wants to have an impact on member retention, it needs to have a service culture that is focused on creating and sustaining experiences that exceed the expectations of members. In that regard, two critical issues arise: what is meant by the term "an experience" and what role does service culture have in driving these experiences. In order to address those issues, the first step is to understand the relationship between service and experience. Both factors are defined as follows:

If a club wants to have an impact on member retention, it needs to have a service culture that is focused on creating and sustaining experiences that exceed the expectations of members.

❏ *Service.* Service is the process by which a club's people and systems are able to deliver the club's facilities, programs, and other amenities to the member. Service is the process that the club employs to deliver its product. Service requires people and systems that can repeatedly deliver the club's product, with minimal sacrifice on the member's part. The following example can help illustrate the differences between service and experience. A club offers yoga classes for novices, beginners, and advanced members. The classes are the club's product. The manner in which the club's instructors teach those classes and interact with the members is the service the club provides. If the service provided by the club enables members to participate freely, with minimal inconvenience, and enjoy the class, then the club is servicing the members with minimal sacrifice by the members. If instead, the yoga class instructors require members to say a pledge, ask beginners to perform advanced work, and never smile, the club's service in this instance would be requiring the members to make some degree of sacrifice to participate. In other words, in the context of service, the club should think of it as the delivery mechanism for all of the experiences it provides to members. Great service occurs when members sacrifice the least, and poor service exists when the club makes its members exert a considerable sacrifice.

❏ *Experience.* An experience involves the interplay of a club's product, the service process, the expectations and needs of the member, and finally, the club's ability to create the desired circumstances around a theme. In essence, an experience is what members receive or perceive they receive based on how the club themes the service it provides and how it impacts the members' expectations. It should be noted that experiences can be good or bad. Accordingly, the goal of the club should be to create experiences that require minimal sacrifice on the part of the member and enhance the member's sense of member delight.

One positive example of creating a desired experience is a class offered by one of the various Crunch clubs in New York City. This particular Crunch club offers an aerobic class called cardio striptease. The theme of the class is, of course, striptease. The club's product is an aerobic class. The service is the manner in which the instructor delivers the class, hopefully with passion, dressed in full striptease attire which is later removed, of course, and encouraging the members to do the same. While the foregoing is an extreme example, other programming efforts, such as Fireman's Aerobics, Hell Week, Antigravity yoga, etc., also illustrate how clubs can create an experience at the micro level.

Creating Club-Based Experiences

Clubs can achieve noteworthy success with their members by creating a service culture that is focused on delivering unique experiences that not only exceed member expectations, but also help facilitate member delight and loyalty. Among the relatively simple steps that a club can take to become more experience-oriented are the following:

❏ *Establish a Theme.* The first step in creating a unique and differentiating membership experience is to identify a unifying theme. By establishing a theme for the experience that the club intends to provide, it can focus each aspect of its business toward the fulfillment of that particular theme. For example, the Telos Fitness Center, based in Dallas, Texas, is operated around providing an Athenian theme. Each aspect of its design, product mix, and service culture is focused on reinforcing this Athenian theme, from the Greek columns in the lobby, to the God and Goddess awards for members, and finally the Spartan training based on the ancient Greek approach to fitness as medicine. Another example of theme building is Crunch Fitness, based out of New York, which has developed a theme that is designed to deliver out-of-the-box, non-judgmental experiences. When an individual enters a Crunch club, that person can easily see that the design of the club, the attire of the staff, the names of the classes and programs, and the service approach of their staff all align with the club's basic theme. Another club that is built around a theme is the Marsh, which is located outside Minneapolis, Minnesota. The Marsh's theme is focused on mind and body, in essence, attempting to make it an out-of-body retreat. The Marsh's facilities, programs, and service culture all center on creating experiences based on that particular theme. At a more micro level, numerous clubs have developed classes and programs around a highly recognizable theme, such as Boot Camp, Fireman's Aerobics, SWAT Classes, etc.

❏ *Add the "ING."* According to Gilmore and Pine in their insightful book, *The Experience Economy*, when a club takes a particular product and service and thinks of that item in the context of adding an "ING," then the club is

> Clubs can achieve noteworthy success with their members by creating a service culture that is focused on delivering unique experiences that not only exceed member expectations, but also help facilitate member delight and loyalty.

more likely to generate the desired experiences. An excellent example of this concept in practice occurred when Johnny G. created Spinning. What was once just riding a stationary bike (e.g., taking a spin) became a hot experience. By creating Spinning, he made the class more appealing as an experience. The key point for clubs to consider in this regard is for the club to think about the action-oriented aspects of its products and services.

❏ *Build the Proper Stage*. Creating experiences is like putting on a play. In the first act, the club needs to construct the proper stage or set design. Clubs who want to create positive experiences have to first develop an appropriate theme and then make sure the stage for acting out that experience has been established. For example, at the Rochester Athletic Club in Rochester, Minnesota, an area of the club, called the Neighborhood, was established. To make the theme come alive, the operators of the facility took what were formerly indoor tennis courts and constructed a replica of an old Midwestern town, complete with ice cream shop, storefronts, pedestrian street, and a miniature golf course. As a result, The RAC's facilities are designed to look and feel like an old-time neighborhood. Another industry group that focuses on building the proper setting is Crunch clubs, which feature a theme that is non-judgmental and out-of-the-box. When an individual enters the Crunch club in West Hollywood, for example, they will notice that as they walk to the locker rooms, they can see the profiles of people in the showers or that when members are on the exercise floor, that all the mirrors are round and on stands. Crunch also places signs throughout their club with off-the-wall expressions that support their theme. As intended, the members of Crunch clubs definitely get the sense they are immersed in an unusual experience.

❏ *Have the Right Props*. Just as a stage is normally needed to put on a play, clubs also need the right props. From a club perspective, the props are the equipment, the signage, the physical amenities, the classes and programs, and even the staff attire. It is critical that the club's props align with the designated theme of the facility. At Crunch clubs, for example, several outrageous signs are posted throughout the club. Most members stop and read the signs and have a laugh—a process that is part of the intended experience. The Crunch staff can be found wearing cut-offs, earrings, and other unusual items, all of which reinforce the predetermined theme of Crunch clubs. Each Crunch club also offers classes such as cardio striptease and cardio funk, both of which align with their theme. At the Marsh in Minnesota, its theme of a mind/body retreat is reinforced by props such as curtains, chairs, candles, and other items that make the members feel as if they are escaping from the world.

> Just as a stage is normally needed to put on a play, clubs also need the right props.

❏ *The Club's Staff Must See Their Job as Acting*. Actors are adept at stepping into a character and creating the feeling desired by the director. For a club's staff, they too need to know the club's theme and then be able to "act" in a manner that reinforces that theme. For example, at Oase Health and Sport in Germany, its theme is built around being a "home away from home." Accordingly, the employees at Oase try to act not as staff, but as members of the family, encouraging interactions between individuals that create a

A club's staff needs to find ways to help members experience a change that is consistent with the members' personal expectations and needs.

sense of family. At Crunch, members can definitely expect the unexpected from the staff, but always within the context of taking care of the member. Again, this approach is consistent with the theme at Crunch. The art of acting by the club staff is an essential aspect of what could be considered the club's "service culture."

❑ *The Staff Should Be Focused on Creating Transformations.* Not only must a club's staff members be focused on acting, they should also be prepared to deal with each individual member in a manner that allows them to personalize the experience for the member. Transformations occur when an experience takes on a high degree of personal relevance. In essence, a club's staff needs to find ways to help members experience a change that is consistent with the members' personal expectations and needs. These transformations require a strong "service culture."

9

Creating a Member Service Culture That Drives Member Experiences That Build Retention

Chapter Objectives

The previous two chapters looked at membership retention and how this factor is affected by a club's ability to create memorable experiences for its members. In turn, it was pointed out that a club's success in creating memorable member experiences relies heavily on having a service culture. This chapter details the role of service in creating memorable experiences for the club's members and what steps are needed to establish and sustain a service culture.

The Service Profit Chain

According to Leonard Schlesinger of Harvard University in his article, "How Does Service Drive the Service Company," the "service profit chain" lies at the heart of growing a business's profitability. Like a "chain," the process has several interrelated links. Profitability is driven by customer loyalty, which is influenced by customer delight. Customer delight is affected by outstanding external service to the customer, which, in turn, is driven by delighted employees who are the recipients of great internal service (refer to Figure 9-1). Simply stated, in club terms, profitability is driven by loyal members, who have a sense of delight that is derived by their having engaged in memorable experiences at the club. These member experiences are delivered by a staff with a strong internal and external service culture. It is the aforementioned "service profit chain" that lies at the center of membership retention and the ability of a club to create memorable member experiences.

The "service profit chain" lies at the heart of growing a business's profitability.

The Service Profit Chain

Figure 9-1. The service profit chain

Defining a Service Culture

The key to the club staff providing great service that is focused on delivering memorable member experiences starts with the establishment of a service culture. A service culture is a system of customs, habits, and conventions, the values, words, and works attendant to this culture help create and sustain a long-term environment in which the staff are passionate about and are empowered to deliver whatever is required to provide the club's members with a personally relevant and memorable experience. Establishing a service culture therefore becomes one of the most essential elements in any health/fitness club's operating model.

Creating a Service Culture in the Health/Fitness Club Business

Establishing an appropriate service culture in the club industry can involve a number of steps, including the following:

❑ *Create a Set of Core Business Values Around Service.* The core foundation of all cultures is a set of values. Whether it is a societal culture, such as the ones that exist in England, China, or Germany, or a business culture, such as witnessed at Ben & Jerry's, Starbuck's, Nordstrom's, or BMW. The heart of every culture is based on a set of values that lie behind every decision that is made. If a club wants to establish a service culture, its values must be consistent with the service expectations of its membership.

For example, at ClubCorp, a Dallas, Texas-based private club company, the company's founder, Robert Dedman, established a service culture for the organization that featured several core values that were focused on service. The first value was, "the member and guest are king." With this one precept, Dedman established a framework for how he expected each employee to interact with the members of ClubCorp. Another fundamental ClubCorp value that Dedman constantly referred to was, "warm welcomes, magic moments, and fond farewells." When Dedman spoke of this underlying company sense of purpose, he was referring to the role that each employee plays in making sure all members receive a personalized welcome when they arrive, a personalized farewell when they leave, and a memorable and magic experience when they are in the club. Another core value established by Dedman was to call each member by their name at least four times when they were in the club. This practice was intended to reinforce the culture of personalizing each member's club experience. A final value that Dedman preached was "to deliver a Cadillac for a Chevrolet price." As such, his underlying desire was to overdeliver on the company promise or to deliver a far greater value than for which the member actually paid. Over the years, the company values and attitudes instilled by Dedman have served ClubCorp very well.

In a similar approach, Red Lerelle, of Red's in Lafayette, Louisiana, has established some very basic business values for his company that speak to service. At Red's, every employee understands that they are to smile and say hello and goodbye to every member. At Red's, everyone knows that it is their job to do whatever it takes to take care of the members. These values, established by Red when he founded his club nearly five decades ago, continue to set the framework for the club's service culture.

❑ *Create a Tradition of Service Values by Starting at the Top.* In every culture, the values and traditions that are attendant to that culture are sustained by leaders who embody those values and traditions. These leaders act in a manner that supports the core values of the culture. In the club business, one of the steps that can help create a tradition of great service is to reinforce the values in word and deed at all times. At Red's, for example, Red can be found training new employees on the importance of saying hello and goodbye to members of his club, most often by being seen throughout the club saying hello or goodbye. By the same token, at ClubCorp, when Robert Dedman visited a club, he could often be found talking with members and asking what he could do to help them. In both Red's and Dedman's world, the service values started with them. In other words, they did whatever it took to demonstrate the service values that they wanted to inculcate within their organization's culture.

> In every culture, the values and traditions that are attendant to that culture are sustained by leaders who embody those values and traditions.

❑ *Establish Courses of Action that Reinforce the Values and Service Culture.* In any culture, it takes more than one individual to spread the service culture.

According to anthropologists, a culture is sustained by artifacts, tradition, myths, legends, and heroes. In other words, once an entity has the values of a culture established, it must have the people and stories to keep it alive and vibrant with the individuals who are part of that endeavor. As previously described, not only does it take leaders who will share relevant stories attendant to the service culture and believe in a manner consistent with the core values of the culture, it can require much more.

In the club business, for example, leaders must identify key staff members who embrace the service culture of the club and will "walk it and talk it." These employees become the club's storytellers and heroes. Accordingly, clubs should undertake an effort to collect employee recollections of the company's service culture so that they can be shared with the other employees. At ClubCorp in the 1980s and 1990s, the company encouraged employees and clubs to make note of stories that exemplified the service culture, and then to share those stories with their fellow employees by means of the company's web site and through daily staff lineups at each respective ClubCorp club. Sharing their own stories of a service experience during such a lineup can result in a "magic moment" for those staff who are conveying their remembrances.

In the process, these individuals become one of the service culture's storytellers. In 2008, when I first took the reins as CEO for the Russian Fitness Group, one of the first endeavors that I embarked on was to instill the company's culture at all levels of the organization. To accomplish this objective, a "culture leaders team," composed of 30 team members from the corporate office and clubs, was established. This group of 30 employees was assigned the responsibility of spreading the company culture. The team members were deeply involved in immersing the Group's employees in the culture of the company. One particularly potentially helpful step that team members took was to visit the various clubs in the Group and to share personally relevant stories that spoke to what the company culture was all about. Among the other steps that can help reinforce the service culture within a club are the following:

- *Create a service recognition program.* Employees are far more likely to embrace a service culture when they are recognized for actions that align with the club's service culture. At ClubCorp, for example, this recognition program was called STAR Recognition. Other clubs have different names for their recognition programs. The key, however, is to recognize employees who live the service culture, regardless of the term utilized to acknowledge the effort.

- *Develop an education program.* Clubs need to initiate an ongoing education program for all of their employees. At the heart of that training program should be a module dedicated to both the club's service culture and how employees can become the apostles for that service culture. At ClubCorp, the first educational effort an employee is exposed to is a video that explains the service culture at ClubCorp. At the Russian Fitness Group, a course entitled, "Culture; the Ultimate Competitive Advantage," was conducted annually. All company and club leaders were expected

> Employees are far more likely to embrace a service culture when they are recognized for actions that align with the club's service culture.

to attend. Furthermore, it's essential that the club's educational program on its service culture is an ongoing one, not just a one-time delivery.

- *Loosen the knot*. One of the most common complaints from customers is that when they need something done, that employees have to ask their supervisors for instructions or permission to act. In reality, however, if a club wants to have a genuine service culture, it should empower its employees to act according to the culture. It should trust its employees to make the right decisions. At Nordstrom's, for example, employees are given the freedom to deal with customers, based solely on the company's service values. Fortunately, many clubs give its employees the freedom to make the right decision, based on an environment of trust. The key point that should be noted is that the process should be grounded in the clubs' service culture and how the clubs educate and support that culture.

- *All decisions need to be founded in the club's service values*. Many businesses establish service values, but then act outside them. For example, ClubCorp, at least up until the early part of the 21st century, had a core philosophy that was based on the precept that the "member is king." If a situation subsequently occurred where the employee had to make a choice with regard to a particular action, that person's choice had to be consistent with the value that the "member is king." If the employee's decision ran counter to that value, then the first link in ClubCorp's service culture chain had been broken.

- *Document the core values and practices of the club's service culture*. It is critical that the values and practices of the club's service culture be documented and shared with each of its employees. ClubCorp, for example, gave each of its employees the "basics card," which was a small, wallet-sized card on which are noted the values and philosophies that are at the heart of the company's service culture. The card that each employee of Red's receives lists eight specific values that are at the heart of Red's service culture. The card utilized at Red's serves as a statement of the service-culture standards at Red's. Not only does it help all Red's employees know the service culture expectations at Red's, it also furnishes them with a constant reminder of those expectations. The eight values listed on the Red's card include:

  ✓ The members are number one.
  ✓ Make eye contact, smile, and say "hello" and "goodbye."
  ✓ Show up on time and ready to work.
  ✓ If a member has a problem, solve it. Keep them happy.
  ✓ If you've got time to lean, you got time to clean.
  ✓ I don't know the answer; I'll find out, so check back with me.
  ✓ Have a positive attitude; be enthusiastic about your job.
  ✓ Stay in shape.

At the Russian Fitness Group, organizational values were documented through various media. For example, a screen saver was developed for all of the company's computers that displayed the company's values. Another step that was undertaken was to give coffee/tea mugs to each employee,

> It is critical that the values and practices of the club's service culture be documented and shared with each of its employees.

Members must feel like they can share both their praise and their concerns openly and know that management and employees will respond to the members' efforts to communicate with them in a manner that helps ensure a better member experience.

on which were listed the company's core values. The point to keep in mind is that like ClubCorp and Red's, a way was found to put the core values in front of each employee on a daily basis.

❑ *Provide a Means for Members to Communicate with Management About Their Experiences at the Club.* A service culture requires a high degree of openness by management. As such, management must be open to listening to the members and fostering an environment of trust between the members and the staff. Members must feel like they can share both their praise and their concerns openly and know that management and employees will respond to the members' efforts to communicate with them in a manner that helps ensure a better member experience. Among the approaches that clubs can utilize to elicit and enhance feedback from their members are the following:

- *Open door/open floor.* This approach to listening involves management leaving time for members to drop in and talk. It also mandates management should spend a portion of each day out in the club talking with members. The combination of getting out and talking with members and also leaving time on the schedule for members to walk in and meet with club staff allows the club to foster an environment of trust.

- *Member committees.* At ClubCorp, the ClubCorp clubs have committees made up of members. These committees serve dual roles. Not only do they provide valuable feedback on the experiences of the members, they also allow the members to become involved in identifying experience solutions. The number of committees varies from club to club. Some clubs only have a few committees, while others have more than a dozen, such as a social committee, racquet sport committee, membership committee, group-exercise committee, etc.

- *Focus groups.* Focus groups are an effective way for clubs to learn more about what their members feel. Focus groups allow a club to bring together groups of members in a non-intimidating environment and identify what they feel and believe about their experiences in the club.

- *Surveys.* Surveys are a practical method for assessing how members feel about the club experience. In this regard, surveys should be conducted at least once annually. Within the industry, numerous clubs, such as the Maryland Athletic Club in Timonium, Maryland; the Sports Club/LA Clubs in NY, Boston, Washington, and San Francisco; Club One in California; and the Russian Fitness Group in Russia on at least an annual basis, and often more frequently, administer surveys to determine how their members feel about key factors involving their experiences at the facility, particularly those that might affect their decision about maintaining or foregoing their club membership.

- *Comment box system.* Every club should offer members some version of the comment-box system that their members can use to share their concerns and praises. This effort could range from having boxes with comment cards left available throughout the club, to web-based feedback systems. Clubs, such as the MAC in East Lansing, Michigan; the ACAC in Charlottesville, Virginia; Club One in California; Western Athletic

Clubs in California; Fitness First in England and Germany; Virgin Active in England; and Intenso in Germany, all offer some type of a feedback system that their members can use to share their thoughts, concerns, and praises.

❏ *Eliminate the Sacrifices That a Member Has to Make*. The process of creating and sustaining a service culture requires that a club look at its operations and identify the sacrifices that members must make in order to use the club. In that regard, a member can sacrifice in a number of ways, including a loss of convenience, self-esteem, results, friendships, etc. When a club identifies sacrifices that its members must make, it should remove them. For example, many clubs require members to hand over their keys and ID just to get a towel. All factors considered, these clubs are asking members to make some degree of sacrifice just to use a towel. On the other hand, if members can obtain a towel without all of that inconvenience, it could easily be argued that they would feel much better. In reality, too many club operators construct barriers, thinking they will save money, but instead, they create member sacrifices that eventually help drive members away.

The process of creating and sustaining a service culture requires that a club look at its operations and identify the sacrifices that members must make in order to use the club.

❏ *Create a Service Recovery Approach That Can Patch the Gaps*. Even in the best service culture, mistakes occur. According to the data shared by Dr. Leonard Schlesinger in his article, "The Service-driven Service Company," customers who have a bad experience can be turned around with the proper service-recovery process. The data on customer service indicates that up to 95 percent of customers will make a repeat purchase if their experience problem is addressed promptly and correctly. This type of information makes it imperative that a club's service culture includes a service-recovery process. In developing a service-recovery process, clubs should make sure to address each of the following steps:

• *Listen*. The first element of a service-recovery process is to listen to the member. This endeavor begins with having a system, featuring elements such as those discussed previously, that allows a club's members to voice their issues. It is imperative that the members be allowed to express their concerns either anonymously or not. Employees should be willing to listen attentively when members bring up an issue of concern to them. If the issue is brought up through a survey or other medium, then management needs to contact the member and hear what that person has to say. Over the past few years, many clubs have found that social media sites, such as Facebook or even company-sponsored social sites, can provide an outstanding forum for listening to members and conducting a two-way dialogue with them.

• *Empathize*. Whenever a member shares an issue with the club's employees, they need to empathize and show that they understand the member's perspective on the issue. This attitude needs to be communicated clearly to the member.

• *Apologize*. It is imperative that the member with a relevant issue over their experience in the club receives an apology from the individual employee with whom they shared their concern. The apology from the employee should be imparted on behalf of the club, indicating that the club staff regrets the situation. The apology should be made promptly. If the concern is expressed to an employee in person, then the apology should occur at that time. If the issue comes to light at a later time (e.g., by a letter or other communication medium), then the apology needs to be delivered verbally and in person, if possible, as soon as the issue has come to the attention of management.

- *Respond.* Once the club has become aware of the issue and has apologized, it should take action to address the matter. As indicated on the aforementioned values card utilized at Red's, "solve it and keep them happy." If the issue has been brought to the attention of a line employee, the employee should be empowered to solve the issue. If the issue is beyond that person's scope of responsibility, then it should be immediately brought to the attention of an employee or supervisor who can solve the issue. If the issue cannot be resolved immediately, the club should make sure that someone gets back to them as soon as possible. The employees at Red's are instructed to respond to such a situation by stating, "I don't know the answer; I'll find out, so check back with me." If an issue is raised anonymously, management still needs to act promptly to address the situation. The key in service recovery is to empower the employee team to respond to issues promptly with solutions and when the employee does not have a solution to a particular problem, the club should make sure that the employee knows where to go for the solution. Finally, whenever and however the club is responding, the club should inform the member that it is taking action to address the situation.

- *Communicate the response.* When an issue occurs that needs to be addressed, management should begin the process of solving the matter by letting the member know what action the club is taking, something that should be done at the time it learns of the issue. When the issue is raised anonymously, a note can be placed on a communication board in the club or on the club's website or its social media page, informing the membership in general of an issue that has come to management's attention and of the action the club plans to take concerning the situation. If the issue is raised in person, members should immediately be informed of the action the club is taking. Members need to have prompt feedback that the club understands their issues and how it plans to deal with them.

- *Follow up.* The final critical aspect of the service-recovery process is for a club to make sure that once it has taken action on a member issue, it clearly and promptly communicates to the member what the outcome of the action is. If the issue was raised anonymously, then the club should post the resulting action on a comment board at the club or on the club's website or its social media page.

It should be noted that the service-recovery process applies just as much too employee-related issues, as it does to member issues. Clubs that can properly and effectively address an employee-related issue are far more

> **Members need to have prompt feedback that the club understands their issues and how it plans to deal with them.**

likely to have employees who are able to act in an appropriate manner when member-related problems occur.

Implementing Service Culture Values and Standards

Creating and sustaining a service culture is not an easy process. Examples of possible service values and standards that club operators might consider as they create their own service values and culture include the following:

❏ *Greeting Members*:
  • Always smile and make eye contact.
  • Call the member by name.
  • Personalize the greeting by saying more than just "hello."
  • Always greet members by standing and extending a hand.

❏ *Professionalism and Education*:
  • Make sure the staff has the appropriate certifications and education and post that information for members to view.
  • Always have the staff share information of value with members when the opportunity arises.
  • Always have a solution or know how to find the solution.
  • Instill in all employees the understanding that their number one job is to be there for the members, no matter what.

> Instill in all employees the understanding that their number one job is to be there for the members, no matter what.

❏ *Social Engagement and Member Interaction*:
  • Never have staff walk by a member without saying hello and introducing themselves.
  • Make it a practice to introduce members to other members.
  • Ask members in a genuine fashion if they need assistance.
  • Foster a relationship with the members and learn something unique about them.
  • Focus on listening and empathizing with the members before responding.

❏ *Programming of the Club*:
  • Offer a variety of programs for a variety of needs.
  • Be flexible in the club's program offerings.
  • Find ways to determine the program interests of the members.

❏ *Justice and Safety for Members and Employees*:
  • Don't play favorites; treat every member and employee as an equal.
  • Become aware of the personal interests of both the members and employees and have the staff act appropriately.
  • Talk about "we" and avoid using "me."
  • Create an environment that is not intimidating for the members or employees.

❑ *Self-Esteem of Members and Employees*:
- Focus on knowing everyone's goals and make an effort to provide what it takes for them to be achieved.
- Never let a member or employee feel like their needs are a burden; instead let them know they are important.
- Provide an environment that speaks to greater perception of body and mind awareness and comfort.

❑ *The Facility*:
- Keep it clean and make it everyone's job to keep it clean.
- Keep all equipment in working order unless an alternative is provided.
- Make the facility convenient to use.
- Make the facility seem like a second home or office.

Creating and sustaining a service culture is an absolutely essential aspect of a successful health/fitness club.

Creating and sustaining a service culture is an absolutely essential aspect of a successful health/fitness club. As such, this factor should be the first and foremost issue that club operators address if they want to create memorable member experiences and enhance their club's level of membership retention.

10

Programming for Health/Fitness Clubs

Chapter Objectives

According to consumer research on why people either join or leave a health/fitness club, programming plays an important role in both decisions. Since prospective members, current members, and former members all tend to view programming as a critical part of the health/fitness club membership equation, it is essential that club operators understand the dynamics involved in programming the activities that their club offers. Initially, this chapter explores the role that programming plays in membership. It then provides an overview of the variety of program opportunities that exist for clubs. Finally, the chapter concludes by detailing the key steps involved in successful programming.

Programming: Understanding the Basics

Programming involves engaging members in the club experience and creating opportunities for members to become actively involved in the club. Research indicates that individuals join clubs for a variety of reasons, including social engagement (women), group activities (women), challenge and competition (men), and achieving fitness goals (both genders). By the same token, research has also been able to identify some of the primary reasons members give up their club membership, including not being able to make social connections with other members, not feeling engaged by the club, losing the motivation, not having a training partner, and not using the club frequently enough. When those factors that affect the decisions concerning both joining and leaving are examined more closely, it becomes evident that programming lies at the heart of many of them. As a result, a club that is interested in driving its level of membership sales and membership retention needs to become adept at programming.

A club that is interested in driving its level of membership sales and membership retention needs to become adept at programming.

    All factors considered, clubs should look at programming as the "play" or "theatre" that they put on to create the memorable experiences that members want to have. Hypothetically, creating such experiences is like putting on a play, with the facility being the stage for the play, the equipment serving as the play's props, and the staff as the actors in the play. In this scenario, programming becomes a series of one-act plays that the club's staff puts on to entertain and engage the members. Programming has the ability to create connections between members, help motivate individuals to achieve their personal goals, help members establish training partnerships, offer competitive challenges for members, and entertain the members. Programming is the club's most viable option for meeting and exceeding the expectations that most members have about being a club member. Furthermore, effective programming is also one of the best strategies a club has for differentiating itself from its competitors.

Program Offerings of the Health/Fitness Club Industry

Research shows that the health/fitness club industry makes a wide variety of program options available to its members. In that regard, according to the published report, the *IHRSA 2010 Profiles of Success*, clubs offer over 65 different types of major programs to their members. A sampling of the top programs in 2003, 2006, and 2009 are included in Figure 10-1.

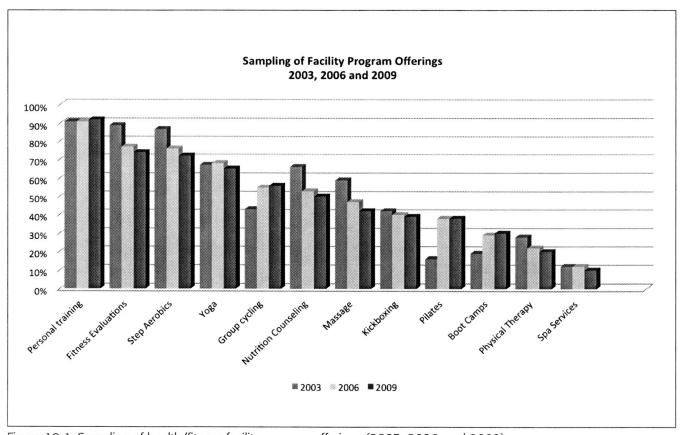

Figure 10-1. Sampling of health/fitness facility program offerings (2003, 2006, and 2009)

Several important observations can be made by reviewing the data presented in Figure 10-1. First, in 2009, the program offerings of clubs tended to lean more toward group-driven programming that serves a relatively small segment of membership (e.g., step/bench aerobics, group cycling, dance, yoga, competitive sports, etc.), as opposed to more individual-oriented programs (e.g., personal training, massage, etc.). This state of affairs is a shift from the industry's programming approach in the earlier part of the 21st century, when individual programming took precedence. Second, the programs offered by most health/fitness facilities have changed little over the past several years, with the possible exception of boot camps, Pilates, and wellness programs. Third, while the U.S. and other nations are experiencing a dramatic increase in obesity and lifestyle-related diseases, the percentage of clubs offering special-population programs, although such programs have increased over the past five years, still represents a relatively small segment of the programming blend, with less than 10 percent offering programs for lifestyle conditions, such as diabetes, arthritis, etc. As such, based on the information reflected in Figure 10-1 and the data contained in the published report, the *IHRSA 2010 Profiles of Success*, health/fitness facilities have still not fully grasped the importance of creating and delivering programs for niche audiences who are not typically part of the health/fitness market.

> Health/fitness facilities have still not fully grasped the importance of creating and delivering programs for niche audiences who are not typically part of the health/fitness market.

Programming Options in the Health/Fitness Club Industry

A review of the various program categories and the types of programs that are currently offered by clubs indicates that clubs have an extensive array of programming opportunities. Among the various options that clubs have with regard to programming are the following:

❑ *Aquatic Area*. A number of club operators see the pool as a loss leader that can help sell the club. Beyond that limited perception, however, they tend to view pools as an operational challenge. Fortunately, many operators have chosen to make their pool(s) an asset, instead of a liability. In the process, they have developed dynamic programs around their aquatic facilities. In that regard, some of the most successful clubs at aquatic programming include the Baylor Tom Laundry Center in Dallas, the Michigan Athletic Club in East Lansing, Michigan, the Maryland Athletic Club in Timonium, Maryland, and Franco's in Louisiana. Among the more successful and interesting programs that are offered in aquatics are the following:

• *Masters swimming*. Masters swimming involves competitive swimming and training for older adults. Masters swimming is usually restricted to those individuals who are over the age of 25. A strong masters swimming program not only provides adults with a competitive outlet for their interest in swimming, but also a chance to meet others of a similar age. One of the best masters programs in the country is offered at the Baylor Tom Laundry Center in Dallas, Texas. One of the masters programs offered at this center, the Lone Star Masters, which was developed by Jim Montgomery, has over 200 participants.

- *Swim lessons.* Swim lessons are extremely popular, especially in a family-oriented market. The YMCA is probably the most successful in the industry in this programming area. The YMCA's program features multiple levels of skill acquisition, which enables children to acquire the necessary skills and then be recognized when they move up to the next higher level of skill. The American Red Cross also offers a structured format that clubs can utilize in a fashion similar to the YMCA's approach.

- *Aqua-exercise.* Providing opportunities to engage in physical activities that place a minimum of load force on the body's musculoskeletal system, aqua-exercise classes have grown in popularity over the years. In fact, multiple types of aquatic exercise options are currently being offered at clubs throughout the country, including water-step classes, water-based stretch classes, water-based Tai Chi classes, water-based yoga classes, water-based kickbox fitness classes, water-based Pilates classes, and most recently aquatic Zumba. Lending credence to the value of aqua-exercise, the National Arthritis Foundation offers a certification for one type of water-based exercise class.

- *Flick-n-float parties.* "Flick-n-float" is a common term used by many clubs for a party-themed, aquatic event. Flick-n-float refers to the practice of offering film viewing at poolside, while also including such activities as swimming, floating on the pool, and having food delivered poolside. Arguably, this particular program offering can be thought of as a "party at the pool." These events are particularly popular with families that have young children.

- *Scuba and snorkeling classes.* Numerous clubs exist in the marketplace that have leveraged the public's interest in adventure-oriented programming and use their pool to deliver classes in snorkeling and scuba diving. The more creative clubs often tie in an adventure outing at the end of the scheduled classes so that their members can utilize their newfound skills to experience an out-of-the-club event.

- *Swim team.* Many clubs with pools leverage their efforts to target the family market by offering competitive junior swimming. Some clubs, for example, have as many as 200 to 400 kids who are actively involved in the club's swim teams. One of the keys to success with conducting a swim-team program is to be able to offer competition against other clubs. It is interesting to note that many health/fitness club teams will often find themselves in competitive leagues with teams sponsored by country clubs.

Group-exercise programming represents the most significant opportunity for achieving programming excellence in the health/fitness club industry.

❏ *Group-Exercise Programs.* Group-exercise programming represents the most significant opportunity for achieving programming excellence in the health/fitness club industry. At one time, group exercise was somewhat limited in the opportunities it provided as a programming option when it was simply referred to as "aerobics." Since moving toward a group-exercise and group-fitness orientation, however, this area of programming has assumed a significant role for many clubs. For example, some clubs report that nearly 50 percent of their daily visits are driven by participation in their group-exercise programs. In a recent unpublished study conducted by the author of the top health/fitness clubs in the U.S., the facilities that responded indicated that 25 percent to 40 percent of their daily visits were for group-exercise classes. A study released by Les Mills International in the first quarter of 2011 indicates that group-exercise participation contributes to a significant portion of the daily participation in most clubs. In fact, as reported in the Les Mills study, some clubs generated over 50 percent of their daily visits from group exercise. Clubs that have established a reputation as offering great group-exercise programming include Crunch, Equinox, Sports Club/LA, and Healthworks. Among the most successful program offerings in group exercise are the following:

- *Group cycling.* Originally known as Spinning, group-cycling programming has evolved to include other licensed programs, such as Precision Cycling and RPM (a Les Mills program), along with a host of other club-oriented names. While the group-cycling juggernaut has slowed down somewhat in recent years, it is still one of the most popular program options in the industry. An example of group cycling's strong following is the growing popularity of boutique cycling studios, such as SoulCycle, a popular chain of group-cycling studios that is based in New York.

- *Yoga.* Since the 1990s, yoga has been one of the two fastest-growing forms of group exercise. In fact, in some clubs, yoga constitutes nearly 50 percent of their group-exercise programs. Yoga's popularity grew as a by-product of the focus that baby boomers had on mind-body exercise. Initially, yoga just involved Hatha yoga. Currently, however, there are over 20 varieties of yoga offered in clubs, including Hatha, Astranga, Ishevanya, Bikram, Power Yoga, and most recently, AntiGravity Yoga, a class offered at various Crunch facilities. As such, the yoga of today and the future will continue to evolve as an integrated form of the original Eastern art and the desires of western culture.

- *Pilates.* Pilates has been the fastest growing group-exercise program in the industry since the early part of the 21st century. Pilates, first introduced in the 1920s by Joseph Pilates, has undergone several western modifications in the last few years. In the process, it has been integrated into the group-exercise arena. Formerly offered only on special equipment, Pilates is now offered in multiple formats for group exercise, including mat Pilates, prop Pilates, tower classes, and allegro Pilates.

- *Resistance-driven classes.* Over the last 10 years, the concept of resistance training in a group format has exhibited significant growth. Initially, resistance-training programming involved classes such as body sculpting, using resistance tubes and free-hand exercises, and then progressed into classes that utilized hand weights and weighted bars. One of the most popular classes of the latter type is taught with the body bar. In recent years, the industry has started to offer more structured or choreographed resistance-training classes, such as Body Pump, which is marketed by Les Mills International.

- *Core and functional-fitness classes.* Programming involving core stability and functional-fitness conditioning is another highly popular form of group exercise. The introduction of the exercise ball created an entire series of exercise-ball classes that focused on developing the individual's core. In addition to exercise-ball classes, another highly popular and

Pilates has been the fastest growing group-exercise program in the industry since the early part of the 21st century.

effective format for conditioning the core and enhancing an individual's level of functional fitness were classes that were created using foam rollers, an approach based on practices in the physical therapy arena. Other examples of core and functional-type classes include medicine-ball classes, Bosu-ball classes, and core-board (a Reebok program) classes.

- *Theme classes.* A recent trend in programming, which has been popularized by club groups such as Crunch and Sports Club/LA and modified by other club operators, are classes that are designed around a specific theme. The basic underlying concept of a theme class is to remove members from the ordinary and take them on escapist adventures. Theme classes often make use of props and costumes to create a greater sense of theme-related reality. Examples of commonly conducted theme classes include:

  ✓ *Fireman's class.* This class offers exercise movements based on the activities that a fireman typically carries out. Some clubs even use props, such as hoses, stairs, etc. The first club group to popularize this type of class was Crunch.

  ✓ *S.W.A.T. class.* This class offers exercise movements that are based on the activities and physical requirements of police SWAT units.

  ✓ *Boot camp class.* This class is structured around the activities that the military uses to train its recruits in basic training. At Red's in Lafayette, Louisiana, for example, the boot camp classes are held in an outdoor training area that includes obstacles employed in many basic training programs.

  ✓ *Cardio striptease class.* This class, which is offered by Crunch in New York, is an extreme example of a theme class that appeals to a targeted audience that is looking for a real escape. The class would feature movements that might typically occur in a striptease establishment, for example, minor disrobing.

  ✓ *New York ballet workout.* This type of class was popularized at several New York clubs by a former ballet dancer. These classes incorporate the movements and conditioning exercises used by ballet dancers.

  ✓ *LA cheerleaders' class.* This class was popularized by the Sports Club/LA based on the dance movements and routines of the Los Angeles Lakers cheerleaders.

  ✓ *Pole dancing.* Over the past five years, some clubs have begun to offer pole-dancing classes to their members. These classes take have taken the forbidden aura of pole dancing (an activity heretofore only seen in gentleman's clubs) and adapted it as a form of entertaining and fitness-enhancing, group-exercise class.

- *Fusion classes.* Over the past several years, fusion classes have moved to the forefront of the industry's interest in group exercise. Fusion refers to the blending of dissimilar cultures and dissimilar class structures. This movement toward offering fusion classes is, in part, driven by the changing demographics in America and the desire to offer classes that provide a blend of styles and themes. Examples of fusion classes that are currently popular in the health/fitness industry include:

> Over the past several years, fusion classes have moved to the forefront of the industry's interest in group exercise.

✓ *Yoga/spin classes*. These classes offer a blend of group cycling with yoga movements. Participants are given a chance to mix mind/body with intense cardiovascular movement.

✓ *Pilates/spin classes*. These classes offer the mix of high-intensity cardiovascular conditioning with the stretching and strengthening of Pilates.

✓ *Bosu/step classes*. A new twist on the step class is offered by incorporating the core conditioning benefits of a Bosu ball with the cardiovascular benefits of a step class.

✓ *Aqua tai chi*. This class, first offered in the New York market, blends the mind/body benefits of the ancient Chinese martial art with the enhanced resistance provided by exercising in the water.

✓ *Kickbox yoga*. This class, offered in some of the more progressive club markets, blends two martial arts, resulting in an activity that combines soft movement with more intense cardiovascular movement.

✓ *Cardio funk*. First offered at Crunch, this class blends the movements of basic "aerobics" with the music and movements of funk.

✓ *Salsa step*. This class offers a blend of the Latin American dance steps of salsa with the more basic movements of "aerobics." These classes often include the use of band music (either live or recorded) to extenuate the theme of the class.

✓ *Chocolate and yoga*. This class combines yoga movements and positions with breaks that involve consuming small amounts of chocolate. The concept was originally introduced by David Romanelli, founder of At One Yoga, and chocolatier Katrina Markoff. As of 2011, the two founders continue to offer workshops throughout the U.S. to help clubs interested in offering this unique fusion class to their members.

✓ *Wine and yoga*. This is similar to chocolate and yoga, only it involves consumption of wine instead of chocolate. The concept for this class was first introduced in California, by David Romanelli, who was one of the pioneers of chocolate and yoga. Not long after the introduction of wine and yoga classes, entrepreneurs introduced a spin-off class entitled, Pilates and yoga.

• *Equipment classes*. Equipment classes, which have been popular since the mid 1990s, are based on offering classes that are structured around the use of standard fitness equipment in a group setting. Among the equipment classes that clubs offer to its members are the following:

✓ *Trekking*. A registered program of Star Trac, trekking involves walking/running on a treadmill in a group format, choreographed to music.

✓ *Rowing*. These classes, featuring a group-exercise class format, involve the use of rowing ergometers.

✓ *Stairclimbing*. The company that manufactures StairMasters developed a registered program called, "stomp," which involves having individuals exercise on a stairclimbing machine in a group format.

✓ *Gravity*. Gravity classes involve the use of Total Gym equipment, which resembles Pilates equipment.

Equipment classes, which have been popular since the mid 1990s, are based on offering classes that are structured around the use of standard fitness equipment in a group setting.

Personal training has become the most popular fitness program in the industry, as well as the leading source of incremental revenue for many clubs.

❏ *Fitness Programs.* Fitness programming refers to a generic blend of program activities that target members who tend to only use the club for cardiovascular or resistance training. As a rule, these members use the club on a more personal basis while pursuing their fitness goals. By offering fitness programming, clubs can provide avenues that allow those members to make connections with other club members who have similar interests and be better positioned to achieve their personal fitness goals. The primary goals of fitness programming are to create personal connections, stimulate competition, enhance motivation, and support the pursuit of each member's fitness goals. Among the examples of fitness programs that are currently offered in the health/fitness club industry are the following:

• *Personal training.* Personal training has become the most popular fitness program in the industry, as well as the leading source of incremental revenue for many clubs. Personal training can be offered either on an individual basis or in a group format, an option that has increased in popularity over the past few years. Personal training allows a member to work individually or in a small group with a fitness professional who provides instruction and motivation. In some instances, personal training programs are developed around a particular theme, such as "women on weights."

• *Sports-performance training.* One popular fitness offering is to offer sports-specific conditioning programs in either a group or individual format. This type of programming targets members who have an interest in enhancing their level of performance in a specific sport. The most popular of these sports-performance programs include golf fitness, football conditioning, speed and quickness training, jump training, tennis fitness, and ski conditioning.

• *Special population fitness.* Over the past few years, with the aging of the baby boomers, clubs have begun to be aware of the value of offering fitness programs that target the needs of individuals who have certain health conditions. Examples of such programs include cardiac rehabilitation, arthritis exercise, physical therapy, senior exercise, and exercise for the obese.

• *Fitness games.* One of the most effective methods that clubs can use to increase member participation in their fitness programs is to provide games and challenges that allow the members to exercise independently, yet be part of a social and competitive event. Fitness games are often based on board games or more large-scale sports events. Examples of some of the more popular fitness games include:

  ✓ *Race across America.* This type of fitness event allows members to earn miles for the time they exercise. These miles then go towards their efforts to cover a certain distance, such as crossing America. Some clubs pair members up in teams in an effort to introduce members to other members.

  ✓ *Clue.* This particular fitness game involves having members move across a Clue board, based on the time they accumulate exercising. This game is the same as the board game, except that it requires that a participant perform a predetermined amount of exercise to move, rather than based on numbers derived from the roll of a dice.

✓ *Monopoly*. This fitness game is based on the board game of Monopoly, with members getting the opportunity to move and buy and sell properties, based on their fitness activities.

✓ *Football challenges*. A popular theme for fitness games is to recreate a specific football classic, such as Texas vs. Texas A&M or Michigan vs. Ohio State. The game involves having members choose a particular team, and then having each team earn yards for the activities of the members on their teams. The game is held over a specific time period, and the team that crosses the goal line most often wins.

❑ *Health Promotion Programs*. Health promotion programs, often called "wellness" programs, are specialty programs that focus on activities and interventions intended to benefit the health and well-being of the individuals who participate in a given program. Health promotion programs can range from personal programs, such as nutritional counseling, to group programs such as stress management. The following examples illustrate several of the most common health-promotion programs that are offered by health/fitness clubs:

- *Health screenings*. Health screening programs can range from blood-pressure screening to mammograms. Most clubs coordinate with other healthcare institutions to offer these programs for their members and the community. The most popular health screenings include cholesterol screenings, blood-pressure screenings, cancer screenings, coronary risk-factor screenings, bone-health screenings, and diabetes screenings.

- *Health fairs*. Health fairs feature a more comprehensive form of health screening that is extremely popular among corporations and local communities. There are endless programs that clubs can include in their health fairs, including multiple offerings such as blood-pressure screenings, postural screenings, cholesterol screenings, massage, nutrition education, cooking demonstrations, body-fat appraisals, and exercise demonstrations. As a rule, health fairs are best offered once or twice a year.

- *Health education seminars and classes*. Members are often attracted to seminars and classes that focus on specific health-related themes. Such seminars usually involve a one-hour offering, in comparison to classes that might constitute a series of several sessions. The most popular health-education seminars and classes include:

  ✓ *Back care classes*. Back care classes, such as the YMCA's Healthy Back Program, are extremely popular with members and offer an opportunity for members to get professional instruction in dealing with their back problems.

  ✓ *Weight-loss classes*. Weight-loss classes and seminars are among the most popular programs offered by health/fitness clubs. Some clubs offer franchised programs, such as "Healthy Inspirations" or "Weight Watchers," while others design their own weight-loss programs that mix exercise, nutrition education, and monitoring.

> Health promotion programs, often called "wellness" programs, are specialty programs that focus on activities and interventions intended to benefit the health and well-being of the individuals who participate in a given program.

As a rule, seminars and classes that focus on smoking cessation are very attractive to a club's corporate members, because most corporations are aware of the fact that smoking is one of the most costly health behaviors in which employees can engage.

✓ *Women's and men's health seminars.* Another popular health-education program offering involves seminars and classes that are targeted at gender-specific health concerns, such as prostate cancer, breast cancer, osteoporosis, heart disease, and diabetes.

✓ *Smoking cessation classes.* As a rule, seminars and classes that focus on smoking cessation are very attractive to a club's corporate members, because most corporations are aware of the fact that smoking is one of the most costly health behaviors in which employees can engage.

✓ *Alternative medical practices seminars.* Clubs have found that seminars in such medically-related endeavors as chiropractic care, acupuncture, herbal medicine, and physical therapy can be appealing to many members.

❑ *Recreational Programs.* Recreational programs refer to program activities that are structured around the various recreational facilities of a club. Recreational programs can be offered in a variety of competitive arenas, such as basketball, volleyball, racquetball, squash, handball, softball, soccer, badminton, tennis, and (for those clubs fortunate enough to have a course) golf. Most recreational programs are offered in one or more of the following formats:

• *Intra-club leagues.* An intra-club league is based on organizing teams from among the club's members and then having the teams compete among each other over a specified period of time. In sports such as racquetball and tennis, the competition can be held between individuals or teams.

• *Inter-club leagues.* An inter-club league is based on establishing teams from the club's members and then organizing competition against teams from other clubs. Such competition can be held between individuals or teams.

• *Tournaments.* Tournaments are normally one-day events that are conducted at the club level, but can also be conducted for a larger audience. Most tournaments are offered in a single-elimination, double-elimination, or round-robin format. A tournament can involve competition between individuals or teams.

• *Mixers.* Mixers are popular in tennis, but offer a great program structure for other recreational activities as well. In a mixer, members or teams of members are scheduled to play other members/teams in a less-competitive format. One of the keys to a successful mixer is to include a social component in the event, such as providing a meal, serving drinks, or including a dance.

• *Ladders.* Ladder competition is a popular format in both tennis and racquetball. In a ladder, the members' names are placed on a ladder, and the members schedule games with those above them on the ladder. The primary goal of this type of recreational programming is for a member to move up the ladder by defeating the members who are above them on the ladder.

❑ *Adventure Programs.* Many clubs have found that programming can move outside the four walls of their club's facilities and, in the process, address the outdoor interests of their members. With the emerging growth in the number of echo boomers and the increased focus of many Americans to connect with the outdoors, the value of adventure programming has increased in recent years. In England during the mid-1990s, Cannons—a large club operator—offered an incredible array of adventure-driven programs for which members can register. While individual adventure programs may not attract comparatively large audiences, when taken as a whole, adventure programs represent an exceptional opportunity to provide members with greater membership value. The most common types of adventure programs offered by health/fitness clubs include:

> While individual adventure programs may not attract comparatively large audiences, when taken as a whole, adventure programs represent an exceptional opportunity to provide members with greater membership value.

- *Bike tours.* Some clubs offer these events as one-day adventures, while others might schedule bike tours with a theme. For example, some clubs in California, such as the Western Athletic clubs, offer wine-tasting bike tours. World Class Fitness, based in Moscow, Russia, conducts bike tours which often take groups as large as 200 to various parts of Europe for one- to two-week outings.
- *Ski outings.* Ski outings are extremely popular among members. Clubs can schedule these events for small-member groups and offer them multiple times during the year.
- *Scuba outings.* Many clubs, particularly clubs in the South, have found that scuba and snorkeling outings are extremely popular with members.
- *Whitewater rafting.* Whitewater rafting is one of the more popular adventure programs offered by clubs. In most parts of the country, there are outside groups that will work with clubs in scheduling whitewater outings.
- *Rock climbing.* The popularity of rock climbing has driven many clubs to schedule special one-day or weekend rock-climbing outings.
- *Golf tournaments.* While golf might not be considered an adventure outing, many clubs have found that offering an annual club golf outing brings high member and guest participation.

❑ *Social Programs.* Some club operators feel that because they are in the health/fitness club business, that their programming efforts should be focused entirely on fitness. What these operators don't seem to understand is that many members of a club are interested in making connections with other members. One of the best ways a club can support the interests and needs of members to create connections with other members is to develop social programs that place an emphasis on getting individuals together, rather than focusing almost entirely on exercise and health programming. Among the most successful social programs that clubs can offer include events that feature the hobbies, cultural interests, and sports interests of their members. In this regard, some of the most popular social programs include:

- *Beer, wine, and food tasting events.* Beer, food, and wine tastings are among the most popular social events that clubs can schedule for its members. Clubs can offer these evening beer, wine, or food tasting events as a means of bringing members and their guests into the club. In fact, a number of clubs combine these tasting experiences with other club activities as a means of prospecting for new members.

- *Theatre nights.* Many clubs have found value in coordinating special social events that involve taking a group of members to a particular cultural activity, such as a theatre event, symphony, play, or opera.

- *Sporting-event outings.* One of the most popular social events that a club can schedule is taking group outings to local sporting events. Furthermore, clubs can coordinate organized activities where members meet at the club, travel to a sporting event, and then return to the club afterwards for dinner or a reception. These outings involve attending a variety of sports-related activities, such as professional sports, college sports, or special sporting events.

- *Charity events.* Clubs can organize special events at their clubs to support a local charity. These events can be receptions, auctions, or dinners, using the club's facility areas, such as group exercise rooms or sport courts. For example, the Met in Houston, Texas takes a tennis court and converts it to a large ballroom for its annual charity event. Clubs can also consider hosting special runs for charity that begin and end at the club.

- *Clubs within a club.* "Clubs within a club" refers to the creation of special interest groups within the club. The basic concept underlying "clubs within a club" is to create small-niche interest groups that appeal to the interests of the club's members. In most cases, clubs within a club are built by identifying members with a passion for a particular hobby or activity and then working with those individuals to establish a club based on that activity. The best clubs within a club are those in which the members lead the clubs, but for which the club provides a degree of administrative and financial support. Among the types of "clubs within a club" that might be organized are the following: dancing club, photography club, gardening club, mountaineering club, running club, biking club, yoga club, card club, skiing club, swimming club, wine club, theatre club, bowling club, tennis club, golf club, etc.

The Keys to Great Club Programming

A number of critical steps are involved in the efforts by health/fitness clubs to develop and execute an effective program strategy that enhances membership retention and sales. Among the essential steps that can help provide club operators with a simple process for achieving successful programming are the following:

The club's first step in developing its programming approach should be to establish a purpose and vision for its programming.

❑ *Have a Purpose and Vision.* The club's first step in developing its programming approach should be to establish a purpose and vision for its programming. This purpose and vision need to align with the club's overall mission. The purpose and vision should be based on its answers to the following questions:

- Is the club's programming designed to drive member involvement and participation?

- Is the club's programming designed to enhance the sale of memberships?
- Is the club's programming an integral part of the club's brand differentiation process?
- Is the primary purpose of the club's programming seen more as providing incremental revenue?
- Is the club's programming part of its experience theme?

At best, every club needs to establish a purpose and vision for its programming that can be stated in one paragraph and serve as the framework for its programming efforts. At ClubCorp clubs, for example, the purpose of programming is to drive member involvement in the club and create memorable experiences that can help enrich the lives of the members and build relationships.

❏ *Understand the Market Served.* Once the club has established the purpose and vision for its programming efforts, its next step should be to make sure that it understands enough about its members to provide the programming strategies that will enable it to successfully address the club's purpose and vision. The discovery process for a club to understand its members should begin with the club opening the lines of communication with its members and determining their interests, needs, and wants. In this regard, conducting focus groups and surveys on a regular basis can help provide clubs with the basic information it might need. At a minimum, every club should ask a series of questions of all of its new members that enables it to determine what the program and activity interests of these individuals are. Another excellent step in this regard is to keep track of what activities members participate in when they are in the club. As this information is collected, the club should create a file on the interests and participation level of each member, as well as a record of the programs in which each individual is engaged. Subsequently, this information may help to facilitate efforts by clubs to provide member-centered programming.

❏ *Get the Members Involved.* One of the best-kept secrets about programming is that the more a club's members take ownership in its programming efforts, the better it will be for the club. When members take a sense of ownership in a club's programming, those individuals will be more likely to help the club design its programming efforts to meet their personal interests and needs and assist the club in getting other members to participate in the club's activities. Among the steps that clubs can employ to successfully get their members involved in their programming are the following:

- Establish member committees that act as liaisons with the membership and serve as ideation centers for programming.
- Identify member loyalists and get them involved in the programming at a volunteer level.
- Provide recognition and rewards for the members who become involved in the club's programming efforts.

> One of the best-kept secrets about programming is that the more a club's members take ownership in its programming efforts, the better it will be for the club.

❑ *Get the Employees Involved.* The club's ability to get its employees involved in its programming efforts is an essential factor with regard to whether it will be able to deliver exceptional programs. All factors considered, employees who participate in the planning and execution of the club's programming are more likely to assume an enhanced sense of ownership and responsibility for the success of the club's programming. Each club should initiate its programming efforts by having the staff assigned to the task brainstorm about program ideas. Subsequently, the club should appoint employee teams to flush out the various possible programs in more detail. Finally, the club should assign particular programs or program initiatives to specific employees and hold them accountable for their efforts. Most importantly, clubs should never make programming a one-person show.

❑ *Create an Annual Program Business Plan for the Club.* Once the club understands and executes the aforementioned steps, it then needs to develop an annual program plan for itself. An annual program plan allows the club to establish goals, timelines, schedules, and accountability for its program offerings. The annual program plan serves as the club's roadmap for programming success. The essential components of such an annual program plan include:

• *Address specific "S.M.A.R.T. objectives."* As such, the club should begin the process of developing an annual plan for its programming efforts by identifying specific objectives that should be achieved yearly that are simple, measurable, attainable, realistic, and trackable. These objectives should be consistent with the club's overall objectives and values. Examples of S.M.A.R.T. objectives include:

  ✓ Achieve an average of 3,000 participants each week in group exercise

  ✓ Increase member retention from 65 percent to 70 percent by the end of the year

  ✓ Generate an additional $30,000 each month over the prior year in program revenue

• *Establish a blended mix of programs.* The club should ensure that the success of its programming efforts is not dependent on just one type of programming, such as group exercise. Rather, its programming efforts should incorporate a variety of program options, including fitness programs, group-exercise programs, health-promotion programs, social programming, etc. Furthermore, the club's annual program plan should feature a mix of ongoing programs (i.e., programs that are offered on a daily or weekly basis, such as personal training, group-exercise classes, etc.) and special-event programs (i.e., programs that are conducted once a month or at certain designated times, such as fitness games, adventure outings, etc.).

• *Create a program booklet and calendar.* Most highly successful clubs develop both an annual program calendar and a quarterly program calendar. Program calendars serve to provide a club's members with a timetable of the facility's programs so the members can arrange their personal and business calendars to participate in the programs that are

Most highly successful clubs develop both an annual program calendar and a quarterly program calendar.

of interest to them. Producing a program booklet that can be given to its members is another productive step that clubs can take. These booklets feature a description of the offerings on the club's program calendar, thereby making it easier for the members to select the programs in which they are interested. These program calendars and booklets can be made available to the members through a variety of possible platforms, for example, the club's website, its newsletters, and the various distribution channels that the club uses to interact with its membership, including its social media sites.

- *Establish core marketing and promotional strategies for each program.* As part of its annual program plan, the club should identify how it plans to market its programs to its members. The top three to five strategies should be detailed in the plan and then implemented to the degree possible. For example, some clubs employ posters and flyers to promote their programs, while others utilize their club's newsletters and websites. A number of clubs use displays and interactive media to promote their programs. Because most clubs will not be able to use every possible marketing tool, they should make a concerted effort to identify the strategies that it plans to use and then do the best it can to execute them.

- *Assign each program to an employee and include a timeline for its implementation.* As part of its annual program plan, the club should assign an employee to be held accountable for the delivery of the program. As such, many larger clubs have program directors who have overall responsibility for the club's entire programming efforts. Unfortunately, however, many smaller clubs cannot afford a program director. In these instances, the club should appoint someone who is held accountable for each program.

- *Build a basic financial plan for programs as part of the program plan.* Another aspect of a club's program plan that should be included is itemized revenue and expense goals for the overall program and for each of the programs offered. While the financial portion of the program plan does not need to be detailed, it should, at a minimum, provide a framework for which employees can be held accountable.

❑ *Market, Promote, and Sell Constantly.* Some clubs develop a plan for programming, get their members and employees involved, and have all the materials that they need to offer the various programs, and yet their members still don't participate in the programs. A question arises concerning how such a scenario could occur. In this regard, one of the biggest pitfalls for club programming is the failure of many clubs to let their members know what programs are being conducted and when they are offered. Too often, clubs feel that if they simply put a poster up, that their members will sign-up for the activity. In reality, nothing could be further from the truth. Because members are constantly exposed to a variety of marketing materials, clubs need to be creative and disciplined in their approach to marketing and selling their programs. Among the steps that clubs can take to successfully market and sell its programs are the following:

Because members are constantly exposed to a variety of marketing materials, clubs need to be creative and disciplined in their approach to marketing and selling their programs.

- *Touch all of the senses with its marketing efforts.* Most members of a facility will respond to the club's marketing efforts if the club blends the media it uses to promote its programs and these efforts touch the various senses of its individual members. For example, the club can stir a person's visual senses by employing flyers and posters. It can affect an individual's sense of hearing by using audio marketing through the club's audiovisual mediums. It can also market a particular program by addressing a person's sense of smell, through the use of such contrivances as lighted incense or scented candles. Still other clubs might appeal to the member's sense of touch by using an interactive display to promote their programs.
- *Think about targeting marketing efforts toward specific member audiences.* Instead of using generic posters, videos, or displays, clubs should develop direct-mail pieces, invitations, targeted text messages, email blasts, and social media page postings to enhance member awareness. By using its records of member interests and activity patterns, clubs can create special invitations that are targeted to provide information on specific programs to specific member groups.
- *Create sales goals for each program.* The club should ensure that each program has a measurable target and then should share that information with its employees. Creating measurable targets for each program will make it easier to hold employees accountable for each program's success.
- *Teach employees the importance of leveraging their relationships to sell the club's programs.* For whatever reason, most employees are uncomfortable with "selling" and shy away from it. As a result, many clubs find that even the best-planned sales goals and marketing efforts often fall short. In reality, clubs need to educate their employees to understand the fact that the relationships that they have with the club's members is often the best avenue for program sales. Accordingly, clubs should establish incentive and reward programs that support the sales efforts of their employees. Such programs can have a meaningful impact on a club's efforts to market and sell its programs.

❏ *Feedback Is the Breakfast of Champions.* Even after the club has undertaken each of the aforementioned programming steps and the club's members have responded by participating in the activities offered in numbers never anticipated, the club has one more critical step to complete—obtain feedback from its members about its programming efforts. The most effective programmers in the health/fitness club industry make a concerted effort to get feedback from the members and employees at the conclusion of every program. By soliciting feedback from all parties involved, the club will help lay a framework for continuous growth in its programming efforts, as well as continued success in those endeavors. Feedback provides information concerning what everyone really thinks about the club's programming. It also offers an objective look at the successes, opportunities, and possible limiting factors that may exist within a club's programs.

> Clubs need to educate their employees to understand the fact that the relationships that they have with the club's members is often the best avenue for program sales.

THE HEALTH/FITNESS CLUB BUSINESS

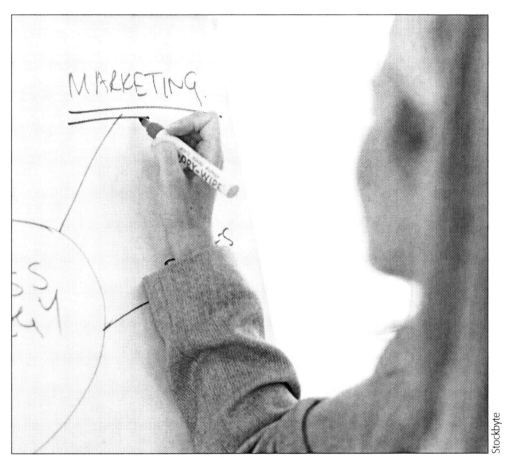

Stockbyte

Part Four

11

Establishing a Health/ Fitness Club Business

Chapter Objectives

The process of establishing a health/fitness club business can be relatively complicated. This chapter reviews the basic legal and business requirements for establishing a health/fitness club business entity and then examines how to develop the proper plans and systems that can help to insure that the business is successful. Initially, the chapter looks at the legal options for creating a health/ fitness club. Next, the chapter discusses the types of club business models that are commonly employed. Finally, the chapter details the key steps that are necessary to help turn a business venture into a great business organization.

The Legal Business Structure: Understanding the Options

The first step in establishing any business is to determine which legal business structure makes the most sense for that particular business. The business structure selected will play a significant role in the degree of legal liability, taxability, distribution of profit, and ability to solicit investment capital that the new business will face. Not a decision to be taken lightly, it should always be pursued with the professional advice of both legal council and a certified public accountant. As a rule, individuals have five basic options concerning which legal business structure should be employed for a particular business: a sole proprietorship, partnership, corporation, sub-S corporation, and limited liability corporation.

❏ *Sole Proprietorship (SP)*. A sole proprietorship is the simplest form of business structure that can be established. A sole proprietorship has no formal legal requirements and involves a single owner, the individual who is forming the business. As a sole proprietorship, the individual can reference the business under their own name or indicate that they are doing business as (d.b.a.) under a specified name. If the decision is made to establish a sole proprietorship and operate under a d.b.a., then the owner will be required to file for a certificate "for doing business as" with the state government.

> As a rule, individuals have five basic options concerning which legal business structure should be employed for a particular business: a sole proprietorship, partnership, corporation, sub-S corporation, and limited liability corporation.

The advantages and disadvantages of a sole proprietorship include the following:
- *Advantages*:
  - ✓ The business is owned an operated by one person who has complete control of the business.
  - ✓ The net profit of the business is taxed only once, and all expenses involved in operating the business can be deducted from the revenues by the owner.
  - ✓ The owner can file to operate under another name other than that of the owner.
- *Disadvantages*:
  - ✓ No insulation exists from liability, and all liability and debt are the responsibility of the owner.
  - ✓ The assets of the owner are left vulnerable to the business, and therefore, the personal assets of the owner can have a lien placed on them.
  - ✓ The business will terminate upon the death or incapacity of the owner.

The sole proprietorship structure might be an appropriate option if an individual was establishing a personal training business and chose not to have any employees beside themselves. For a business such as a health/fitness club, however, it is not the recommended option.

> A general partnership can consist of two or more persons carrying on business as co-owners. In a general partnership, each partner is an agent of the partnership and can legally bind the other partner to any agreement entered into by the other partner on behalf of the business.

❏ *Partnerships*. Partnerships are another basic form of business structure. Partnerships can exist in several structural arrangements—general partnerships, limited partnerships, and limited liability partnerships:
- *General partnership (GP)*. General partnerships can be written, oral, or implied and are intended to generate a profit. A general partnership can consist of two or more persons carrying on business as co-owners. In a general partnership, each partner is an agent of the partnership and can legally bind the other partner to any agreement entered into by the other partner on behalf of the business. In a general partnership, each partner has joint and severable liability, meaning that one individual or all of the individuals can be held accountable for the debt and legal liability of the business. In a general partnership, either partner has the ability to dissolve the partnership at any time. One common type of general partnership is a joint venture in which the partnership is intended to carry out a single business transaction.
- *Limited partnership (LP)*. Limited partnerships require a formal agreement between the involved parties and a certificate of limited partnership. A limited partnership has a general partner who usually manages the business and typically has the largest financial stake in the business. This type of business structure also has limited partners who have a financial stake in the business, but who are not involved in managing it. In a limited partnership, the partners can be individuals or corporations. Limited partnerships are similar to general partnerships in that the partners have joint and severable liability, meaning one or

all partners can be held liable for the actions of the business. A limited partnership exists as long as the general partner is involved or until all partners agree to terminate the arrangement. Limited partnerships are commonly employed by such organizations as law firms, physician groups, and accounting firms. In the health/fitness club industry, limited partnerships can be created that can have ownership of the physical assets of club and then be operated as a management company under another type of business structure.

- *Limited liability partnership (LLP)*. In a limited liability partnership, the general and limited partners are protected from liability beyond a collective limit of $100,000. To register as a limited liability partnership, the partners have to demonstrate that they have insurance to cover the $100,000 limit and must file a formal application with the state. In certain instances, the partners in a limited liability partnership are not always liable for the debts and obligations of the business. The registration for a limited liability partnership expires after one year.

> In a limited liability partnership, the general and limited partners are protected from liability beyond a collective limit of $100,000.

When looking at each form of partnership, it should be understood that with the exception of the limited liability partnership, that each partner assumes liability for all obligations of themselves and the other partners. Furthermore, in this particular business structure, only the general partner has control of the business. The upside to such a partnership is the opportunity for a limited partner to participate in the success of a business without having to be involved in management. As was previously discussed, limited partnerships are an appropriate option for those individuals or businesses who are interested in owning a health/fitness club and do not want the responsibility of managing the business.

❑ *Corporations (C-Corp)*. Corporations, also known as C-Corps, are legal entities created to conduct business and authorized to act with the rights and liabilities of a person. Such business entities can exist as general, professional, and non-profit corporations. Of the three options, general corporations are the most commonly found type in the health/fitness club industry. In a general corporation, the business is organized for profit and distribution of earnings to the officers and owners (stockholders). When a corporation is formed, it must file articles of incorporation, which include a listing of the owners, directors, and officers, with the state in which the business is incorporated. A corporation is required to have both bylaws and annual meetings of its directors and officers, with the directors and officers representing the owners. A corporation may also issue stock, both common and preferred. Such an issuance enables numerous individuals and organizations to have an ownership stake in the business. A corporation may exist for perpetuity.

A corporation insulates its owners from personal liability and loss, which is much different than the situation that sole proprietors and partnerships encounter. In essence, a corporation allows the owners to walk away from the business with minimal liability for the company's liabilities and debt. The downside of the corporation is that earnings are taxed at both the corporate level and again at the individual level, based on the individual's stake in the business. In addition, a corporation requires a majority decision of its directors and officers for major business decisions, which is considerably different from other legal business structures. In the future, as registration and licensure of health/fitness professionals occurs, a time might come when personal trainers might incorporate as professional corporations, similar to physicians, lawyers, and architects.

❏ *Sub-S Corporations (Sub-S).* A sub-S corporation is a hybrid corporation that has certain features that do not exist with the typical corporation. For example, a sub-S corporation is restricted to a maximum of 35 stockholders and can only issue one kind of stock. Another unique aspect of a sub-S corporation is that it insulates the owners from personal liability associated with the business. At the same time, it avoids the double taxation of a typical corporation by allowing all earnings of the business to be distributed to the owners without any corporate taxation. As a result, all earnings are passed on to the owners, who are then taxed on their vested earnings. For many single-unit health/fitness clubs, the sub-S is an attractive legal alternative for structuring the business.

> For many single-unit health/fitness clubs, the sub-S is an attractive legal alternative for structuring the business.

❏ *Limited Liability Corporation (LLC).* The limited liability corporation is a relatively new corporate structure that is seen as providing its investors and owners with a combination of benefits from the other legal entities previously described. For example, an LLC provides comparable, if not better, insulation from liability than a corporation, while at the same time offering the favorable tax advantages of a partnership or S-corp. An LLC must create articles of organization with the state in which it forms and assign managers. Instead of stockholders, an LLC has members. An LLC can consist of a single member or multiple members. LLCs can have individuals, partnerships, or even corporations as members. Furthermore, one caveat of the LLC is that it can last no longer than 30 years and in states such as Texas, it must provide the appropriate funding to cover a specified dollar level of liability coverage.

As is evident, health/fitness club owners have numerous options concerning their choice of which business structure to employ—each of which has its benefits and risks. As such, potential business owners need to weigh the council of lawyers, accountants, and other professionals to determine what structure will work best for their business. Figure 11-1 presents a comparison of some of the primary advantages and disadvantages attendant to each of the various types of business structures.

Business Operating Models

Once a decision has been made from a legal and tax perspective on the type of business structure under which the club will function, the next step is to identify which operating model the club prefers. In the health/fitness club industry, there are three basic models from which to choose: an independent club operator, a part of a multiple-club operation (regional or national), or a franchise (single or regional). A review of each of the three types of models can help reveal the benefits and risks associated with each option:

	Sole Proprietor	Partnership	Corporation	Sub-S Corporation	LLC
Personal Risk	Unlimited	Share of total investment	Amount of personal investment	Amount of investment and loans	Amount of investment up to a cap
Taxation	One time on business earnings	One time on share of earnings	Company earnings and then again on personal earnings	One time on all personal share of business earnings	One time on personal share of business earnings
Control of Business	Very high	Moderate to limited	Depends on stock position	Moderate to limited	Moderate
Capital for Growth	Owner's money	Loans from partners	Stock sale, bonds	Sell stock or loans	Sell stock or loans
Staffing	Poor	Poor to fair	Good	Fair	Fair to good

Figure 11-1. A comparison of the advantages and disadvantages of selected types of business structures

❑ *Independent Club.* An independent club model involves a business that operates independently of any other club or business association. As such, the development and operation of the club is solely dependent upon the club's ability to build the systems needed to operate itself. Over 50 percent of the health/fitness clubs operating in the U.S. are independently owned and operated, including industry leaders such as Red's in Lafayette, Louisiana, Franco's in Mandeville, Louisiana, the Maryland Athletic Club in Timonium, Maryland, the Gainesville Health and Fitness Center in Gainesville, Florida, the Rochester Athletic Club in Rochester, Minnesota, and the East Bank Club in Chicago, Illinois. Among the benefits of establishing the business as an independent club are the following:

- The club can be designed and operated as part of the local community, thereby creating a product unique to the demographics of the market in which it is located.
- The ownership group of the business has control of the club's destiny as a business and can create the systems and structures it deems necessary.
- The club can establish a brand for itself in the local community that is built on the values and goals of the ownership group.
- The club will not be burdened with some of the overhead costs normally associated with being part of a franchise or multiple-club operation.
- Concurrent with the aforementioned benefits, the owner and operator of an independent club also faces several challenges that the other operating models do not have, including:
- Independent operators will not have access to the capital, operating, and marketing resources that the other operating club models can offer.
- Independent operators may find themselves at a disadvantage with the other club models when it comes to purchasing power, marketing clout, and talent recruitment.

While the health/fitness club industry was founded by independent operators whose talent and passion helped forge the $20 billion U.S. industry that presently exists, the current landscape portrays an environment that is less friendly to those individuals who operate independently.

❏ *Multiple-Club Operation.* The multiple club business model exists today because it affords owners and operators several distinct advantages when it comes to accessing capital, recruiting talent, and controlling a particular market. Multiple clubs currently occupy about one-third of the entire club market. A multiple-club operation can be national, such as 24 Hour Fitness, LA Fitness, Lifetime Fitness, or Bally; regional, such as Town Sports International (Northeast corridor), Western Athletic Clubs (California), or Sport and Health (Washington, Maryland, and Virginia); or local, such as Wisconsin Athletic Clubs (Milwaukee), Fitness Formula (Chicago), Healthworks (Boston), or DMB Sports (Phoenix). In the current global economy, multiple-club operations can also position themselves as multi-national or global club companies, such as Fitness First (United Kingdom, Germany, Australia, India) or Virgin Active (United Kingdom, Italy, South Africa, Spain).

Being part of a multiple-club operation offers several business advantages when compared to being an independent club operator, including:

* Access to capital for growth
* Business systems and programs that can assist in operating a club more profitably
* Talent sources and intellectual capital that can enhance the opportunities in a given market and help grow local talent
* Cost efficiencies driven by volume purchases
* Branding and marketing as provided by the parent company

Concurrent with the aforementioned advantages, being part of a multiple-club operation also has several potential downsides about which a business operator should be aware, including:

* The business operator will normally have less control of their destiny and less freedom to operate their business as they desire, because they will need to fit their efforts into the systems, policies, and procedures of the parent company.
* The business operator may find that the club is less unique to its market than it would prefer or expect since it must function according to the branding and operational model established by the parent company.
* The business will most likely have to assume the name of the parent company and thereby forfeit any direct identity with its local market (e.g., 24 Hour Fitness, LA Fitness, Bally's, Virgin, Fitness First, etc.). Some multiple-club operations, however, such as Wellbridge and Tennis Corporation of America, allow their clubs to have individual identities.

❏ *Franchised Club Operation.* Owning and operating a franchised club provides some of the advantages of both an independent operation and a multiple-club operation. The franchising model is based on the principle

> While the health/fitness club industry was founded by independent operators whose talent and passion helped forge the $20 billion U.S. industry that presently exists, the current landscape portrays an environment that is less friendly to those individuals who operate independently.

that local business owners will have greater success connecting their club to the local community and making it successful if they have an ownership stake in the business. At the same time, these individuals will benefit from being associated with a recognized brand that provides operational and marketing assistance. The most established and possibly most recognized health/fitness club franchises are Anytime Fitness, Gold's Gym, World Gym, and Powerhouse Gyms. Since 2000, specialty franchises, such as Curves, Anytime Fitness, and Snap Fitness, have established themselves as leading franchise operations and have helped to reshape the industry by establishing greater value to the franchise model. Multiple-club operations, such as Bally's in the U.S. and Fitness First based in the U.K., also provide franchise opportunities, especially on an international basis, for individuals and companies wanting to get involved in the health/fitness club industry.

A franchise can be purchased for one club or an entire region. Most franchisers, such as Gold's, require potential investors to meet certain financial expectations before they can assume a franchise. These expectations include the requirement that the franchisee must demonstrate the level of financial backing that would be needed to build and operate the franchise. Most franchisers charge the franchisee an up-front franchise fee that can range from as low as $5,000 to as high as $25,000 and an annual fee that can run between $3,000 and $6,000 annually. In addition, there are other costs associated with having a franchise, including the cost of purchasing the operational and retail products needed for the club through the franchiser's business system.

> Most franchisers charge the franchisee an up-front franchise fee that can range from as low as $5,000 to as high as $25,000 and an annual fee that can run between $3,000 and $6,000 annually.

The advantages to a health/fitness club operator who chooses to become a franchised operation include:

- Obtaining the rights to a nationally recognized brand that will immediately position the new business in the marketplace
- Access to the business systems created by the franchiser, such as design plans, equipment discounts, operations manuals, marketing templates, etc.
- Access to national marketing programs and the ability to share costs on marketing and advertising programs
- Access to educational programs and conventions operated by the franchiser
- Ability, as a local owner, to control the destiny of their business as long as they meet the criteria established by the franchiser

Concurrent with the aforementioned advantages are some disadvantages, including:

- Upfront capital for the franchise fee, something the club would not have if it operated independently or was part of a multiple-club operation
- The annual cost of maintaining the franchise
- An association with a specific brand, especially if that brand proves to be the wrong one for the club's particular community. A club should

be aware of the fact that the consumer will associate it with a specific brand, even if it operates differently than most of the others who use that franchise brand.

- Limitations in the club's flexibility to operate the business as it desires, because of the requirements of the franchise agreement

As the aforementioned discussions point out, the options for a club business model are as varied as are the legal options for setting up the business. Figure 11-2 provides a simple comparison of the three basic models for opening a club.

Deciding Whether to Buy or Build a Club

Once individuals have successfully navigated the decision-making path of what legal structure to assume and what type of club model under which they want to operate, the next major business hurdle they face is to decide whether they want to build a club or purchase an existing club. All factors considered, this decision is as important as any they will make and more than any other will impact their initial capital requirements and their ability to achieve profitability. It is essential that the individuals who are making these critical decisions (whether to build or buy) fully understand the various factors that affect each choice. Such an understanding can help them decide which option is the best course of action for them.

- ❑ *Building a Club.* If the decision is made to build a club, two standard courses of action can be taken. One is to purchase land, and then proceed to build a free-standing club structure. This approach to building requires not only that the land be purchased, but also that the club operators have the capital to build a free-standing building. This course of action is normally the most capital intensive, because it requires the funds both to purchase the property

	Independent Club	**Multiple Club**	**Franchisee**
Branding	Local brand that has to be built by owner	Aligned with a national brand, but still some branding required	Instant brand recognition and marketing support of the brand
Operating Support	Entrepreneur; owner has to develop all the systems	Based less on entrepreneur and more on systems administration	Entrepreneur focus, but systems provided
Marketing Support	None, except what is developed locally	Varies according to the parent company; can range from high to very low	Excellent support with templates and tie-in to national campaigns
Sense of Community	Very high	Low to moderate	Moderate to high
Cost Advantages	Few to none	Moderate to high	Moderate
Educational Support	None	Moderate to high	Low to moderate

Figure 11-2. A comparison of selected club operating models

(ranging from $2 to $20 a square foot), and also to build a free-standing structure (ranging from $75 to $400 a square foot). By the time the process is completed, anywhere from $2 million to $20 million could be spent on the club. (It should be noted that some operators have spent over $30 million for clubs that exceed 100,000 square feet in size.) Besides the large outlay of cash, when a club is built from scratch, the membership also has to be built from scratch. As a result, the cash flow from the club's operations at its opening will normally not support the facility's operating expenses. It is common in the industry for free-standing clubs to not reach profitability until the end of their second or third year of operation and not begin to provide any return on their assets until at least their third year. Of course, exceptions to this rule exist.

It is common in the industry for free-standing clubs to not reach profitability until the end of their second or third year of operation and not begin to provide any return on their assets until at least their third year.

Another option concerning building a club that operators have is to lease space in a strip mall, office park, or office building. In this instance, the club will still have to build out the facility, but the costs will be less. In this scenario, the landlord usually provides the shell structure, along with an allowance for tenant build out (usually ranging from $15 to $50 a square foot). A typical tenant finish-out will range from $50 to $150 a square foot, which is considerably less than building from the ground up. This contribution of the shell and core by the landlord reduces the amount of up-front capital that is needed by the club's owner. Similar to a free-standing club, the time needed to generate enough membership to reach profitability will often take approximately two to three years. In this scenario, the owner's initial level of debt will not be as great. However, some additional built-in overhead—e.g., rent—will exist if this option is chosen.

❏ *Buying a Club.* An attractive alternative to building a club is to purchase an existing club. When individuals purchase a club, they have two options—one is to purchase the entire business and the other is to purchase only the assets of an existing club's business. Most attorneys will advise individuals to purchase only the business assets, an option that will allow them to avoid assuming the liabilities of the existing business. The primary advantage of purchasing an existing club begins with the cost of purchase. As a general rule of thumb, most clubs will have an enterprise value (the value of the business before accounting for debts and related liabilities) equal to four times to six times their EBITDA (earnings before interest, taxes, depreciation, and amortization). As a result, the majority of clubs normally sell for far less than they would cost to build. Another benefit of purchasing an existing club involves the fact that purchasers are also getting an existing membership and an existing cash flow. In other words, the time it will take a club to reach profitability and gain a return on assets or equity will typically be far shorter. On occasion, an existing club can reach profitability immediately and provide returns on the purchased assets as early as the first year. (It should be noted that the process of purchasing is far more complicated than the aforementioned discussion indicated and will be covered more thoroughly in Chapter 14). Figure 11-3 provides an overview comparison of buying an existing club versus building a club.

	Free-Standing Building	Building in Leased Space	Purchase Free-Standing Club	Purchase Club in Leased Space
Upfront Capital Required	Very high—land costs and structure costs	Moderate to high, depending on landlord allowance	Moderate; depends on club's earnings performance	Low to moderate
Range of Cost All In	$150 to $300 s.f.	$50 to $200 s.f.	4x to 6x EBITDA	1x to 4x EBITDA
Time to Profitability	1 to 3 years, with average closer to 3 years	1 to 3 years, with average closer to 2 years	Immediately to 1 year	Immediately to 1 year
Risks	High capital costs; time to profitability; cost of taxes	Capital costs; limitations set by landlord; time to profitability	Capital costs moderately high; unknown liabilities not uncovered during due diligence	Condition of the space; unexpected liabilities or costs; restrictions set by landlord

Figure 11-3. Comparison of buying vs. building a club

Getting the Business Started

To this point, the chapter has addressed the primary challenges facing a prospective club owner, which revolve around the legal structural framework for the club, the type of club model employed, and whether to buy or build the club. The final critical step in starting a health/fitness club involves establishing the business framework that will enable the club to be successful. In that regard, several key steps can be undertaken by club owners that can help them establish an appropriate framework for their business, including:

❏ *Establish a Clear Vision of the Business.* The vision of any business revolves around three distinct narratives—the mission statement, the promise, and the theme. The mission statement is a succinct statement that clearly communicates to both a club's customer and its employees who and what the business is. At ClubCorp, their mission statement articulated the fact they would be the "world class leader in delivering the private club experience." This simple statement makes it clear what the intentions of the business are and whom they intend to serve. For any business, it is imperative that they provide a mission statement that allows their team and customers to understand the overall focus of the business.

The second essential narrative is the club's customer or brand promise. The promise is the commitment that the club makes to each and every customer of its business. At ClubCorp, that promise was to "build relationships and enrich lives." The promise not only lets a club's customers know what to expect, more importantly, it enables the club's staff to be aware of what experience they are expected to deliver to the club's members.

The final piece of the vision puzzle is the theme. The theme is the driving force behind the experience the club intends to provide its members. Many businesses forget to establish a theme. As a result, their business tends to lose focus on the experience it is trying to create. An example of where a club is using a predetermined theme in an appropriate manner is at Crunch. Their theme speaks to "making no judgments." When individuals visit one of their clubs, they definitely can pick up on the fact that the Crunch employees are making an effort, with the help of their facilities and programs, to act out that theme.

❑ *Create a Culture and Strive to Maintain It.* Culture is often defined as the traditions and practices that make a country, business, or people unique. With regard to a business setting, its culture is what makes a business unique from any other. Culture for a business is like culture for a country; it speaks to what is unique and special about the business and in what each and every employee can take pride. Culture begins with the establishment of core values and traditions, which are then sustained through stories told by the "leaders and heroes" of the business. Over time, these stories become the myths of the business, and the heroes become the legends.

> **Culture for a business is like culture for a country; it speaks to what is unique and special about the business and in what each and every employee can take pride.**

The first step that a business must take in order to create a culture is to identify its core values. The core values serve as the foundation behind every decision a business makes. They are the roots of the business that nourish it and sustain it. At ClubCorp, their core values included a philosophy where the member/guest is king, a mandate for every employee to plan their work and work their plan, an unwavering commitment to integrity, and a firm belief in the necessity to exhibit character at all times. At Red's in Lafayette, Louisiana, their core values reflected such precepts as "greeting each member with a smile," "saying hello and goodbye," and "if you have time to lean, you have time to clean." Although simple, the aforementioned values are powerful influencers of positive business behavior.

The second step in creating a business culture is to establish specific philosophies and practices that, when replicated over time, will become traditions. At the Ritz Carlton, for example, they speak of "ladies and gentlemen serving ladies and gentlemen." Similarly, at ClubCorp, the discourse of "creating a refuge for the member, a home away from home" is commonly expressed. The philosophies of both companies serve as a framework for the actual practices in which their employees engage. Over time, as employees repeat these mantras and engage in these practices, they become traditions. Even more importantly, over time, employees will tell stories about how certain employees carried out these practices in a special way. When this occurs, myths and storytellers have been created, which are critical to sustaining the culture the business has developed.

❑ *Establish Long-Term and Short-Term Business Objectives.* Before the club ever opens its club doors to serve its future members, it needs to establish both long-term objectives (e.g., 10 to 20 years out) and short-term objectives (e.g., one-year, three-year, and five-year). Together, these objectives can help establish a road map for the club's business journey and help inform the club's investors and employees where it is planning to go and how it plans to get there.

The long-term business goals are often referred to as BHAG's (big hairy audacious goals). These goals represent what the club ultimately wants to achieve. While these goals should be clear and succinct, at the same time, they should not be as specific as those the club establishes for the short-term. An example of a BHAG for a health/fitness club might be "to be recognized as the premier health/fitness club in the market, as reflected by capturing 15 percent of the market." If this goal were part of a club's plan, then it should be relatively clear to everyone what the club planned to accomplish in the future. Just as importantly, it could also serve as a marker for the club's progress over the years.

The club's short-term business goals need to be S.M.A.R.T. (simple, measurable, attainable, realistic, and trackable). All factors considered, short-term goals serve as the benchmarks for the beginning of a club's business journey. Examples of short-term business goals might include:

- Achieve 2,000 members at the end of year one
- Achieve revenues of three million dollars at the end of the first year and seven million dollars by the end of the fifth year
- Achieve an annualized return on assets of 12 percent for each of the first five years
- Open up a second club by the end of the third year of business

By establishing its goals, the club is attempting to provide a meaningful framework for its success.

> **By establishing its goals, the club is attempting to provide a meaningful framework for its success.**

❑ *Establish Replicable Operating Standards and Systems.* When a business is young, the club owner can often oversee every step that is taken. As time passes, however, the business' success will not depend on the ability of a single person. Rather the club's staff must be able to replicate the practices that drive the club's success. In that regard, the club must have clearly defined standards and systems.

Standards set the expectations for how a specific practice should be carried out. Standards need to be simple and clear. In essence, standards convey a description of the outcome that the club expects from an operational practice. Standards do not tell employees the "how," but rather the "what" and "when" a particular practice/action needs to be achieved. An example of a standard might be, "Every member will receive an orientation to the fitness floor that includes an exercise prescription." As such, this standard communicates the expectation, but not the path to be taken.

Systems are the processes and resources that the club provides to its employees that enable them to achieve the standards. More importantly, systems create consistency in the club's service delivery across space and time. Systems can include such factors as employee education programs, procedural documents for the handling of membership sales, procedural documents for accounting practices, etc. If the club does not establish business systems, even simple ones, it may find that its employees will tend to take the steps that are best for them and not necessarily the best for the business. Figure 11-4 helps illustrate the connection between standards and systems.

❑ *Establish an Accountable Organizational Model.* Every business, especially a health/fitness club business, needs to have an organizational structure

Standard: The Expectations	System: The Process
"Every new member will receive an orientation."	"Every new member will be scheduled for an appointment at the time of joining the club."

Figure 11-4. The relationship between a standard and a system

that brings decision-making relatively close to the member or customer. This scenario involves creating a flat organization where as few layers as possible exist between the customer or member and the employee who is making the decision concerning what should be done. This process of creating an accountable organizational structure requires the following key steps:

- Create a clear structure showing the relationships of each position to the members and to the other employees. Make sure to have as few layers between the customer and the owner as possible.
- Create a job description for each position that is based on accountability and not on tasks.

Establish a model for open communication up and down the organizational structure. Eliminate communication holes and traps by doing away with positions of power.

By addressing these issues up front, the club can create an organizational structure where every employee takes a sense of ownership in the success of the business. Samples of organizational charts and job models are included in the appendices.

❑ *Hire the Best and Then Provide a Continuous Learning Environment.* The truest indicator of how successful a particular club business will become lies in the talent of the people it employs. As a consequence, club owners and operators need to hire the best people. According to Jim Collins, author of *Good to Great,* the best employees are those individuals who embrace the company's values and culture and have disciplined focus, disciplined thought, and disciplined action. As such, it is imperative that business leaders take the time to select and hire the best individuals. Furthermore, to keep the best, the club needs to provide an environment that promotes continuous learning and growth. In addition, the club needs to establish a culture that encourages employees to learn new skills and provide the support, both financially and time-wise, for employees to take advantage of learning opportunities. In addition, clubs should budget for educational efforts and programs, bring in outside speakers, establish regular in-house education, expose employees to other job roles, and promote those individuals who demonstrate that they are leaders and achievers.

❑ *Remember That Service Delivery Stays Close to the Member.* Many businesses create hurdles and barriers that force their customers to sacrifice something as part of their experience. When individuals create a business, they should establish a framework that eliminates member sacrifice. More importantly, the framework should enable its frontline employees (i.e., those employees who directly interact on a daily basis with the members) to do the delivery and, if necessary, the recovery of the services. For example, if a member comes to a fitness instructor and has a concern about an issue, the member should not be made to wait while the instructor chases down a supervisor. Instead, the club should have a policy of empowering instructors to act on their own.

❑ *Create a Standard Financial Model and Budgets.* A final key to achieving success in a business is to create a financial model that everyone can understand and work with. The financial model should be based on establishing budgets that the respective club staff can work from and by which they can monitor the club's financial performance. As a matter of practice, club owners/operators should make the budget available to the appropriate staff members so that they know what has to be achieved and how they have performed over the course of the budgetary period, financial-wise. The club's financial model should also include simple reporting tools that enable the club to monitor the key financial indicators on a daily, weekly, monthly, quarterly, and annual basis.

Qualities of Great Clubs

A great club is one that, year in and year out, generates success for everyone involved in the facility—members, financial stakeholders, employees, and the community. In this regard, some of the most significant indicators are:

A great club is one that, year in and year out, generates success for everyone involved in the facility—members, financial stakeholders, employees, and the community.

- Continuous growth in membership each year
- Continuous growth in revenues and earnings each year
- High levels of membership retention (well above the industry average)
- High levels of employee satisfaction
- Low employee turnover (less than the industry average)
- Tenured senior staff
- High levels of member satisfaction and member loyalty
- High levels of respect in the community
- Have been in business for at least 10 years, exhibiting the ability to sustain itself for an extended period
- Documented return on investment for the equity holders of at least 10% annually

Without question, additional indicators of success can be identified. Regardless of the ultimate mix of factors that is ultimately associated with a particular facility prospering, one observation is clear: great clubs always seem to have a full compliment of members and employees with tenure. More importantly, great clubs seem to perform well, year after year, even during periods when other facilities are struggling. As such, great clubs in the health/fitness industry tend to exhibit certain characteristics, including:

❑ *Location, Location, and Location.* Similar to the real estate business, location is one of the best predictors of success in the health/fitness club business. More often than not, great clubs are located in areas that are close to the right demographics and convenient to access. It is also important to note that while some of the current great clubs did not always have a great location, they did know that in the future their location would be an outstanding one. In reality, location involves more than just having the right demographics or even just the right street address. Rather, location involves building the club in a place where its visibility to the public is enhanced. Without the proper location, the process of achieving greatness can take considerably longer.

❑ *The Owners Constantly Reinvest in the Facility.* Great clubs invest their earnings into their facilities. By engaging in such activities as purchasing new equipment, repairing worn areas, adding the newest services, and making sure that the facility is never outdated, great clubs show their members and their staff that they are committed to providing a positive experience for everyone involved. According to statistics reported by IHRSA, most clubs devote approximately three percent of their revenue in capital upgrades. Great operations spend nearly double that. As a result, these clubs continue to grow and prosper.

❑ *Clean Facilities.* Really great clubs are incredibly clean. Just as importantly, all of the employees, including the manager, feel a sense of personal accountability for keeping every aspect of the club clean. From the top on down, all levels of staff should focus on cleanliness.

❑ *Vision, Values, and Strong Culture.* Great clubs have a clearly defined vision that identifies and articulates the target toward which they are channeling their resources and energies. Vision is what defines the future of the organization. It is the standard of excellence by which the efforts of everyone within the organization can be judged. It is the benchmark that keeps every staff member on track. An appropriate vision meets several criteria, including being achievable, tangible, and meet the expectations of the club's staff and members.

Great clubs also have a values-orientation. They exhibit a moral core that is based on ethically grounded principles. Their values inspire confidence and help rally staff to achieve a common purpose. Great clubs know the difference between doing their best and doing what is right. From top to bottom, employees in great clubs exhibit high levels of integrity, honesty, trustworthiness, loyalty, and pride in their mission and their accomplishments.

Great clubs know the difference between doing their best and doing what is right.

In addition, great clubs have a unique culture that is often easily distinguished from the other clubs in the market. A club's culture is similar to the culture of a country. It involves an integrated pattern of beliefs, behavior, customs, knowledge, and traditions. When a facility's leadership makes an effort to maintain a strong culture, everyone associated with the club benefits.

❑ *Investment in People.* Great clubs see their employees as their greatest asset. In that regard, great clubs view their staff as the heart of the organization. As such, they make a concerted effort to provide a work environment that enables their employees to achieve at their maximum level of productivity and potential. One step that great clubs employ to help attain that objective is to develop and support a program of ongoing education for their employees. Such a program can include such activities as bringing in outside speakers to address the staff, encouraging employees to attend professional meetings, requiring staff to be certified by an accredited organization, recognizing and rewarding employees for their efforts at lifelong learning, providing financial support for learning-related endeavors, etc. The key point that should be noted is that great clubs are aware of the fact that an investment in their staff is an investment in the facility's future.

❑ *Teamwork.* Every great club is a unified team. A team is another name for a group of two or more individuals who are interacting in pursuit of a common goal. In that regard, great clubs have an enhanced level of esprit de corps. They feature a workplace environment that, all factors considered, is more "worker friendly." This atmosphere helps reinforce parochial attitudes in the staff. Employees are more willing to do whatever it takes to do the job that needs to be done. Furthermore, they are more likely to accept responsibility for their efforts (personal accountability) and take pride in the final outcome. In team-oriented situations, an aura of collected responsibility is ingrained. If the team succeeds, everyone succeeds. On the other hand, if the team fails, everyone fails.

❑ *Tenured Staff.* Great clubs typically have employees who have been with them for an extended period of time. Having a tenured staff can benefit a club in a number of ways. First and foremost, tenured staff tend to know the nuances of their jobs and fulfill their roles within the club very well. Retaining staff means time and resources don't need to be devoted to attracting and training new employees. Tenured staff are more likely to be team-oriented and less likely to act in a self-interested manner. Perhaps most importantly, tenured staff tend to inspire loyalty from the club's members. The members know them, like them, and trust them. Such loyalty enhances the experience a member achieves at the facility, as well as improves the club's membership retention levels.

❑ *Two-Way Flow of Communication.* Great clubs are able to communicate effectively with both their members and their employees. They appreciate and understand the need for a two-way flow of communication. In that regard, they develop systems that allow members to easily communicate with management about their experiences at the club, good or bad. They also make it a practice to always respond to member's feedback within at least a 48-hour time period, if not before. As such, these clubs are constantly seeking feedback from their members through the use of such tools as focus groups, surveys, and one-on-one discussions. Great clubs clearly communicate their policies, rules, and related practices to their members, as well as their employees. Furthermore, they understand that the ability to communicate effectively involves more than just verbal skills.

Great clubs are able to communicate effectively with both their members and their employees.

They are able to utilize their entire array of communication skills (including listening, feedback, memory, and non-verbal), depending on the situation, to reinforce their message

❏ *Everyone Knows the Numbers*. Great clubs share their important "numbers" with their staff. They understand that a key factor in achieving the desired results is to have employees who take ownership of the numbers. Sharing this information sends a very positive message to staff members. It enhances their feelings of importance and self worth. It helps inspire loyalty and commitment to the club's mission/vision. In that regard, such proprietorship can serve as an exceptional catalyst for inspired performance. Great clubs ensure that the department heads and other employees know the key numbers. As a result, these department heads know what their performance targets are and how they have performed against them. Their employees are aware of how membership sales are going. One step that some clubs take to share their numbers with the staff is to have a scoreboard in the employee break room that reflects all of the club's key performance indicators.

❏ *Member Apostles*. Member apostles are individuals who are very loyal to the club and believe so strongly in the value of the club that they enjoy referring friends and associates for membership. Creating these member apostles is a by-product of a culture that focuses on treating each member the same by treating them differently. Great clubs embrace the belief that once a member joins a facility, it is the responsibility of every employee of the club to do everything in their power to create a positive experience for that person. When this attitude is put into practice, members are more likely to take a sense of ownership in the club and fervent advocates (i.e., become the sales people) for the club. Great clubs obtain many of their new members from member referrals.

Great clubs embrace the belief that once a member joins a facility, it is the responsibility of every employee of the club to do everything in their power to create a positive experience for that person.

12

The Health/Fitness Club Financial Model

Chapter Objectives

Initially, this chapter reviews basic accounting methodologies, followed by a review of the basic financial tools that are used to measure financial performance in the health/fitness club industry. The chapter concludes by presenting an overview of benchmark financial data from the industry.

Accrual Versus Cash Accounting

In general, the business world employs two methods for accounting for the financial performance of a business—cash accounting and accrual accounting.

❑ *Cash Accounting.* Under cash accounting, a business accounts for all revenues and expenses as they are incurred by the business. This method is sometimes referred to as "checkbook" accounting. When using the cash accounting method, a club must record every revenue collected and every expenditure incurred on the day on which it occurred. This approach to accounting is typically used by smaller organizations that need to closely manage their cash flow. All factors considered, this "check book" approach provides them with the control that they need.

❑ *Accrual Accounting.* Accrual accounting is the method employed by most businesses. In accrual accounting, a business accounts for its revenues not as they are generated, but how they are earned. With regard to expenses, a business using accrual accounting accounts for these outlays not as they may actually be expended and paid for, but as they are represented by the operating practice. For example, a club receives a quarterly rent statement from its landlord for $300,000. In accrual accounting, the business would account for this payment as $100,000 in each of the months covered by the agreement, while in cash accounting, the $300,000 would be accounted for when the bill was paid. Another example might involve a situation in which a club sold $360,000 in annual membership contracts in January. In accrual

> In general, the business world employs two methods for accounting for the financial performance of a business—cash accounting and accrual accounting.

accounting, the club would only allocate 1/12 of that amount ($30,000) to January's revenues, along with any carryover accruals from the previous 11 months. In contrast, in cash accounting, the entire sum of $360,000 would be accounted for at the time it was received. Accrual accounting practices are governed by specific rules. The International Financial Reporting Standards (IFRS) are used around the globe, while Generally Accepted Accounting Principles (GAAP) are employed in the United States. These two standardized systems spell out exactly how a business should account for its expenses and revenues when it's using accrual methodology.

The Basic Financial Tools Used by the Health/Fitness Club Industry

As the health/fitness club industry has matured, the tools for measuring financial performance have also become more sophisticated. The three most important financial tools and the information each provides are as follows:

❏ *The Balance Sheet* (refer to Figure 12-1). The balance sheet provides a quick snapshot of the financial health of the club on a day-to-day, week-to-week, and period-to-period basis. The balance sheet tells the business exactly how healthy its finances are at any point in time. The balance sheet lets the club know what its assets are, what its liabilities are, and what its equity in the business is.

> As the health/fitness club industry has matured, the tools for measuring financial performance have also become more sophisticated.

- *Assets.* The assets of a business are the cash value of its business holdings—property, equipment, land, etc. In turn, its holdings are defined as either short-term (current) assets or long-term (non-current) assets. A club's short-term assets are those assets or holdings of the business that can be turned into cash (e.g., become liquid) over the next 12-month period of time. Examples of short-term assets include:
  - ✓ Cash in the bank and cash equivalents (short term CDs, etc.)
  - ✓ Short-term physical assets that could be sold over the next year, such as small equipment
  - ✓ Accounts receivables that are due and not collected (i.e., the money members owe the club, but have not paid yet, such as dues and personal training fees)
  - ✓ Prepaid expenses (i.e., expenses the club has paid ahead of time to save money, such as utilities or phone expenses)
  - ✓ Inventory items (e.g., merchandise with a shelf life of less than one year)
  - ✓ Deferred taxes

  In most successful health/fitness club businesses, the club's current assets would typically represent between 15 percent and 30 percent of its total assets. According to the published report, the *IHRSA 2010 Profiles of Success*, in 2009, the average club had current assets equal to 20.9 percent of its total assets, with a range of 6 percent to 29 percent. Just as importantly, the majority of its current assets should be either cash or cash equivalents. If the club's current assets are more heavily weighted toward inventory, it may end up having to write that off

	Current YTD	Prior YTD
Assets		
Current Assets		
Cash	$500,000	$450,000
Cash equivelents	$50,000	$25,000
Accounts receivables	$100,000	$150,000
Inventory	$50,000	$60,000
Pre-paid expenses	$25,000	$20,000
Total Current Assets	$725,000	$705,000
Non-Current Assets		
Equipment	$500,000	$525,000
Building	$3,000,000	$3,000,000
Property	$500,000	$400,000
Less accumulated amortization & depreciation	$300,000	$225,000
Net of property and equipment	$3,700,000	$3,700,000
Investments	$250,000	$200,000
Total Non-Current Assets	$3,950,000	$3,900,000
Total Assets	$4,675,000	$4,605,000
Liabilities		
Current Liabilities		
Account payable	$125,000	$120,000
Accured expenses	$75,000	$100,000
Current maturities on long term debt	$200,000	$190,000
Deferred income taxes	$50,000	$25,000
Total Current Liabilities	$450,000	$435,000
Non-Current Liabilities		
Long Term debt	$1,500,000	$1,800,000
Capital lease obligations	$300,000	$400,000
Other long term liabilities	$100,000	$100,000
Total Non-Current Liabilities	$1,900,000	$2,300,000
Total Liabilities	$2,350,000	$2,735,000
Owner's Equity		
Common stock	$1,985,000	$1,670,000
Preferred stock	$0	$0
Retained earnings	$150,000	$100,000
Paid in capital	$100,000	$100,000
Total Owners Equity	$2,325,000	$1,870,000
Total Liabilities and Owner's Equity	$4,675,000	$4,605,000

Figure 12-1. The balance sheet

the inventory as an expense and potentially have to pay taxes on that inventory. By the same token, if the club has a large accounts receivable, then it is in a position of losing a portion of that to bad-debt expense and having to write that portion off. Not having sufficient short-term assets (less than 10 percent of total assets) can result in a club experiencing cash-flow problems, as well as an inability to cover important expenses during seasonal changes in financial performance.

The club's long-term assets are those holdings and financial instruments of the business that are not expected to be collected over the next 12 months. Examples of long-term assets include:

✓ Property (land and buildings)
✓ Leasehold improvements (e.g., the capital the club has placed into a leased space to make it operational, such as new carpeting, new showers, tenant finishes, etc.)
✓ Equipment (e.g., treadmills, resistance training equipment, etc.)
✓ Security deposits and lease deposits
✓ Loan fees
✓ Depreciation (deducted)

The non-current assets of a financially healthy health/fitness club should range between 70 percent and 85 percent of its total asset value. According to the published report, the *IHRSA 2010 Profiles of Success*, the average club had non-current assets equal to 79.1 percent of its total asset value, with a range of 71 percent to 94 percent. Just as importantly, the club's long-term assets should lean toward property, equipment, and deposits because these assets are more easily sold. If the club has substantial dollars tied up in leasehold improvements, it is less likely to recoup them.

> The non-current assets of a financially healthy health/fitness club should range between 70 percent and 85 percent of its total asset value.

• *Liabilities*. The club's business liabilities are the financial obligations it has—in essence, the money it owes to others as part of operating its business. Liabilities are defined as either short-term (current) liabilities or long-term (non-current) liabilities. In the best of cases, the club would prefer that its total liabilities not exceed more than 70 percent to 75 percent of the value of its total assets, with less being better. According to the published report, the *IHRSA 2010 Profiles of Success*, the average club had average liabilities equal to 67.6 percent of its total assets, an increase of approximately five percentage points when compared to three years earlier. According to the IHRSA data, clubs had total liabilities that ranged from 49 percent to 90 percent of total assets. Given those statistics, it is important to note that financial experts on occasion talk about "leverage," which is a reference to the liabilities that a business has. When those liabilities exceed 80 percent of the business's assets, the business is considered to be highly leveraged.

The current liabilities of the club are those obligations that will be due and payable within the next 12 months. Examples of current liabilities include:

✓ Accounts payable (these are invoices that the club has not paid for, but for which the club has already used the service)

✓ Notes payable (e.g., any loans that come due during the current year)

✓ Income taxes that are due

✓ Deferred revenue (this is revenue from contracts or agreements that have been collected, but not earned. For example, if the club sells one-year membership contracts, it must reflect all revenue not attributed to the current operating period as deferred revenue and therefore a current liability.

✓ Deferred rent (any rent the landlord agrees can be paid at a later date)

✓ Deferred taxes

A rule of thumb with regard to current liabilities is that they should never exceed the value of the club's current assets (current ratio) and, ideally, should be equal to 50 percent of the value of the club's current assets (referred to as a club's current ratio).

> A rule of thumb with regard to current liabilities is that they should never exceed the value of the club's current assets (current ratio) and, ideally, should be equal to 50 percent of the value of the club's current assets.

The long-term liabilities (debt) are those obligations and expenses, while not due during the next 12 months, are due some time thereafter. In the health/fitness club industry, it is recommended that the club's long-term debt not exceed a value of 40 percent to 50 percent (e.g., in 2009, the average club had long-term debt equal to 50.4 percent) of its total assets, an increase of several percentage points from several years earlier. In the publication, the *IHRSA 2010 Profiles of Success*, the average long-term debt for clubs ranged from 49 percent to 90 percent of total assets. It should be noted, on the other hand, that some club companies, which are underwritten by private equity and/or venture capital, look favorably on carrying a high debt load (i.e., a situation that is commonly referred to as being highly leveraged), since it is one way to generate business growth. In fact, a number of private equity firms assume debt levels equivalent to 80 percent to 90 percent of assets in an effort to stimulate business growth. The downside of this approach is the liability of such debt and the strain it can place on a club's operating cash flow. During challenging economic times, such as the recession of 2008 and 2009, many of the operators who were highly leveraged experienced loan defaults and bankruptcies because of their inability to cover their debt payments. Examples of long-term debt include:

✓ Future interest and principal payments on loans from financial institutions

✓ Deferred revenue from long-term contracts (an example might be a five-year corporate membership contract)

✓ Deferred rent (oftentimes, a landlord will agree to provide a tenant with a window of no rent with the stipulation that the rent must be paid at a later date when the club is more profitable)

✓ Deferred taxes

- *Owner's equity*. Owner's equity represents the owner's actual investment in the club, which can include any initial dollars invested, as well as any dollars earned over the life of the business. Owner's equity can vary, depending on whether the club was established as a corporation, a limited liability corporation, a partnership, or a sole proprietorship. Owner's equity is determined by subtracting the total liabilities of the business from the total assets of the business. In the case of a financially sound club, the owner's equity will usually be in the neighborhood of 20 percent to 40 percent of the total asset value. In the case of more mature clubs, however, it may be closer to 50 percent of the total assets. In 2009, according to IHRSA data, the average club reported owner's equity of 32.5 percent, down from nearly 38 percent in 2006. Situations also exist, especially in highly leveraged clubs (i.e., clubs carrying a high level of long-term debt), where the owner's equity might be as low as 10 percent. Examples of owner's equity are as follows:

  ✓ *Corporations*. In corporations, the owner's equity can exist in a number of forms, including capital stock (common or preferred), paid in capital (actual cash put into the business), and retained earnings not distributed to the stockholders (money the business makes and then puts back into the business).

  ✓ *Partnerships, limited liability corporations (LLC), and sole proprietorships*. In these business structures, the owner's equity can exist as contributions in cash or kind (sole proprietor or partnership) and cash generated by the withdrawal of assets (partnerships). Investors and lending institutions will look at a club's balance sheet as one way of evaluating its current financial health and its ability to be profitable over the long run.

- *Balance sheet indicators*. A few critical financial ratios or key indicators, based on the information furnished on a club's balance sheet, can be used to provide a quick glimpse of a club's overall financial health. The most frequently used balance sheet-based indicators are current ratio, acid-test ratio, debt-equity ratio, interest-coverage ratio, return on equity, return on invested capital, and return on fixed assets.

  ✓ *Current ratio*. The current ratio is an indicator of a club's financial liquidity (cash in hand) within the next 12-month period. The current ratio is determined by dividing the value of the club's current assets by the value of its current liabilities. For example, if a club had a total of $1,000,000 in current assets and $500,000 in current liabilities, then its current ratio would be two. A current ratio above two is considered excellent; a ratio between one and two is deemed to be good; a ratio between .6 and one is regarded as fair; and a ratio that is less than .6 is considered poor. In 2009, the median current ratio for a club was 1.2. It should be noted that if a club generates a significant portion of its revenue from the sale of annual memberships, then the current ratio may fall below one, because deferred revenue represents a current liability. For example, in my former company in Russia, nearly all memberships were annual memberships. As a result, the company

In the case of a financially sound club, the owner's equity will usually be in the neighborhood of 20 percent to 40 percent of the total asset value. In the case of more mature clubs, however, it may be closer to 50 percent of the total assets.

had a significant amount of deferred revenue reflected on its balance sheet, which resulted in its current ratio being around .5 to .6. If not for the deferred revenue, the current ratio would have been closer to 1.5.

✓ *Acid-test ratio*. The acid-test ratio is a measure of a club's "quick" liquidity or its ability to generate cash immediately. The acid-test ratio is determined by taking the club's current assets and subtracting out that portion attributable to inventory and prepaid expenses, and then dividing by its current liabilities. A financially sound club operation should have an acid-test ratio of one or higher. For example, if the club has $1,000,000 in current assets, of which $300,000 is in inventory and $200,000 is in prepaid expenses, and has $500,000 in current liabilities, then its acid-test ratio would be one.

✓ *Debt-to-equity ratio*. The debt-to-equity ratio is a good measure of a club's leverage (in other words, the value of the owner's equity in comparison to the total liabilities that the club carries). The debt-to-equity ratio is measured by taking the total liabilities of the business and dividing them by the total owner's equity. For example, if a club has $4,000,000 in total liabilities and the owner's equity was $1,000,000, then the debt-to-equity ratio would be four. In 2009 the average debt-to-equity ratio in the club industry was approximately 1.8, although it ranges from .8 to 6.8. The higher the ratio, the greater the debt is in comparison to the owner's equity, and the more likely the club is highly leveraged. A review of the last several years worth of industry data shows that 2009's leverage-oriented ratios (debt-to-equity, interest-coverage, etc.) were higher than in previous years, indicating that in 2009, clubs were more likely to experience debt-related problems.

✓ *Interest-coverage ratio*. The interest-coverage ratio is frequently used by investors as a measure of the balance between a company's ability to grow and pay down its existing debt. It represents the amount of available cash to cover interest payments on existing debt. For example, a club that generates $500,000 in cash annually and has interest payments of $250,000 would have an interest coverage ratio of 2. Ideally, clubs need to have an interest-coverage ratio of at least 2, if they want to be assured of being able to cover their interest payments, and have capital available for growth, as well as for emergencies. According to the publication, the *IHRSA 2010 Profiles of Success*, the average club in 2009 had an interest-coverage ratio of 3.1, with a range of 1.5 to 6.4. All factors considered, if a club has an interest-coverage ratio that is too low (i.e., below 1.5), it is likely to have potential problems with cash flow, while if its ratio is relatively high (i.e., over 4), it may not have sufficient debt to successfully grow its business.

✓ *Return on equity*. Return on equity is a measure that is used by investors to assess the value of their investment. Return on equity is determined by taking the net income (earnings before taxes) and dividing it by the cash or equity invested. In an investor's mind, this ratio tells them how well their investment is working for them in generating cash flow. On average, most venture-capital groups look for returns in excess of 40 percent, while other investors are likely

> The average debt-to-equity ratio in the club industry was approximately 1.8, although it ranges from .8 to 6.8.

to be satisfied with returns of 20 percent to 30 percent. According to the publication, the *IHRSA 2010 Profiles of Success*, the average return on equity in 2009 for the industry was 20.1 percent, down nearly 10 percentage points from earlier in the decade. For owners who reinvest in their own club, such as when undertaking an expansion of an existing facility, they may be satisfied with a return of 15 percent to 20 percent. For example, if a club owner were to invest $250,000 for a fitness-center expansion and, as a result, generated an additional $50,000 in cash flow as a by-product of having more members and spending more money, their return on equity would be $50,000/$250,000 or 20 percent. Another way of looking at return on equity is what is called return-on-invested capital. This measure represents the return an investor generates on the capital that individual invests in a project. If an investor puts in $100,000 for a club expansion and over the next five years, generates, on an annual basis, an additional $25,000 in cash, then that person's annual return-on-invested capital (AROIC) is 25 percent.

✓ *Return on fixed assets.* Return on fixed assets is another measure used to assess the value of an investment. Return on fixed assets represents the profitability of a business measured against the amount the business holds in its fixed (non-current) assets. To some investors, this measure is considered a more valuable indicator of how well their money is working for them than is the return-on-equity ratio. For example, if a club had $2,000,000 in fixed assets and, as a result, produced an additional $200,000 in cash flow for the club, then the return on fixed assets would be $200,000/$2,000,000 or 10 percent. While many club investors look for returns on fixed assets of 20 percent to 25 percent, ranges of 10 percent to 15 percent are considered acceptable. In 2009, the average return on fixed assets for the industry was 9.4 percent, down one full percentage point from three years earlier. The basic reason investors and owners see this measure as a more realistic assessment of their return is because they have their money tied up in the assets of the business. In turn, the cash they generate is a result of how well that equity is doing for them.

As can be seen, understanding the nuances of a club's balance sheet is essential to understanding the value and financial health of that business.

❏ *The Profit-and-Loss Statement or Statement of Income* (see Figure 12-2). The profit-and-loss statement is a financial tool that is used to reflect a club's operating performance over a given period of time. The standard practice in the health/fitness club industry is to produce both monthly and year-end profit-and-loss statements. Several club chains divide the year into 13 operating periods of four weeks each and compile a profit-and-loss statement for each of the four-week periods, as well as an annual statement. Finally, a few clubs actually provide a weekly profit-and-loss statement that reflects their operating performance on a weekly basis. Some businesses refer to the profit-and-loss statement as a statement of income or a statement of operations.

The standard practice in the health/fitness club industry is to produce both monthly and year-end profit-and-loss statements.

Category	YTD Actual	YTD Plan	YTD Variance
Revenues			
Membership department	$2,450,000	$2,300,000	6.5%
Fitness department	$600,000	$550,000	9.1%
Food & beverage department	$125,000	$100,000	25.0%
Spa department	$265,000	$250,000	6.0%
Tennis department	$300,000	$300,000	0.0%
Total Revenues	$3,740,000	$3,500,000	6.9%
Department Expenses			
Membership department	$300,000	$320,000	-6.3%
Fitness department	$600,000	$615,000	-2.4%
Food & beverage department	$90,000	$75,000	20.0%
Spa department	$175,000	$200,000	-12.5%
Tennis department	$250,000	$250,000	0.0%
Total Department Expenses	$1,415,000	$1,460,000	-3.1%
Undistributed & Fixed Expenses			
G&A department	$250,000	$247,000	1.2%
Housekeeping department	$225,000	$217,000	3.7%
Marketing and sales	$100,000	$95,000	5.3%
Property taxes	$120,000	$120,000	0.0%
Utilities	$230,000	$225,000	2.2%
Rent	$200,000	$200,000	0.0%
Total Undistributed Expenses	$1,125,000	$1,104,000	1.9%
Total Operating Expenses	$2,540,000	$2,564,000	-0.9%
EBITDA	$1,200,000	$936,000	28.2%
EBITDA Margin	32.1%	26.7%	20.0%
Depreciation	$130,000	$130,000	0.0%
Interest	$350,000	$350,000	0.0%
Net Income	$720,000	$456,000	57.9%
Principal	$75,000	$75,000	0.0%
Capital replacement	$100,000	$100,000	0.0%
Net Cash Flow before Taxes	$675,000	$411,000	64.2%

Figure 12-2. The profit-and-loss statement or statement of income.

The profit-and-loss statement is designed to show the club operator how well the club is performing financially over the designated time period by providing information on actual performance, planned performance, and the variance-to-plan performance. With each profit-and-loss statement, the club operator can get an accurate update on how the club is performing, both actually and against budget, for the given period, as well as year-to-date. This type of information allows the operator to make decisions regarding such factors as membership sales, revenue strategies, and expense control in a timely and effective manner. It is important to remember that the profit-and-loss statement is typically based on an accrual system. In other words, it measures financial performance based not only on both the cash generated and spent, but also on allocations for cash yet to be received or yet to be spent during a given period of time.

As such, the profit-and-loss statement provides a reflection of both planned performance and actual performance. One of the most useful tools in the health/fitness club industry, for understanding the profit-and-loss statement is the book—Uniform System of Accounts for the Health, Racquet, and Sportsclub Industry—which was developed under the leadership of IHRSA. This document establishes specific categories within the profit-and-loss statement for budgeting and monitoring financial performance in the industry. The key profit-and-loss categories (revenues, department expenses, undistributed expenses, fixed expenses, EBITDA, and EBIT) that the industry employs to monitor and evaluate a club's financial performance include the following:

- *Revenue categories*. The revenue portion of the profit-and-loss statement is intended to provide the club operator with a means of budgeting and tracking the revenue-producing aspects of the business. The primary revenue areas or revenue departments on a profit-and-loss statement include:

  ✓ *Membership*. The membership revenues are those revenues that are generated through the membership dues paid by members on a monthly basis and the initiation fees that members pay upon joining a club. A club must record all revenues from these two areas on the profit-and-loss statement under the category assigned to the membership revenue department. In the instances where a club uses membership contracts, the club can only reflect on its profit-and-loss statement the amount of revenue from the contract that has been earned during the period of time reflected on the profit-and-loss statement. For instance, if a club receives $1,200 from a member upon joining for one-year's dues, then on the monthly profit-and-loss statement, only $100 of those dues can be reflected on the statement. In the health/fitness club industry, according to the publication, the *IHRSA 2010 Profiles of Success*, approximately 63 percent to 80 percent of all club revenues come from the membership department. As such, a number of companies in the health/fitness club industry are trying to reduce their dependence on membership revenue by promoting other revenue sources. In that regard, some clubs, particularly large multi-purpose clubs, report

According to
*IHRSA 2010
Profiles of Success,*
approximately
63 percent to 80
percent of all club
revenues come from
the membership
department.

that they generate closer to 50 percent of their overall revenue from their membership department. An interesting divergence from this trend of decreasing dependency on membership revenues is seen in those clubs that have positioned themselves in the high-volume, low-priced segment of the industry (e.g., Planet Fitness, U.S.; Gym Group, England; and Mcfit, Germany), in which dues can actually represent in excess of 90 percent of the revenue of the business.

According to industry data, the average fitness department contributes in the neighborhood of 10 percent of a club's total revenues.

✓ *Fitness.* The fitness department generates the second largest amount of revenue in the club industry. Revenues earned from personal training, group-exercise classes, Pilates classes, and locker rental are examples of income that could all be attributed to this particular department. According to industry data, the average fitness department contributes in the neighborhood of 10 percent of a club's total revenues. At the Russian Fitness Group based in Moscow, its clubs, on average, generated 16 percent of all revenues from fitness. In reality, in a number of clubs (e.g., Equinox), the fitness department generates upwards of 20 percent of the total revenues. In fact, some clubs claim to generate as much as eight million dollars annually in personal-training revenue.

✓ *Spa.* The spa department contributes revenues by providing such services as massages, facials, pedicures, manicures, and related activities that are delivered in a spa environment. In the last few years, the spa department has developed into a significant revenue source for many health/fitness clubs. In fact, spas can generate as much as $10,000 per treatment room per month. According to the publication, the *IHRSA 2010 Profiles of Success*, the average club generated 8.9 percent (with a range of 2.7 percent to 14.6 percent) of its revenues from its spa. At the Russian Fitness Group based in Moscow, the average club generated 10.5 percent of all revenues from its spa.

✓ *Tennis.* The tennis department generates revenues through court fees, instructional lessons, and programming. In multipurpose clubs, tennis might be the second largest contributor of revenues. Industry data shows a tennis department can easily generate between $25,000 and $50,000 in revenue per outdoor court and $50,000 to $100,000 per indoor court on an annual basis.

✓ *Pro shop.* Financially, the pro shop is the source of the net revenues that are generated by merchandise sales. In most clubs, this contribution is relatively small when compared to total club revenues. According to the published report, the *IHRSA 2010 Profiles of Success*, the average club generated 2.3 percent of all revenue from retail sales (with a range of 1.1 percent to 5 percent). In some clubs, the pro shop may generate as much as $500,000 to one million annually, though, on average, most generate less than $100,000 in annual revenues.

✓ *Food and beverage.* The food-and-beverage department generates revenues through the sale of food and beverages and by conducting special functions, such as parties. In most health/fitness clubs, the food-and-beverage operation is not a comparatively large contributor to the club's revenues because their operations usually don't consist of much more than a snack bar or smoothie bar. According to IHRSA data from 2009, the average club generated 5.3 percent of its revenues from food and beverage (with a range of 2.5 percent to 10 percent). Some clubs, such as the East Bank Club in Chicago, generate millions of dollars in food-and-beverage revenue through multiple outlets, including private parties. On the other hand, most food-and-beverage departments are fortunate if they achieve a 10 percent margin.

✓ *Youth services*. The youth department is a relatively recent undertaking for most of the clubs in the industry, but one that shows promise as a meaningful source of revenue. The youth department generates revenues by holding parties, providing youth programming, and offering childcare services. In 2009, according to IHRSA statistics, youth programs generated between 1.6 percent and 8.7 percent of club revenues.

✓ *Other revenue*. A number of clubs generate revenue from services that do not fall into the standard accounting categories on the profit-and-loss statement. In these instances, these revenues are often reflected under the category of "other revenues." The most significant sources of other revenue in the health/fitness club industry are revenues from space rental, physical therapy, and other medically related services. Some club chains, such as Western Athletic Clubs, lease space to physical therapy businesses. The revenues from these leases are normally reflected as other revenue on the club's profit-and-loss statement.

• *Departmental expenses*. Departmental expenses are that part of the profit-and-loss statement where the expenses incurred by each of the operating revenue departments in the delivery of their respective services and the generation of their respective revenues are listed. According to the publication, the *IHRSA 2010 Profiles of Success*, a club's departmental expenses typically run approximately 25 percent of revenues and may range from 17 percent to 32 percent of revenues. In other words, the departments of membership, fitness, spa, tennis, pro shop, food and beverage, and youth all have expenses that are directly associated with the services they provide and the revenues they generate. On the profit-and-loss statement, the expenses generated by each department are placed in an account that best reflects its activity or function. Examples of the accounts that are reflected in each department include:

✓ *Payroll*. This category of expenses represents the cost of employee wages and commissions. Payroll includes such items as salaries, hourly wages, commissions for employees, incentive pay for employees, etc. For example, the commission that the club pays a personal trainer would be considered wages, just as would the wages paid to a group-exercise instructor by the club, or the commission given to one of the club's sales representatives. Payroll (benefits and payroll taxes included) alone can represent approximately 40 percent

Most food-and-beverage departments are fortunate if they achieve a 10 percent margin.

to 50 percent of a club's total operating expenses and as much as 75 percent to 80 percent of any given department's operating expense.

✓ *Benefits.* This expense category represents the cost of providing basic benefits to the club's employees. These costs will vary, depending upon the benefits a club offers to its employees. The standard benefit package normally includes health benefits (hospitalization, dental, vision) and federally and state mandated payments, such as FICA, FUTA and SUTA (the payments made for Social Security, Medicare, etc.). Additional employee benefits that many clubs offer include such items as club contributions to a company-sponsored savings plan (401 K), life insurance, long-term disability insurance, etc. Normally, the cost of employee benefits can range from as little as 15 percent of a club's total payroll expense to as high as 30 percent of its total payroll expense.

> The cost of employee benefits can range from as little as 15 percent of a club's total payroll expense to as high as 30 percent of its total payroll expense.

✓ *Education and training.* This expense category involves the expenses associated with the ongoing education of the club's employees. This category can include the cost of sending employees to conventions and conferences, funding continuing education credits, providing in-house training, and providing scholarships for pursuing coursework at local colleges. As a whole, the industry does not apply any standard allocation to this area. It would be in the club's best interest, however, for club operators to consider allocating funds equal to one to three percent of payroll for this expense category.

✓ *Total payroll.* Total payroll represents the combined cost of wages, salaries, benefits, education, and taxes (payroll plus benefits). According to the report, the *IHRSA 2010 Profiles of Success,* the average club spent 43 percent of all of its revenues on total payroll, with a range of 37 percent to 48 percent. Clubs that have a brand that depends on delivering a highly personalized, customer service-oriented experience will tend to have a higher total payroll cost (with a range of 40 percent to 50 percent) ,while some of the high-volume, low-price operators that provide minimal staffing tend to have a total payroll that does not exceed 15 to 20 percent of its total revenue.

✓ *Supplies.* This category of expenses varies from club to club. As a whole, this category includes expenses associated with cleaning supplies, general maintenance supplies, paper supplies, locker room amenities, etc. The industry average for this category is approximately two percent of the total revenues generated by a club.

✓ *Advertising/promotions/marketing.* This expense category represents the costs associated with marketing, promoting, and selling a department's products and services. For a particular department, such as fitness, this expense would include such items as the cost of flyers, posters, pamphlets, post cards, and other marketing pieces used to promote the department's services. Expenses emanating from efforts to promote activities in the membership department would involve internal departmental promotions, rather than external club promotions. Normally, the cost of external marketing is allocated to an undistributed expense category for marketing.

✓ *Printing*. This expense category is used to allocate expenses associated with printing efforts by the club, including club brochures, letterhead, envelopes, newsletters, and other hard-copy documents.

✓ *Dues and subscriptions*. This expense category is used by clubs to expense items, such as club subscriptions for newspapers, magazine subscriptions for the club, subscriptions to special-interest publications, etc. The largest part of this expense category would arise from the costs involved with providing professional membership dues for employees (e.g., ACSM, NSCA, etc.), association dues for the club (e.g., IHRSA, ISPA, IDEA, etc.), and dues for local and community associations and groups (e.g., Chamber of Commerce, Rotary, etc.).

✓ *Contract labor*. This expense category is used to allocate the costs associated with retaining the services of outside professionals. For example, contract labor could include such items as attorney fees, accounting firm fees, outside speaker fees, special instructors, etc. In fact, many club operators pay their personal trainers and group-exercise instructors out of a contract-labor account, based on their mistaken belief that these providers are not employees, but rather independent contractors. As a result, they attempt to save on the cost of providing benefits to these individuals. Unfortunately, most club operators are misinformed about what constitutes an independent contractor. As such, they are running a risk in expensing these costs to this particular account. (Note: The issue of independent contractors is addressed in Chapter 15 of this book.)

Many club operators pay their personal trainers and group-exercise instructors out of a contract-labor account, based on their mistaken belief that these providers are not employees, but rather independent contractors.

✓ *Maintenance and repair*. This category of expenses is associated with the general costs of maintaining the club's facilities and providing minor repairs to the facility. For example, if the club hires an exterminator to service the club, this expense would fall under this category. Another example of an expense assigned to this category would be if the club had to purchase some parts to repair a treadmill.

✓ *Cost of goods sold*. This category of expenses only applies to departments that sell retail items. The cost of goods sold represents the cost of an inventory item that is removed as it is sold from the inventory. For example, if the club purchases 500 shirts for $10 each, it would have a total of $5,000 in inventory. Later, if it sold all 500 shirts for $10,000, then its inventory cost for the shirts would be $5,000 (50 percent of the total revenue received from the sales). In most clubs, the cost of sales usually runs between 60 percent and 80 percent for their retail operations (e.g., the pro shop), though the inventory cost at many clubs runs much higher. As a rule, the cost of sales can be relatively high when a club holds too much inventory of an item and is later forced to write it off or it experiences shrinkage of inventory.

While the aforementioned expense categories are the primary departmental expense categories that exist on the profit-and-loss statement of most health/fitness clubs, they are not the only ones that occur. Clubs that want to monitor their costs in detail should create even more definitive expense categories. Establishing such categories can help them maintain an even firmer grasp on their expenses.

- *Undistributed expenses*. Undistributed expenses are associated with the overall operations of the club, rather than for running any specific department. In most club operations, these are expenses that emanate from the successful operation of the club that have no direct association with a specific department. In these situations, clubs allocate such expenses to the undistributed-expenses category. According to the most recent data published by IHRSA in its *2010 Profiles of Success*, the industry average for undistributed expenses was 25 percent of revenues, with a range of 17 percent to 32 percent. The most significant categories for undistributed expenses typically include the following:

  ✓ *Sales and marketing*. The cost of sales and marketing is an expense that is generated by efforts to market the club, such as advertisements in the media, websites, direct-mail pieces, and related sales materials. On average, most health/fitness clubs spend approximately two to five percent of their revenues on sales and marketing (e.g., averaging 2.8 percent in 2009). In fact, major multiple-club operators, such as Bally, 24 Hour Fitness, LA Fitness, and Town Sports International, frequently devote considerably more of their resources to this undertaking, often reaching as high as 10 percent of their revenues.

  ✓ *Utilities*. Utility expenses include the costs of such items as electric, gas, water, and telephones. Most clubs lump these items as an undistributed expense, while some club operators might distribute them as departmental expenses. The industry average for clubs is to spend between four and seven percent of operating revenues on utilities (e.g., averaging 5.7 percent in 2009). For clubs in the Northeast and West, especially California, utility expenses can often run as high as 10 percent of their revenues.

  ✓ *Member services*. The cost of member services is an undistributed expense that is associated with the delivery of special member services and member relations. Expenses that fall into this category might include the cost involved in conducting focus groups, surveys, member-reward programs, and member-appreciation functions.

  ✓ *G and A (general administration and accounting)*. G and A is an undistributed expense that entails the costs involved in running the accounting department and in providing general management (e.g., manager, assistant manager, office assistant, etc.). It should be noted that in many clubs, the management and accounting areas are actually set up as departments, with their own expenses, and are treated as a separate department. Besides payroll, costs, such as postage, credit-card charges, bad-debt expense, and EFT (electronic funds transfer) charges are normally debited to this accounting category.

  ✓ *Capital replacement and repair*. This undistributed expense involves the costs associated with funding the ongoing upkeep and repair of the club's facilities. In most instances, capital costs involve items that either cost more than $500 or have a depreciation period of at least three years. Examples of capital replacement costs include such expenses as the funds allocated for buying new exercise equipment, buying computers for the staff, replacing carpet, expanding an area within the club, or replacing or repairing a piece of equipment (e.g.,

> On average, most health/fitness clubs spend approximately two to five percent of their revenues on sales and marketing.

an air conditioner). On average, in the club industry, a facility spends approximately three to five percent of its total revenues on capital replacement and repair. As a rule, some clubs may find that they need to allocate up to 15 percent of their revenues every five to seven years to handle their larger capital needs. In reality, many successful club operators handle this situation by accruing expenses over a few years to make sure that the funds are available for these larger capital requirements.

• *Fixed expenses*. Fixed expenses are considered those expenses that are not directly impacted by a club's operation, but rather the expenses that are recurring and relatively consistent year in and year out. According to the publication, the *IHRSA 2010 Profiles of Success*, fixed expenses in the industry typically range from five percent to 20 percent of revenues, with an average of approximately 14 percent. The standard fixed-expense categories for the profit-and-loss statement include:

  ✓ *Insurance*. This particular category includes the costs associated with providing property, general liability, key-man, and professional liability insurance. In the health/fitness club industry, these costs average between one percent and three percent of the club's total operating revenues In 2009, the average club expended 1.5 percent of its revenues toward insurance payments. In fact, a few club operators feel insurance is not a fixed expense, but rather an expense that can be controlled through risk-management practices. As a consequence, in their operations, insurance is categorized as an undistributed expense.

  ✓ *Rent*. Rent is probably the largest single expense for most clubs, other than payroll. The industry average for rent in 2009 was 9.3 percent, ranging between .3 percent and 16 percent of the club's total operating revenues. In some markets, such as Los Angeles, London, New York, Moscow, etc., the high cost of real estate can drive rent costs as high as 25 percent to 35 percent of revenues. In order for a club to be profitable, it should make every effort to keep its rent payments below 15 percent of its total revenue. In most instances, rent is derived from the lease a club operator enters into, many of which run at least five years and more often for 10 years. A number of landlords also include what are called CAM costs into the rent. CAM costs are the landlord's costs for common area maintenance. In fact, class A office spaces (i.e., office space located in highly desirable locations and newer buildings) in many large, urban markets can have CAM costs that run as high as $10 to $15 a square foot. As such, it is essential that club operators get clarification of the CAM costs for a particular space and not make an operating or lease decision purely on the quoted rent cost.

  ✓ *Real estate/property taxes*. Real estate/property taxes contribute the fee that the club pays local government for occupying its property. If the club owns its land and building, then its property taxes are based on the assessed value of the property and building. On the other hand, if the club leases its space, its property tax will be based on an assessment of the leasehold improvements on the facility.

The industry average for rent in 2009 was 9.3 percent, ranging between .3 percent and 16 percent of the club's total operating revenues.

✓ *Management fees.* Management fees are expenses that usually only occur in clubs that are part of a multiple-club operation. In a multiple-club operation, the ownership group or the management parent normally charges a management fee for the expertise, services, and guidance that it provides to each particular club. In addition, in some independent clubs, ownership creates a separate management company for the business that then charges a fee to the club for the services of the owner. The majority of multiple-club operators charge a base management fee, which typically ranges from three to six percent of a club's total operating revenue.

✓ *Depreciation.* Depreciation is the actual cost that a business incurs as a result of the loss in value of its fixed assets. Most clubs utilize a standard depreciation table to determine the depreciation schedule for its fixed assets. For example, property and buildings are depreciated over 20 years and equipment over 5 to 10 years. According to IHRSA's data from 2009, the average club annually expended 6.8 percent of its revenues toward depreciation and amortization.

✓ *Principal and interest.* Principal and interest represent the costs associated with paying down debt and include the interest on the loan balance, as well as the amortized amount of principal. The interest portion of this expense line averaged 3.7 percent of revenue in 2009 according to the published report, the *IHRSA 2010 Profiles of Success.*

• *EBITDA (earnings before interest, taxes, depreciation, and amortization).* EBITDA is determined by taking the total revenues of the club and deducting the departmental expenses, undistributed expenses, and fixed expenses. The only expenses not counted in this expense category are the costs of depreciation, capital replacement, and capital repair. An indicator of a club's profitability and earnings, this number is used by investors and owners as a benchmark for valuing a company and benchmarking its operating efficiency. For example, if a club that generates four million dollars in revenue has two million in department expenses, $500,000 in undistributed expenses, and $500,000 in fixed expenses, its EBITDA would be $1,000,000 or 25 percent of revenues.

As a rule, the club industry utilizes broad EBITDA benchmarks to indicate the operating effectiveness of a club (refer to Figure 12-3). In 2009, according to IHRSA's research, the average club had an EBITDA margin that was equal to 17.8 percent, with a range of 13 percent to 23 percent. Lifetime Fitness, a publically held company, has consistently reported EBITDA margins in its public documents in excess of 25 percent, and during its first few years of being listed, it reported EBITDA margins approaching 28 percent to 30 percent. Equinox, which is privately held, has reported that its EBITDA margins are in the range of 23 percent to 25 percent. At McFit in Germany, reports have circulated of EBITDA margins approaching 35 percent. Under most circumstances, a club that is leasing space will find it a challenge to ever exceed an EBITDA margin of 25 percent, due to the impact that its rent has on its overhead.

As a rule, the club industry utilizes broad EBITDA benchmarks to indicate the operating effectiveness of a club.

Efficiency	EBITDA Range
Fair	10% to 15%
Good	15% to 22%
Excellent	22% to 30%
Extraordinary	30% or above

Figure 12-3. EBITDA benchmarks in the health/fitness industry

- *EBIT*. EBIT stands for earnings before interest and taxes and represents the net cash flow before interest and taxes that the club owner is able to earn. EBIT is derived by taking the calculated EBITDA and then deducting the expenses associated with capital replacement, depreciation, interest on loans, and amortization of a loan (the principal that is paid). On average, a club operator can expect this factor to range between 2 and 10 percent of the total revenues, with a range of six to eight percent the most likely scenario. In 2009 the average reported EBIT in the health/fitness club industry was 7.4 percent.

❑ *The Departmental Income Statement.* The departmental income statement is a detailed profit-and-loss document for a specific department. While the profit-and-loss statement provides a look at the financial performance of a club for a specified period of time, a departmental income statement provides each operating department within a club a comprehensive summary of the revenues, expenses, and net cost of operating that particular department. For the club operator, the departmental income statement can be a useful tool for helping evaluate the performance of a specific department and holding the respective department head (supervisor) accountable for the financial performance of that department. Many of the top club operators in the industry expect their department heads and supervisors not only to develop a departmental income budget, but also to then use the departmental income statement as a tool for monitoring the success of their department.

The IHRSA book, *Uniform System of Accounts for the Health, Racquet and Sportsclub Industry*, provides a detailed description of the various departmental income statements that are employed in the industry. A list of the most common departments within the health/fitness club industry includes membership, aquatics, fitness, spa, pro shop, racquet sports, food and beverage, and children's programs. For each of these departments, a complete accounting of the revenues, expenses, and net cost of the department can be determined and then compiled in a departmental income statement. Figure 12-4 provides a sample departmental income statement for a fitness department. Having such detailed accounting for each department can help a club operator hold each department head accountable for the financial success of that individual's respective department.

Departmental Income Statement
Fitness Department

Category	Actual - to - Date	Plan - to - Date	Variance
Revenues			
Personal Training	$750,000	$710,000	$40,000
Classes	$50,000	$20,000	$30,000
Activity Programs	$100,000	$75,000	$25,000
Locker Rental	$100,000	$100,000	$0
Other	$10,000	$12,000	($2,000)
Total Revenues	**$1,010,000**	**$917,000**	**$93,000**
Expenses			
Wages	$250,000	$248,000	$2,000
Commissions	$375,000	$360,000	$15,000
Bonuses	$60,000	$56,000	$4,000
Total Wages	**$685,000**	**$664,000**	**$21,000**
Payroll Costs	$76,000	$71,000	$5,000
Hospitalization	$20,000	$16,000	$4,000
Workers Compensation	$20,000	$17,000	$3,000
Related Benefits	$10,000	$10,000	$0
Total Payroll and Benefits	**$811,000**	**$778,000**	**$33,000**
Advertising and Promotions	$50,000	$58,000	($8,000)
Printing	$15,000	$17,000	($2,000)
Postage	$7,000	$6,000	$1,000
Dues & Subscriptions	$5,000	$5,100	($100)
Supplies	$76,000	$75,000	$1,000
Maintenance	$23,000	$20,000	$3,000
Education	$5,000	$4,000	$1,000
Total Other Expenses	**$181,000**	**$185,100**	**($4,100)**
Total Department Expenses	**$992,000**	**$963,100**	**$28,900**
Department Net Contribution	**$18,000**	**($46,100)**	**$64,100**

Figure 12-4. Sample departmental income statement for the fitness department

Benchmarks for Financial Performance in the Health/Fitness Club Industry

A summary of the key industry benchmarks for financial performance is provided in Figure 12-5. The data reflected in Figure 12-5 is based on material from the published report, the *IHRSA 2010 Profiles of Success*, which summarizes the results of a comprehensive survey of the health/fitness club industry. (Note: Individuals who would like to obtain a more detailed compilation of the basic financial indicators for the health/fitness club industry should contact IHRSA.)

Benchmark Category	All Clubs (IHRSA)		Multipurpose Clubs (IHRSA)	
	2008	*2009*	*2008*	*2009*
Revenue	$2,107,600	$2,193,l00	$2,589,000	$2,465,300
Revenue per Member	$732	$763	$759	$845
Non-dues Revenue as a % of Total Revenue	26%	26%	25%	23%
Payroll as a % of Revenue	44%	45%	44%	45%
EBITDA as a % of Revenue	17%	14%	17.5%	14%

Figure 12-5. Key financial performance benchmarks for the health/fitness club industry

13

Budgeting, Forecasting, and Driving Profitability in the Health/Fitness Club Industry

Chapter Objectives

The previous chapter reviewed how the industry keeps score of its financial performance, but not how it establishes its financial targets or drives the achievement of those financial targets. This chapter initially offers an overview of the budgeting and forecasting process, and then concludes with an examination of the most effective industry practices for driving profitability and achieving budget targets.

Budgeting in the Health/Fitness Club Industry

The practice and process of budgeting exists in every business. Creating a budget is the first step in driving a successful financial plan and achieving profitability. Budgeting is simply the process of creating financial targets for the business, based on an understanding of the underlying forces that shape the operations of the business. In the club industry, budgets are done on an annual basis, usually beginning three to four months prior to the start of the next fiscal year. A club budget is a best estimate of its future financial performance, based on a thorough knowledge of the current year's financial performance and the market and the operational forces that will impact its financial performance going forward. At all times, a budget is a living, breathing document that serves as a roadmap for a club's financial targets.

> Creating a budget is the first step in driving a successful financial plan and achieving profitability.

Most clubs initially create a five-year budget prior to opening for business and then once they're open and operating, develop an annual operating budget. Two primary approaches to budgeting exist in the industry: zero-based budgeting and trend-line budgeting.

❑ *Zero-Based Budgeting.* Zero-based budgeting involves the process of building a budget from scratch, using such factors as information on pricing, market forces, expected usage levels, expected staffing levels, etc. When a club develops a zero-based budget, it uses its knowledge of the market and market conditions to build a template of what it expects to occur and what these circumstances will mean from a financial perspective. Zero-based budgeting is used most often when developing a new club or making a significant change in the operation of an existing club. When a club uses the zero-based approach to budgeting, it must take into consideration a host of assumptions, examples of which are shown in Figure 13-1.

Revenues	Expenses
1. What will be the expected number of members or memberships at the beginning of the year and the end of the year?	1. What will be the club's total hours of operation?
2. What will be the net gain in membership each accounting period?	2. What will be the total number of FTE (full-time equivalents) that will be required for each area of club operations (fitness, spa, front desk, classes, etc.)?
3. What will be the average monthly and annual dues for each membership?	3. What will be the average hourly rate for each FTE by area?
4. What will be the average enrollment fee collected with each membership?	4. What percentage of revenues, based on industry averages, will be allocated to payroll?
5. What percentage of memberships will participate in personal training services?	5. What will be the cost of benefits as a percentage of total wages?
6. What will be the average fee collected for personal training services?	6. What will utilities be, based on square footage and an average cost per square foot?
7. What percentage of membership will participate in services such as massage, athletic leagues, court reservations, group classes, special events, etc.?	7. What are the expected unit costs for various expenses, such as supplies, uniforms, printing, etc., as a percentage of revenue?
8. What will be the average price for each service at the club (e.g., massage, classes, leagues, court fees, event fees, etc.)?	8. What are the expected unit costs for insurance, property tax, capital repairs, etc., per square foot for the club?
9. How many guests will use the club and what will be the average guest fee?	9. What is the total club square footage?
10. What percentage of the revenues does the club want to derive from dues, personal training, etc.?	10. How many members will the club have?
11. What revenues does the club expect per member or per square foot of the facility?	11. What is the club's target for EBITDA and EBIT as a percentage of revenue?

Figure 13-1. Examples of basic assumptions and questions used in the zero-based budget proces

The questions included in Figure 13-1 are the types of queries that club operators must ask and be able to answer if they want to pursue a zero-based budget process. Figure 13-2 presents an example of a zero-based budget for a fitness department.

Assumption	Volume	Unit Cost	Weekly Budget #	Annual Budget #
Level of membership	2,000	NA		
% of members taking personal training each week	5% (100)	$50	$5,000	$260,000
Average fee for personal training	$50	NA		
% of members taking paid exercise classes each week	5% (100)	$10	$1,000	$52,000
Average fee for classes	$10	NA		
% of members taking other fee-based services each week	10% (200)	$5	$1,000	$52,000
Average fee collected for other services	$5	NA		
Total Revenue			**$7,000**	**$364,000**
# FTE for department	10 (400 hours)	$10	$4,000	$208,000
Average hourly rate for FTE	$10	NA	NA	
% of commission on personal training	50%	50%	$2,500	$130,000
Benefits as a % of payroll wages	15%	15%	$600	$31,200
Other expenses as a % of department revenues	25%	25%	$1,000	$52,000
Total Expenses			**$8,100**	**$421,200**
Department Net				**-$57,200**

Figure 13-2. An example of a zero-based budget for a fitness department

As can be seen in Figure 13-2, a zero-based budget requires that the club operator make accurate assumptions with regard to several factors, including membership levels, pricing, volume of traffic for services, and selected other categories. Many club operators believe that using zero-based budgeting forces them to stay attuned to the factors that are impacting their market and business. As a consequence, they are more likely to achieve their budgetary predictions or estimates.

❑ *Trend-Line Budgeting.* Trend-line budgeting is the most commonly used budgeting practice for multiple-club operations and independent-club operations. The trend-line budget process is based on the principle of clubs building their next year's budget off the past financial trends of their business and then extrapolating forward, based on those trends. This method of budgeting is assumed to be more accurate and predictable, because it relies on a known history of financial-performance trends and then applies certain assumptions to those trends. A downside of this approach is its overreliance on past performance trends and its shortsighted view of current and future market forces. In any event, trend-line budgeting is an effective approach to budgeting, one that is much easier to apply when working with multiple-club entities. Figure 13-3 illustrates the revenue, payroll, and EBITDA trends, in millions, for a club over a three-year period.

As can be seen in Figure 13-3, the club's revenues have grown consistently over the past three years at a rate of approximately $100,000 annually. At the same time, payroll has decreased slightly, and as a consequence EBITDA has increased slightly each year. For the next calendar year, using the trend-line budgeting process and assuming that its revenues and expenses will increase in proportion with the results of prior years, the club could assume that its EBITDA will drop as a result of the trends in revenues and expenses. When using the trend-line budgeting process, club operators need to consider a number of assumptions and questions (for ease of understanding, the data in Figure 13-3 serves as a reference for the assumptions and questions). Figure 13-4 lists several of these assumptions and questions.

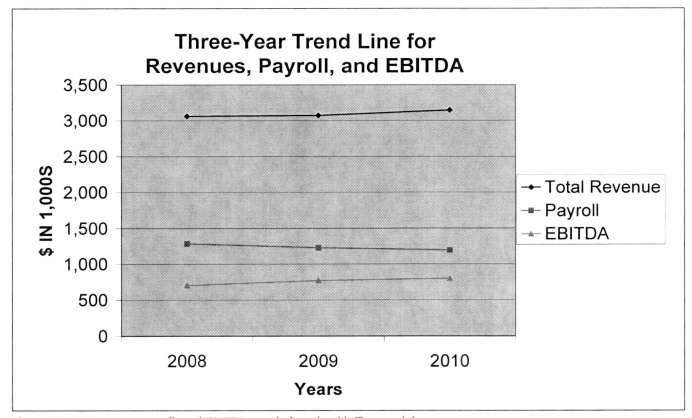

Figure 13-3. Revenue, payroll, and EBITDA trends for a health/fitness club

Revenues	Expenses
1. What is the average percentage rise in revenues for each of the last five years?	1. What has been the average percentage increase in expenses each of the last five years?
2. What is the expected or assumed percentage increase for revenues in the upcoming year due to CPI?	2. What is the expected or assumed percentage increase in payroll and other expenses due to CPI?
3. What is the expected or assumed percentage increase in revenues due to either pricing or usage increases?	3. What is the expected or assumed percentage increase in payroll due to merit increases or the addition of new staff?
4. Is the club adding a new service that will bring new revenues?	4. What are the expected or assumed percentage increases in other expenses, such as utilities, benefits, hospitalization, etc., due to unexpected or rumored market conditions?
5. Is a new competitor moving into town that might pull members from the club?	5. Does the club have any outstanding liabilities that are expected to come due?
6. Is there an indication of a new business or residential development coming in that would cause a higher-than-expected bump in membership levels?	6. Does the club have any delayed capital repair that it must address in the coming year?

Figure 13-4. Examples of basic assumptions and questions used in the trend-line budgeting process

As Figure 13-4 illustrates, the trend-line budgeting process requires both an understanding of a club's prior year's financial-performance trends and the ability to foresee both the expected and unexpected with regard to external and internal business forces. For example, when the 2008 financial crisis hit the global marketplace, club operators preparing for their 2009 budget had to reconsider their past financial performance and apply new thinking to those trends in order to establish a realistic budget for the upcoming year. If club operators tried to extrapolate their financial performance from 2007 and 2008 (trend-line budgeting) to 2009, they most likely would have had unrealistic forecasts. Instead, operators had to adapt their approach to using trends and reconsider some of their most basic assumptions. For example, at the Russian Fitness Group, the company had experienced over 10 percent growth in cash revenues in 2006, 2007, and during the first six months of 2008. When preparing the 2009 budget, the company could have assumed the same basic revenue trends would continue, and therefore it could have budgeted for a 10 percent revenue increase in 2009. Instead, the company took into consideration the impact of the economic downturn and budgeted for flat revenue growth (and concurrently for lower expenses), the result of which was an EBITDA plan for 2009 that was only slightly higher than forecasted for 2008.

Forecasting in the Health/Fitness Club Industry

Forecasting is an extension of the budgeting process. It is normally undertaken to more accurately predict financial performance over a shorter period of time than an annual budget, such as on a quarterly or monthly basis. The process of forecasting is a mainstay of both the public market and those club operators desiring to enter the public market. In recent years, many, if not most, multiple-club operators have moved toward quarterly forecasting as a means to create more accurate financial predictions than they normally obtain from their annual budgets. The main difference between budgeting (an annual process) and forecasting (normally a quarterly process) is that with forecasting, the club is looking at its budget, then taking the most recent external and internal business events, and finally using those factors to create a more accurate estimate of its financial performance for the upcoming period (usually a quarter). By forecasting, the club can better predict its future financial performance and cash position. Forecasting is also an excellent tool for developing club leaders who are able to take greater accountability for the club's financial performance. Figure 13-5 illustrates a club budget, examples of recent business events, and their application to a quarterly forecast.

As Figure 13-5 indicates, the forecast for the next quarter has been adjusted from the original budget, because the operator has taken into account several recent external and internal business changes. As a result of the forecast, the operator is better prepared to manage the club's cash flow for the upcoming quarter and to make adjustments in the club's operations, if they're needed, to compensate.

Category	Annual Budget	Next Quarter's Budget	Recent Events	Quarterly Forecast
Membership dues	$2,000,000	$500,000	In the last quarter, the club lost 50 members at annual dues of $50,000.	$487,500
Gross operating revenues	$3,000,000	$750,000	Price increase occurred in all services of 10%.	$762,500
Payroll	$1,200,000	$350,000	Wage increases go into effect at 5%.	$367,500
Other expenses	$1,000,000	$250,000	As predicted	$250,000
Total expenses	$2,200,000	$600,000	See above	$617,500
EBITDA	$800,000	$150,000		$145,000
Loan payment	$300,000	$75,000	No payment for quarter	$0
EBIT	$500,000	$75,000		$145,000

Figure 13-5. An example of forecasting, using an existing annual budget

Industry Practices for Driving Revenues

Personal training
is the second
largest source of
revenue in the
industry, with
the possible
exception of
tennis revenue in
those clubs that
offer tennis.

❑ *The Sources of Revenue.* Research conducted by IHRSA indicates that the largest source of revenue for clubs comes from membership dues. In the publication, the *IHRSA 2010 Profiles of Success*, it was reported that between 64 percent and 80 percent of a club's total revenue is derived from membership dues. As a result, it can be seen that membership sales and retention play a critical role in driving a club's overall revenue. The other 20 percent to 30 percent of a club's revenue is normally provided from a number of sources, including:

• *Personal training.* Personal training is the second largest source of revenue in the industry (e.g., based on data reported by IHRSA in 2007, it accounts for approximately 5 to 20 percent of a club's revenues), with the possible exception of tennis revenue in those clubs that offer tennis. According to anecdotal research, most clubs report that between 5 and 10 percent of their membership participates in personal training on a weekly basis. In fact, with regard to personal training, a few club companies (e.g., Equinox, U.S. and World Class, Russia) indicate that they are able to attract close to 20 percent of their members for personal training. In other words, if the club has 1,000 members, it can expect to see 50 to 100 sessions involving personal training a week, and if the club has 5,000 members, it can expect to see 250 to 500 personal-training sessions a week. As a rule, personal training fees tend to range from $40 to $120 an hour, with the highest U.S. rates found in New York, Los Angeles, and San Francisco. With these types of numbers, it is not unreasonable for a club of 1,000 members to generate as much as $7,500 a week in personal-training revenues or $360,000 annually, while a club of 5,000 members can derive as much as $37,500 a week or $1,950,000 annually from personal training. The Eastbank Club, based in Chicago, generates over $3 million in personal training annually, while the Reebok Club in New York generates over $8 million annually. Equinox, which operates approximately 50 clubs throughout the U.S., and World Class, which operates approximately 28 clubs in Russia, both report facilities that generate over $2 million in annual revenues each from personal training.

• *Tennis services.* In clubs that have tennis courts and tennis services, tennis is often the largest source of revenue after membership. In clubs with tennis, the largest single generator of revenue is providing tennis lessons (individual and group). Lesson revenue can account for as much as 80 percent of all tennis revenues. Other sources of revenue for tennis include court fees (indoor courts), youth programs, leagues, tournaments, and pro-shop sales. A club with outdoor courts can annually expect to generate between $25,000 and $50,000 in revenue per court, with the best clubs approaching $75,000 per court, while a club with indoor courts can expect to derive $35,000 to $100,000 per court. Club operators usually generate an average of $40,000 for an outdoor court and $75,000 for an indoor court. The reason indoor courts generate significantly more revenue is due to court fees. As previously indicated, lesson revenue is the top source of tennis revenue, with the average fee charged for a one-hour private lesson ranging from $40 to $60. Court fees range from a low of $10 per court hour to as high as $100 per court hour, depending upon the market in which the club is located. It should be noted that 10 percent to 40 percent of a club's members may be actively involved in tennis lessons on either an individual or group basis.

- *Spa services*. Spa services have grown into a prime source of revenue for the health/fitness club industry. According to the publication, the *IHRSA 2010 Profiles of Success*, in 2009, the average club generated approximately 8.9 percent of its revenues from spa services, with clubs that were part of a chain generating approximately 9.5 percent of revenue from their spa services. In some clubs, this source of revenue might only involve the delivery of massage, while in other clubs, it might involve a number of activities, including massage, facials, body treatments, pedicures, manicures, and even hair service. According to research conducted by ISPA (the International Spa Association), massage is the leading revenue source in the spa-service category, followed (in order) by facials, pedicures, manicures, and body treatments. In most instances, massage will account for at least 50 percent of the spa-service treatments. Research conducted by the spa industry shows that a typical treatment room could generate as much as $10,000 a month, while a pedicure station usually generates approximately $3,000 a month. In the club industry, anecdotal research indicates that a club can expect to generate about $3,000 to $10,000 a month from a single treatment room. This same research also shows that between one percent and five percent of a club's members will be active users of its spa services. With regard to pricing, a one-hour massage can range from as low as $40 in some midwestern clubs to as high as $120 in some of the high-end clubs in the more affluent markets. In fact, some club-based spas, such as those operated by DMB Sports headquartered in Phoenix, generate over $2 million annually.

> Research conducted by the spa industry shows that a typical treatment room could generate as much as $10,000 a month, while a pedicure station usually generates approximately $3,000 a month.

- *Youth programs and services*. In the last several years, the children's program and activity areas have become a significant source of revenue for many health/fitness clubs. In 2009, according to the publication, the *IHRSA 2010 Profiles of Success*, youth programming generated approximately five percent of a club's total revenues. Activities conducted in these areas, such as birthday parties, sports camps, dance classes, martial arts, tumbling, after-school camps, holiday camps, swim lessons, and swim teams can provide significant revenues. In fact, youth programs in suburban clubs, such as the Pacific Athletic Club in Redwood City, California, Franco's in Mandeville, Louisiana, and ACAC Fitness & Wellness in West Chester, Pennsylvania, all contribute significantly to each club's overall revenue numbers.

- *Pilates*. One of the newest sources of revenue for the industry has evolved from offering Pilates to club members. By combining both private instruction and group instruction, many clubs have seen Pilates become their second largest source of revenue. For example, Health Works, a women's-only chain of clubs located in Boston, has a Pilates center that grosses close to a half a million dollars a year. One multiple-club company, Equinox, has Pilates studios that occupy 600 to 800 square feet per studio, each of which (according to sources at Equinox) generates between $20,000 and $50,000 a month in revenue.

- *Other revenue-generating programs.* In addition to the aforementioned four sources, clubs have developed a variety of services that can contribute to revenue growth. For example, ClubCorp's Rivers Club in Pittsburgh, Pennsylvania generates over $200,000 annually in locker-rental income. The East Bank Club in Chicago derives over seven million annually in food and beverage revenue. Many clubs (e.g., Western Athletic Clubs, etc.) have found that leasing space to a physical therapy operator can bring in as much as $100,000 annually from fixed leases and revenue sharing. Still other clubs have leveraged activities, such as special events, leagues, adventure programs, and social events into significant sources of new revenue.

❑ *Increasing the Revenue Stream from Each Revenue Source.* As a rule, clubs have three core strategies that they can employ to increase their revenue output from the aforementioned revenue sources: increasing the pricing, increasing the usage rate of the services that they offer, and adding new products and services.

- *Price increases.* Many club operators assume that the best approach to driving revenues is to increase the price of a service. While price increases can generate significant bumps in revenue, especially if applied to membership dues or personal training, such increases can also have a negative impact if club operators do not take into consideration their club's market position and the value of the club's product offering. Many clubs make it a practice to increase their dues or personal training fees two to three percent every year, irrespective of market conditions, while others carefully consider the dynamics of the marketplace and their club's niche before passing on any price increases. In reality, if the club is delivering a great product and its members are satisfied, then an annual price increase equal to the consumer price index (CPI) or slightly higher can usually be accommodated.

  Operators need to understand that pricing is generally influenced by two primary forces. The first factor is the influence of competitive market conditions. For example, if a club's competitors in a particular market are continually decreasing their pricing, it will make it challenging for that club to increase its prices, even if it offers a fantastic experience. The second major influence on pricing is related to supply and demand. For example, if a club has more people requesting a service than it can serve, then the facility is in a position to raise its prices. On the other hand, if far more of a supply of a service existed than what the market was demanding, it is likely that the club would be unable to increase its prices.

- *Increasing volume.* Another effective approach for driving revenues is to increase member and guest participation in fee-based services. While the health/fitness club industry, as a whole, tends to shy away from this approach, all factors considered, it is the most effective strategy for generating relatively large increases in revenue. For example, multiple-

As a rule, clubs have three core strategies that they can employ to increase their revenue output from the aforementioned revenue sources: increasing the pricing, increasing the usage rate of the services that they offer, and adding new products and services.

club operators, such as Equinox, 24 Hour Fitness, and Bally's, focus most of their non-dues revenue efforts on internal selling. To effectively increase member usage of fee-based services, clubs should consider the following approaches:

✓ *Sales management.* The best clubs closely manage the sales of their primary revenue sources, such as personal training, massage, and other services, just as they do membership. The top revenue-producing clubs establish sales targets for their teams and each individual employee, and then closely monitor each entity's sales performance. Not only do these clubs establish challenging sales goals for both the sales teams and individuals, they then hold the teams and employees accountable for their performance against these goals. All factors considered, Equinox, based in New York, may do this better than anyone else in the industry.

✓ *Sales training.* Fitness staff (e.g., trainers, instructors, therapists, etc.) tend to be relationship people who often shy away from sales. As a rule, many individuals view sales in a negative light. Accordingly, many top club operators make a concerted effort to provide continuous sales training for their employees that can help make them more comfortable about selling themselves and the services of their clubs. During my tenure as the CEO of the Russian Fitness Group, targeted sales training was provided for our trainers and therapists.

✓ *Selling upfront.* The top revenue-producing clubs have learned that the best time to sell a service, such as personal training or massage, is when the member first joins the club. Many club groups, such as Equinox, 24 Hour Fitness, and Sports Club/LA, bundle special-service packages that the membership sales team makes new members aware of when they join the club. This process is often referred to as up-selling the club's services. Club operators should keep in mind that, all factors considered, new members represent the best audience for sales.

✓ *Internal marketing.* All too often, some clubs believe that by putting a poster on the wall, their members will automatically sign-up for the offering. In reality, to effectively make members aware of the services it offers, the club should utilize a variety of marketing tools, such as interactive displays, direct-mail invitations to members, web-based marketing, newsletter messages, and audio-visual messages, utilizing the club's internal audio-visual entertainment equipment.

✓ *Relationships and making the call.* Members who respect and trust the employees of the club are much more likely to purchase a service from those employees. The same can be said about members who know and respect other members. The top revenue-producing clubs make an effort to utilize their employees and members as sales people. Having employees make sales contacts or extend invitations to the members that they know can contribute significantly to revenue generation. Members who are provided an incentive will often serve as apostles for the services offered by the club and invite their friends to join them to participate in a fee-based service.

The top revenue-producing clubs have learned that the best time to sell a service, such as personal training or massage, is when the member first joins the club.

• *Adding new products and services.* The third strategy for effectively driving revenues is to introduce new products and services to the club's members. For example, if the club does not offer spa services, adding these services can generate new revenue streams. By the same token, if the club does not offer Pilates, including a Pilates center in the facility can help drive revenues for the club. In reality, the opportunities for adding new products and services are virtually endless. One proven strategy for identifying new sources of revenue is to create a club-based revenue team, consisting of employees from different areas of the club. This revenue team should then be empowered to meet on a regular basis and brainstorm new ideas for generating revenue. When the revenue team identifies a revenue idea that has consensus, then management can work with them to develop an execution strategy.

Industry Practices for Controlling Expenses

While driving revenue is critical to growing a club's profitability, controlling expenses also plays a vital role. The process of controlling expenses involves having systems and practices in place that can help prevent the club from needlessly wasting money. At the same time, the process can help the club invest its money more wisely in its people and assets.

> **Wages and salaries comprise approximately 38 percent to 48 percent (a figure that includes employee benefits and taxes) of every dollar in revenue that the club generates.**

❏ *The Leading Expense Categories.* According to the publication, the *IHRSA 2010 Profiles of Success*, the top expense categories for clubs are wages and salaries, benefits, utilities, lease costs, and capital replacement and repair costs.

  • *Wages and salaries.* According to the most recent industry studies, wages and salaries comprise approximately 38 percent to 48 percent (a figure that includes employee benefits and taxes) of every dollar in revenue that the club generates. If the related benefit costs are subtracted, then payroll is probably closer to 30 percent to 35 percent of gross revenues. This figure approximates the total of all other departmental undistributed expenses combined. Wages and salaries include the salaries of supervisors, the hourly wages of the non-exempt employees, commissions paid to personal trainers and other instructors, wages paid to group-exercise instructors, and bonuses provided to any employee of the club. For most clubs, the wages paid to group-exercise instructors and the commissions paid to personal trainers and others constitute the largest single payroll expense.

  • *Benefits.* Benefit costs can range from 15 percent to 25 percent of the actual wages and salaries. These costs include club contributions to social security taxes, hospitalization benefits, disability insurance, retirement type accounts, and education. The single largest contributor in recent years has been hospitalization costs, which have grown at rates over 12 percent annually the last several years.

  • *Utilities.* Utility costs normally range between 5 percent and 10 percent of a club's operating revenue, depending upon its geographic location. The largest contributors to utility costs are heating, and air conditioning, and expenses attributed to the operation of the pools and whirlpools.

- *Leases.* For clubs that rent space, the cost of rent can be a club's second largest expense after wages. According to the publications, *IHRSA's Uniform System of Accounts* and the *IHRSA 2010 Profiles of Success*, lease rates can run as high as 20 percent of a club's revenue (it should be noted that in some global urban markets, such as New York, London, and Moscow, rent can consume as much as 30 percent to 35 percent of a club's revenues). Successful club operators look to keep their lease rate under 15 percent of revenues and preferably closer to 10 percent of their operating revenue. According to the publication, the *IHRSA 2010 Profiles of Success*, in 2009, the average lease for a healthy fitness club was 9 percent of revenues. Many clubs get lulled into a state of complacency by assuming that they have a fixed based rent and they fail to consider the common area maintenance (CAM)—costs that landlords pass through, which represent the club's share of the building operating costs assumed by the landlord. In most markets, landlords like to offer triple-net leases, which means the club pays the landlord a base rent, CAM costs, utilities, and property taxes. In most markets, the lease rates for class "A" space run approximately $30 to $60 a square foot per year, while the lease rates for class "B" space tend to be in the neighborhood of $15 to $25 a square foot per year. CAM costs can run another $6 to $15 a square foot, depending upon the market in which a club is located. In smaller markets rent rates for space in strip malls run in the neighborhood of $15 to $20 a square foot.
- *Capital replacement and repair.* According to industry surveys, clubs should allocate approximately three to six percent of their gross revenues on an annual basis to capital replacement and repair. Every fifth year, the percentage should be increased to as much as 15 percent of the club's gross revenues. These numbers represent a significant amount of a club's revenues and, if not budgeted for correctly, can have dire consequences for the club. Many club operators try to save money by not spending the capital replacement dollars. In the long run, however, such an approach almost always results in poorly kept facilities and lost revenues. According to the publication, the *IHRSA 2010 Profiles of Success*, clubs who invest more into their club have the highest membership retention rates. Capital replacement dollars are used to purchase new equipment, repair worn areas of the club, and fund expansion efforts when they are needed.

Controlling the Leading Expense Categories

Achieving profitability requires that the club operator put systems in place for controlling the large and small expenses that can often erode the revenue gains that a club makes. Among the most effective strategies that the industry employs to help monitor and control operating expenses, thereby facilitating growth in profitability, are the following:

❑   *Managing Wages and Benefits Expense.* Since wages and benefits contribute, on average, close to 45 percent of all operating expenses, it makes sense that by effectively managing its payroll, the club can also better manage its

> Achieving profitability requires that the club operator put systems in place for controlling the large and small expenses that can often erode the revenue gains that a club makes.

expenses. Examples of the most effective strategies for managing payroll include:

- *Scheduling for less than 40 hours.* Smart operators avoid scheduling their full-time employees for 40 hours and instead schedule them for 35 to 37 hours a week. This approach has two advantages. First, it provides leeway if an employee is asked to serve a few more hours, and second, it allows the clubs to avoid both overtime and overlapping schedules.

- *Not scheduling employees during low-usage periods.* Many clubs save wages by limiting their level of scheduling during low-usage times. While it is important to be fully staffed during peak-usage periods, during times when members are not using the facility, management can limit their scheduling of employees to only provide the necessary level of employee coverage. As needed, if additional staffing is required when special functions are held, these situations can be handled with salaried supervisors.

- *Monitoring and avoiding overtime.* Since overtime costs a club 50 percent more than regular time, wise club operators make it a practice to carefully monitor employee hours to avoid overtime. In this regard, software programs are available that will provide the club with reports that indicate when its employees are approaching overtime. In which case, the club can make whatever adjustments are necessary in its employee schedules to avoid overtime situations.

- *Going to flat rates versus percentage commission.* Personal trainers and massage therapists are often paid a commission on the revenue they generate. The industry norm for commissions tends to vary from 40 percent to 60 percent. Instead of paying a commission, many clubs pay a flat rate for personal training and/or massage. This approach enables the club to avoid providing wage increases every time the fees for services offered by the club are raised.

- *Group-exercise classes.* For many club operators, the cost of offering group-exercise classes can be very substantial. The average wage for a class instructor can vary from an average as low as $18 a class in some mid-western markets to $75 per class in the large urban markets, such as New York and San Francisco. When the fact that some clubs offer as many as 100 classes a week is considered, the enormity of the potential costs involved becomes apparent. At the Russian Fitness Group, the group-exercise payroll often ran has high as 10 percent of membership revenue. The top club operators make it a habit to establish specific attendance requirements for a class to continue and when attendance falls below those specified levels, the class is eliminated. The primary goal of most clubs is to offer only the classes that appeal to members and thereby only pay the wages for those classes that bring value to each club's program offerings.

❑ *Managing Operating Supply Costs.* In most clubs, the costs associated with operating supplies, printing, and other miscellaneous supplies can run as high as 10 percent of revenue and, if uncontrolled, much higher. The most effective approaches to managing these expenses include:

> **Instead of paying a commission, many clubs pay a flat rate for personal training and/or massage.**

- *Using a purchase-order system.* A purchase-order system requires that before employees can purchase an item for the club, they need to obtain a price quote and submit it to management for approval. If subsequently approved by management, the purchase order becomes the basis for an order. This approach allows management to monitor expenses against budget to insure that funds are not expended for unnecessary items.

- *Par stock and inventory.* A par stock is a term that connotates a process that involves purchasing sufficient quantities of supplies and creating an inventory of those items for the club to pull from in times of need. In reality, many clubs unfortunately wait until they run out of an item before attempting to restock the item by purchasing it. With a par-stock process, the club purchases items based on its usage experience and keeps an inventory sufficient to cover a particular period of time. Under the par-stock process, when the club's inventory drops to a certain level, it purchases the standard reorder quantity. This approach is similar to an open-to-buy system in retail. The par-stock method allows the club to buy in bulk, which saves money, but it also allows it to closely monitor the usage of products and control its shrinkage (e.g., inventory loss due to theft).

- *Preferred vendor arrangements.* Clubs can negotiate with vendors to obtain preferred status and thus gain discounts. If a club is willing to purchase its supplies from one or two vendors, it can often negotiate a discounted price schedule. In large multiple-club operations, this approach can involve a significant savings opportunity. In this regard, independent-club operators, should consider using industry-association programs, such as the programs offered by IHRSA.

❏ *Utility Costs.* As previously discussed, utility costs can amount to as much as 10 percent of a club's operating revenue. Most clubs can save on their utility costs by incorporating one or more of the following strategies:

- *Converting electric heating appliances to gas.* Gas is usually less expensive than electric, especially when it comes to heating pools, water heaters, whirlpools, and washers.

- *Using light-saver switches.* Many clubs use automatically controlled lighting systems that turn off lights in rooms when they are not in use. Far too many clubs waste money by keeping lights on in particular areas, even though those rooms are not in use. These clubs rely on their employees to turn off the lights as appropriate, an approach that is not always as effective as automated systems.

- *Installing water restrictors in the showers.* Water restrictors are devices that can be added to showers that reduce the total volume of water that is dispensed. Over time, these implements can save considerable costs in water bills.

- *Insulating the club.* Most utility companies will provide the club with incentives if it upgrades the level of insulation in the club. In many cases, utility companies will even cover most of the cost for such improvements. The upside for the club comes with the reduced cost of heating and cooling.

> **If a club is willing to purchase its supplies from one or two vendors, it can often negotiate a discounted price schedule.**

- *Negotiating with the utility company for a flat rate.* Club operators can often negotiate with the utility company to establish a flat utility rate that is reviewed on a semi-annual basis. Not only can this practice save money, more importantly, it can also enable the club to more accurately forecast its utility costs.

- *Installing low-energy lighting.* Many utility purchasing groups offer incentives to businesses that install low-energy lighting systems. Such incentives allow a business to spend less in the conversion process, with savings subsequently being realized on their monthly utility bill.

❑ *Leases.* In most cases, leases are non-negotiable once they're in place. At least, this situation is what most operators assume. As a result, many club owners pay higher-than-needed rent and CAM costs. The first step for the club in managing its lease expense is to know its lease terms inside and out. By knowing the terms of its lease, the club can identify when unnecessary costs are passed through, such as high CAM costs and rent increases, when none exist in the lease. Even more important than knowing its lease, the club should be fully aware of a situation when the opportunity exists to renegotiate its lease. Landlords are open to renegotiating leases under several possible circumstances, including: when a new building owner becomes the landlord, when the landlord is looking to extend leases, and when lease rates for other spaces are going at a lower rate than what the club currently pays. For example, during the economic downturn of 2008 and 2009, a number of landlords provided temporary lease relief to their tenants. At the Russian Fitness Group, for example, the company was able to negotiate rent reductions on several of its properties, saving the company hundreds of thousands of dollars in the process. All factors considered, if the club has established itself as a worthy and reliable tenant and has built a good relationship with the landlord, then the club is in a better position to renegotiate more favorable lease terms.

> By allocating three to six percent of its revenues to capital repair and replacement and then using it, the club is investing in its physical assets, an approach which, in turn, helps to drive revenues and prevent costly operational maintenance costs.

❑ *Capital Repair.* In the publication, the *IHRSA 2010 Profiles of Success,* it is noted that in 2009, clubs, on average, spent $113,700 on reinvestment, a statistic that represents on average four percent of revenues. As indicated previously, this outlay represents a significant allocation of cash for most club operators. Some operators feel that by limiting their allocation for capital reserve that they can bring more of their existing revenue to the bottom line. At first glance, this attitude might make sense, since it decreases the out-of-pocket cash that a club has to spend, thereby increasing the EBIT of the club. Unfortunately, this reasoning ends up costing clubs money, both in the short-term and even more so in the long-term. By allocating three to six percent of its revenues to capital repair and replacement and then using it, the club is investing in its physical assets, an approach which, in turn, helps to drive revenues and prevent costly operational maintenance costs. By investing the full capital replacement on an annual basis, the club can also help prevent having to spend much larger sums in future years, when a particular physical asset reaches a point where it requires major renovation and repair.

Key Points to Consider

By incorporating annual budgeting and quarterly forecasting, a club operator can develop realistic and achievable financial targets for its revenues, expenses, and earnings. These financial targets can then be used to foster individual and team accountability for the club's financial performance. Once in place, these targets can assist the club operator in determining which revenue-enhancement and cost-control strategies are needed to achieve particular financial targets.

By incorporating annual budgeting and quarterly forecasting, a club operator can develop realistic and achievable financial targets for its revenues, expenses, and earnings.

14

The Art of the Deal: Buying, Leasing, Selling, and Raising Capital for a Health/Fitness Club

For independent-club operators just starting a club or an experienced multiple-club operation looking to expand its business, raising capital is an important factor in achieving success.

Chapter Objectives

As the industry continues to evolve and become more financially sophisticated, club owners and operators need to acquaint themselves with as many of the overriding issues surrounding the purchasing, financing, and sale of health/fitness clubs as possible. In that regard, this chapter will review the information and processes that a club operator should know concerning how to raise capital for the club, how to buy a club, how to sell a club, or simply how to properly evaluate a lease for the space that a club might occupy. Initially, the chapter discusses the key issues attendant to raising capital and then concludes by examining several of the most relevant factors involving buying, leasing, and selling clubs.

Raising Capital for a Health/Fitness Club

For independent-club operators just starting a club or an experienced multiple-club operation looking to expand its business, raising capital is an important factor in achieving success. As a rule, club owner/operators have three primary options for raising capital for their business: bank financing, private investor financing, and private equity-firm investment (venture capital). Besides the aforementioned sources of funding, larger multiple-club operators, with a proven track record of success, can also pursue an initial public offering (IPO), a process that raises capital through the issuance of public stock (e.g., Lifetime Fitness and Town Sports International). Clubs that own their land and building also have a fifth option—selling the land and building to raise capital and then leasing the property back from the investors to whom they sold the land and building (i.e., a sale leaseback).

❑ *Private Investor Capital* (e.g., angel investor capital). Many independent-club operators pursue this approach to raising capital. This method involves having the owner of the proposed business venture (club) develop a business model that is subsequently presented to private investors for raising capital. In most instances, the owner needs to form a limited partnership, limited liability corporation, or corporation to serve as the legal entity for raising the capital. In attracting private-investor equity, the club operator must offer the investor stock, membership shares, or a similar ownership position. In essence, the club operator must allow the investors an ownership stake in the business if they intend to provide the capital.

Private investors look for a minimum annual return on their invested capital (AROIC), a form of return on equity invested (ROE). In most cases, investors are looking for returns of at least 10% to 15% on their invested capital, though higher return expectations of 20% to 25% are not unusual. For example, if private investors provide one million dollars in capital in a club, they will normally expect an annual return of at least $100,000 to $150,000. This amount is based on the free cash flow of the club after the club accounts for all of its expenses. In addition to expecting a reasonable rate of return on their investment, most private investors also want a preferred position with regard to any dividends that the business might distribute (earnings after all expenses and taxes are paid). A preferred position allows investors to get their initial investment capital returned before future earnings and profits are distributed to the respective shareholders. In raising capital through this approach, club operators may need to consider and attract several private investors, especially if they are looking to raise several million dollars. It should be noted that private investors could be individuals or partnerships (e.g., often referred to as angel investors).

❑ *Private-Equity Investment Firms* (venture capital firms, funds, etc.). Clubs that pursue private-equity firms usually are trying to raise millions of dollars in capital. As a rule, it is not likely that an independent-club operation would pursue this option. Rather, this approach is a method that a multiple-club operation, seeking capital for acquisitions or rapid organic growth, would tend to favor. All factors considered, this option is far more suited to capital requirements exceeding $5 million, and typically more than $20 million. When club operators obtain private-equity investment, they should be aware of the fact that the investors assume an ownership position in the business that is proportional to their invested capital, both in equity and debt. In addition, a PE firm will typically have a shareholder or operating agreement prepared that gives it control over certain aspects of the operations of the business (e.g., control of financial considerations, control over new business decisions and investments, preferential decision-making authority regarding selection of the company's top officers, etc.). As a result, the original owners can often lose controlling interest in their business and, as such, be relegated to more of a management role. Accordingly, clubs should give careful consideration concerning whether to pursue this capital strategy.

Most private-equity firms that invest in a club business do so by investing both cash and assuming additional debt. For example, a private-equity firm

> When club operators obtain private-equity investment, they should be aware of the fact that the investors assume an ownership position in the business that is proportional to their invested capital, both in equity and debt.

may invest $40 million dollars in a club—which consists of $20 million in cash and $20 million in assumption of debt. Many private equity groups invest by leveraging the assets of the business, often putting up as little as 15% of the value in equity, and then leveraging the remaining amount (85%) through debt. Private-equity firms tend to view their investment far differently than a private investor, because their primary goal is normally to either sell their invested stake or take the business public (i.e., exit strategy) in a period of three to five years. Most private-equity firms tend to look for two factors when considering whether to invest. Not only do they expect the club(s) to achieve double digit growth in EBITDA on an annual basis (normally a range of 15% to 25%), they also anticipate cashing out after three to five years, with an internal rate of return (IRR) between 20% and 40%. At an investor forum held in 2010 as part of the IHRSA international convention that took place in San Francisco, several PE firms indicated that after the recent recession, PE expectations for IRR had dropped from the 30% to 40% range sought during the early 2000s to a range of 20% to 25%.

In reality, some private-equity firms still have IRR expectations of 30% to 40%. For example, a private-equity firm invests $40 million in capital (which consists of $20 million in cash and $20 million in debt) for a business that generates $10 million in EBITDA. Over the next five years, they invest another $20 million, through cash and debt, to bring their total capital invested to $60 million. In return, hypothetically, they would expect the EBITDA of the business to grow from $10 million at the time of purchase to $12 million after one year, $14.5 million after two years, $17.3 million after three years, $20.7 million after four years, and $25 million by the fifth year. After the fifth year, they would want to sell the business for approximately six to eight times the club's EBITDA, thereby generating a total of $100 to $200 million in cash. After deducting their $60 million of investment, they would receive $40 to $140 million in cash earnings to distribute to their investors, which would amount to a return in excess of 20%. If a private-equity group does not see the expected EBITDA growth or the possibility of exiting the business with an appropriate level of return on its investment, it will often take control of the business and try to push earnings growth, through cost reductions and potential acquisitions, while also looking for a suitable investor to buy the company.

> **When looking for a bank to finance its business, a club should attempt to find a bank that defaults on no more than .5% of its loans. In other words, it makes the right financing decision 99.5% of the time.**

❑ *Bank Financing* (debt financing). Bank financing is one of the most common approaches employed to raise most of the capital needed to develop and operate a small or large business. Because banks are regulated, they tend to be very careful in their lending practices. When looking for a bank to finance its business, a club should attempt to find a bank that defaults on no more than .5% of its loans. In other words, it makes the right financing decision 99.5% of the time. Clubs should understand several basic factors about banks and financing, including:

• For banks, its loans are its assets, which means that every loan application is reviewed very carefully. Since the recent recession of 2008/2009, most banks have intensified their scrutiny of loan applications.

- Banks look for individuals, partnerships, and businesses with good credit ratings.
- Banks expect to see a business plan that has reasonable assumptions, reasonable budget projections, a qualified leadership team (management expertise and experience), and detailed value of the collateral that will be put up to secure the loan (the collateral must hold value to the lender).
- Banks expect full disclosure from the company to which they are going to make a loan.
- Banks will normally apply covenants to a loan. Covenants help protect the bank's investment in the loan. These covenants can be restrictive (e.g., requiring a specific ratio of earnings to debt, ratio of earnings to interest payments, capital replacement approval, etc.). In turn, if the business breaks the covenants, the bank can demand immediate payment of the debt balance, or take over control of the assets of the business, and even sell the business if necessary.
- Banks prefer that the owner(s) of the business have equity in the company. For new businesses, banks like to see one dollar in equity for each dollar being lent. For mature businesses that have a track record of success and can be secured with real estate, banks will normally loan out four to five dollars for each dollar of equity (in other words, owners are required to provide 20% to 25% equity to secure the loan). For example, if a club wanted to take out a loan for $2,000,000, it would need to put up $400,000 to $500,000 in equity. Since the economic turmoil of 2008 and 2009, banks have often asked owners to put up a larger share of equity, and in many cases, have not even considered approving a loan unless the shareholders have at least 30% equity in the business. Many venture capital groups are able to secure debt with as little as 15% equity, particularly when the debt can be secured by hard assets. In almost all instances, banks prefer that the shareholders put up some form of collateral, typically real estate. Referred to as a collateralized loan, this type of a financial arrangement is much easier to obtain than a non-collateralized or non-secured loan.

> For new businesses, banks like to see one dollar in equity for each dollar being lent.

- In the past, most banks liked the debt-to-EBITDA ratio of the business to fall between three and four (i.e., a club's total debt should not exceed four times its EBITDA). For example, if a club has an EBITDA of $1,000,000, its total debt should not exceed $4,000,000 and should fall between three and four million dollars. If its debt exceeds four times it's EBITDA, then the club would be considered as heavily leveraged, which places a financial strain on the business, not to mention exposes it to the danger of not complying with the bank covenants for the loan. Since the most recent global financial crisis, many international banks have tightened up the debt-to-EBITDA ratio requirements, with lenders often restricting the debt-to-EBITDA ratio to 2.5.
- Cash-flow or non-collateralized loans are loans that banks provide that are not secured by real estate. In these instances, banks tend to limit the amount of the loan to a total that does not exceed 50% of the value of the assets of the business (a value that is determined by a multiple applied to the club's EBITDA).

- The bank expects the club to educate it on both the industry as a whole and on the club's business model.
- In the case of small independent operations, the bank will tend to require full financial disclosure of any stockholders or partners with 20% or greater ownership in the business. Furthermore, these owners will often be required to sign a personal guarantee for the loan amount being pursued. Banks typically frame the interest rate for loans against LIBOR (London Interbank Offered Rate). LIBOR is the interest rate at which banks can borrow funds from other banks. The rate is set each day, based on a multitude of financial indexes, in particular interbank deposit rates for larger institutions. Typically, a large multinational business can get a loan rate that is three to five points above LIBOR, although since the recession of 2008/2009, many banks have offered loans at two or three points above LIBOR. As of June 2011, the LIBOR rate was .74%, compared to being as high as 3.4% just prior to the market crash in September of 2008. It is a common practice for most start-up clubs to obtain equity through private investors and then raise the balance of the funds needed through debt. Larger multiple-club operations, on the other hand, usually utilize private-equity investment firms to raise the equity and even source the debt.

Buying and Selling a Health/Fitness Club Business

The health/fitness club industry is a dynamic enterprise in which clubs and club companies are bought and sold regularly. One approach that individuals use who are considering entering the business is to acquire an existing club. In that regard, for a club that wants to grow its business, acquisition may be a suitable option, rather than building a new club. On the other hand, if investors (or an individual) want to cash out of the business or to become part of a larger business by being the acquiree rather than the acquirer, then selling the club may be appropriate. Among the key factors that should be considered when buying or selling a club business are the following:

> *Clubs that are freestanding and own the land on which they are located will have a projected value that ranges from three times its EBITDA to eight times its EBITDA.*

❑ *Selling a Club.* If owners decide to sell their club, they need to understand some of the basic factors that apply to the sale process, including:

- Most clubs are valued by applying a multiple to the club's EBITDA, which results in a measure that is referred to as the enterprise value of the business. For clubs that are in a leased space, that multiple can range from three times EBITDA to as high as five times EBITDA. In the majority of instances, it will likely be four to five times the club's EBITDA. For example, a club that has an EBITDA of $500,000 would be valued at two to two and a half million dollars. Clubs that are freestanding and own the land on which they are located will have a projected value that ranges from three times its EBITDA to eight times its EBITDA. In the majority of instances, its enterprise value will be five to six times its EBITDA. In other words, a freestanding club with an EBITDA of $500,000 would be valued at $2.5 million to $3.0 million. In most cases, the EBITDA that is used to project a club's value is what is termed "trailing EBITDA" (i.e., the EBITDA for the most recent trailing 12-month time period and not for a specific financial year).

- Even after a club's enterprise value is estimated using the multiple of EBITDA, the seller should be aware that buyers will deduct the value of the liabilities from the calculated EBITDA value before determining its equity value (e.g., purchase price), especially if they are buying the business and not its assets. For example, if a club has an EBITDA of one million and liabilities of $1,500,000, then the buyer will likely value the club at five times its EBITDA minus the liabilities, or a projection that is determined by first multiplying one million by five, and then subtracting $1,500,000 to derive a calculated equity value of $3,500,000.

- If someone sells a club, the preference of most individuals is to sell the business and therefore release themselves from the liabilities of the business. The buyer is more likely to want to buy the assets at the mutually agreed upon price, while the seller remains responsible for the club's liabilities.

- If the seller owns the land on which the club sits, the seller should consider holding onto the land and selling the business, and then leasing the land to the new owner. This approach enables the seller to generate more cash out of the sale. For example, if a business is valued at five million dollars (of which the asset value of the land is one million), an individual might sell the business for $4.5 million, but then lease the land to the new owner for $100,000 a year.

- Sellers should make sure that they complete their own due diligence before selling and have an accurate recording of their assets, liabilities, and EBITDA for the past three years, etc.

- Sellers should have an attorney involved and possibly a broker.

Over the past seven years, several health/fitness clubs have generated a final enterprise value at EBITDA multiples in excess of nine. For example, 24 Hour Fitness was reported to have received a purchase price equivalent to 9.5 EBITDA when a controlling interest in it was sold to Forstmann Little. Similarly, Equinox was reported to have received over 11x its EBITDA when it was sold to Related Properties in 2005.

- ❑ *Buying a Club.* If their goal is to buy a club, then the individuals who are considering purchasing the business should make sure that they understand certain basics of buying a club business, including:
  - Buyers should perform their due diligence and audit the books and operations in their entirety. They should also make sure the accuracy and authenticity of the accounting is correct by having an independent audit made of the club's financial statements. Finally, they should make sure that they are fully aware of any liabilities that the business might have, in particular, any hidden account payables or legal suits against the existing club.
  - Most clubs in leased spaces will sometimes sell for three to five times their EBITDA, with four times more likely. Clubs that are freestanding will usually sell for between three and eight times their EBITA, with a range

Most clubs in leased spaces will sometimes sell for three to five times their EBITDA, with four times more likely.

of five to six times most likely. More often than not, sellers try to start at the high end of the price range, while buyers typically start at the low end and then work up.

- If possible, buyers should purchase the business assets, based on the cash flow value, rather than the business itself. When individuals purchase the assets of a business, they are acquiring both the short-term and long-term assets of the club, as well as purchasing the owner's equity. What they don't buy and don't really want are the liabilities.

- When purchasing a club, the buyers should make sure that the debt they finance does not exceed three times the trailing EBITDA.

- If the individuals purchasing the debt decide to buy the entire business rather than just the assets of the business, they should then make sure to deduct the liabilities from the enterprise value when determining the club's final equity value. In addition, it is important that both parties come to agreement on the EBITDA multiple that will be used to calculate the enterprise value.

- The buyers should remember that if they purchase a club that sells annual membership contracts, that when they purchase the assets and cash flow of the business, they might not be receiving the expected level of dues if the previous owner collected the annual dues before the sale. If the buyers know that a club collects annual dues, then they need to consider lowering the price that they are willing to pay for the business or ask for consideration for those dues already collected in the asking price. All too often, buyers end up purchasing a club that does not produce dues for a considerable period of time because of such a scenario.

- The buyers should retain the right to retain or dismiss employees of the former club.

For most first-time club owners and operators, as well as the majority of existing club operations, leasing space for their club is a common practice.

Leasing and Sale Leasebacks

For most first-time club owners and operators, as well as the majority of existing club operations, leasing space for their club is a common practice. Leasing is usually the option most operators choose, especially since obtaining the land to build a freestanding club is often difficult to find and too expensive to purchase. In most situations, leasing requires less upfront capital. In turn, the club has less of a need to assume debt. On the other hand, on occasion, situations exist where independent and multiple-club operators actually purchase land and build a freestanding club under one company and then lease it back to the actual operating-club entity. By the same token, some clubs will take the land and building they own and sell it to an investor, with the agreement that investor will turn around and lease the building space back to the club operator. Such a practice is called a sale-leaseback and is often used to raise capital. Leasing can involve several factors, including:

- As a rule, leases have minimum time requirements. In most urban markets, the landlords of class A and class B buildings look for a minimum time period of 10 years, while in suburban settings, especially strip-mall centers, leases will usually be for five-year periods at a minimum. Prospective tenants should look for a five-year lease with an optional five-year extension period. If they are confident in their business model, then they should consider a 10-year lease.

- Most leases can be negotiated to include clauses that allow tenants to renegotiate their lease rates at a predetermined timeframe within the lease. It is a prudent business owner who makes sure to negotiate this stipulation as part of their lease. A common practice would be to have a window of time for renegotiation in the second or third year in a five-year lease and the fifth year in a 10-year lease. This negotiating practice could also be employed to establish time periods for extending leases.

- Some landlords will offer a straight lease, which means that the tenant only pays the lease rate and the approved common area maintenance costs (CAM), but does not pay utilities and property tax. This type of lease is less common in today's market because of the high upfront costs and the carrying costs that many real estate owners assume. The more common lease is a triple-net lease, which is a contracted arrangement where the tenant is responsible for the lease, CAM costs, utilities, and property taxes on the space. Accordingly, prospective tenants should make sure that they know what type of lease is being offered and what the costs will be for each type.

- Most leases have a base rate that varies by building type (class A, class B, class C, strip mall), by location, and, of course, by market demand. In most markets, strip-mall space will carry base lease rates of between $12 and $25 a square foot. In urban markets, the base lease rate can range from as low as $10 a square foot for undesirable space (basement or concourse space) to $100 a square foot for desirable retail space. The most common range is between $25 and $40 a square foot. All factors considered, club operators should try to keep their base rent under $30 a square foot or less than 15% of their club's expected revenues.

- Tenants should know what their CAM costs will be. While in most leased spaces, it will range from five to eight dollars a square foot, there are buildings in some cities, such as Chicago and New York, where the CAM rates can reach as high as $15 or more a square foot.

- Most landlords provide tenants with a tenant-improvement allowance (TI) when the tenant moves into a space. As a rule, it is common for these allowances to run between $15 and $25 a square foot. In most instances, tenants will have the option of negotiating a higher TI allowance, especially if they are willing to pay a higher lease rate. For individuals who are having trouble raising capital to build the space, negotiating with the landlord to provide higher TI allowances, in exchange for higher rent, can prove helpful. In some instances, a landlord may actually pay for the entire costs of finishing out a tenant's space in return for a higher rental rate.

- If tenants are paying utilities either as part of their lease or separately, they should make sure that they request separate metering of the utilities for their space. Most landlords prefer to bill their tenants for the cost of their utilities. At the same time, a few landlords will add some overhead and profit to the actual utility costs that they pass through to their tenants.

If tenants are paying utilities either as part of their lease or separately, they should make sure that they request separate metering of the utilities for their space.

- Tenants should make an effort to have their HVAC operated separately from the buildings they lease. In many cases, landlords have set times during which they turn their building's HVAC on and off. Turn-off times are normally based on the operating hours of a typical business. As such, all factors considered, tenants who occupy buildings in which they have independent access to the HVAC for their space and have HVAC, which is independently metered, are better off. In the event that the club's space is tied into the building's HVAC, the tenant should be aware that they would probably need to negotiate after-hours access to the HVAC, which will typically result in higher costs to them.

- Tenants should establish a good relationship with the landlord and the landlord's representatives. Furthermore, they should make it a practice to meet with their landlord's representatives on a monthly basis.

- Tenants should know the details of their lease. Many leases require landlords to provide a certain degree of maintenance on tenant spaces. On occasion, some landlords will try to downplay this factor if they can, especially if their tenants have a relatively large space and pay a lower lease rate. Accordingly, tenants should always be fully aware of all of the conditions in their lease.

- In some instances, landlords may be willing to provide tenants with several months of free rent. Tenants should understand, however, that landlords recover these "lost" revenues in the actual rent that they subsequently charge them. As a rule, individuals who are starting a club would be wise to try and negotiate between six months and a year's free rent as part of their lease. The extent of the period of free rent is dependent upon the length of the lease and what they pay for rent, with those who have higher rents and longer leases receiving a longer period of time before their rent kicks in.

A sale-leaseback is another method that individuals employ to acquire space for their business. In a sale-leaseback, the club owner/operator will sell their property and building to another investor who then leases the space back to the club owner/operator for the business. This strategy is often used by club operators who wish to raise capital for expansion or renovation purposes. One of the primary benefits of this strategy is that it allows club owners to pull their equity out of the assets and use it for growing their business. In fact, several major club companies, such as LA Fitness, Lifetime Fitness, 24 Hour Fitness, and Bally, have all participated in sale-leaseback arrangements for one or more of their clubs.

For many club operators, the financial aspects of the business can be the most challenging. On the other hand, by taking the time to understand the basic issues involved in these factors, individuals who operate health/fitness clubs will be better prepared to address these matters in an appropriate manner.

> As a rule, individuals who are starting a club would be wise to try and negotiate between six months and a year's free rent as part of their lease.

STAFFING ISSUES IN THE HEALTH/FITNESS CLUB INDUSTRY

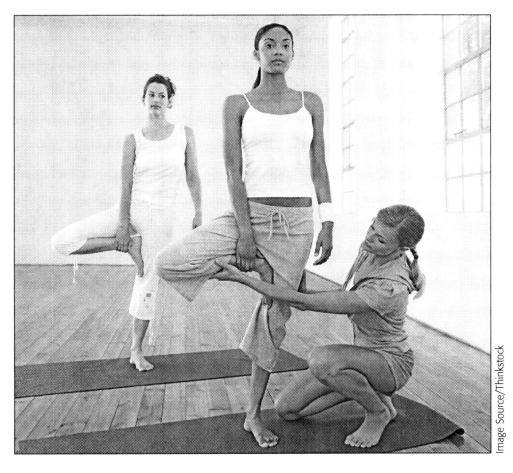

Image Source/Thinkstock

Part Five

15

The People Factor: Employees in the Health/ Fitness Club Industry

Chapter Objectives

The health/fitness club industry is a people-intensive industry. As indicated in the previous chapters on the industry's financial model, most clubs allocate upwards of 40 percent of their revenue towards wages and salaries. When a business allocates 40 percent or more of its resources to one area, that area takes on critical importance to the success of the business. In the health/fitness club industry, the employees create and sustain the experiences that the members have. In that regard, they directly influence a club's overall profitability. One of the most frequently heard comments in the health/fitness club industry is that its employees are the heart of the industry. These essential individuals deliver the services, create magic moments for the members, and foster the relationships that are so vital to a club's success. According to an article written by Leonard Schlessinger, The Service Profit Chain, employees are the key link for any business that desires to deliver great service to its customers.

This chapter initially begins by defining the differences between an employee and an independent contractor, as well as detailing the differences between an exempt and a non-exempt employee. Next, it provides an overview of the various positions in the industry and the role each position has in delivering the club's experience. Then, it outlines the compensation norms and educational expectations for each of these industry positions. Finally, it concludes by reviewing the various organizational structures that independent clubs and multiple-club groups utilize in operating their business.

Employees Versus Independent Contractors

Similar to the separation between church and state, the lines between employees and independent contractors represent a challenge for the health/fitness club industry. All too often, clubs decide to have independent contractors provide a portion of their service delivery, not knowing that they are actually creating an employer-employee environment. It is critical, however, that club operators

> In the health/fitness club industry, the employees create and sustain the experiences that the members have. In that regard, they directly influence a club's overall profitability.

clearly understand the difference between an employee and an independent contractor. Figure 15-1 details several of the basic differences between the two types of workers.

The fundamental differences between an employee and an independent contractor are quite significant. In the U.S., state and federal rules and regulations are very adamant about businesses adhering to the policies and procedures concerning the separation of employees and independent contractors. Clubs that attempt to pay people as independent contractors, but treat them as employees, open themselves to significant fines. If the club identifies someone as an independent contractor, but that person is characterized by any of the factors listed in the employee column in Figure 15-1, then that person is an employee and must be treated as such.

Exempt Versus Non-Exempt Employees in the U.S.

Another potential minefield for club operators involves whether an individual should be treated as an exempt or a non-exempt employee. An exempt employee is a professional who receives a base salary (weekly, monthly, etc.), while a non-exempt employee is an individual who is paid an hourly wage for the provided service. In other words, an exempt employee is normally not eligible for overtime, while a non-exempt employee is almost always eligible for overtime pay. In 2004, federal legislation was passed by congress and subsequently signed by the President that applied tougher rules to the issue of overtime pay, extending overtime eligibility to certain exempt positions at lower pay levels, and extending additional overtime opportunities to hourly non-exempt employees. Historically, the club industry has tried to create exempt positions, in an effort to avoid having to pay overtime, a practice still carried

Employee	Independent Contractor
Schedule is established by the club	Sets own schedule
Expected to follow employee policies and rules, including wearing a uniform	Only required to adhere to contractual obligations
Club can set rates for services the employee provides	Sets own rates for services that are provided
Must punch the clock or otherwise record all hours of work	Keeps own schedule and record of hours worked
Must be paid for overtime (all hours over 40 a week) and for club-recognized holidays	No overtime or holiday pay
Eligible for all club-sponsored benefits, such as holiday pay, vacation pay, insurance benefits, etc.	Not eligible for club-sponsored benefits
Covered by club-sponsored insurance such as disability, liability, etc.	Not covered by insurance and must provide evidence of liability insurance
Receives a W2 at year-end and club pays portion of social security taxes	Responsible for all taxes and receives a 1099 form showing earnings at year-end
Receives compensation via payroll	Receives earnings through a vendor check

Figure 15-1. Selected differences between employees and independent contractors

out by some smaller independent clubs. In most large independent clubs and multiple-club operations, however, the line between exempt and non-exempt employees is very clear. Figure 15-2 provides a basic overview of the factors that delineate exempt from non-exempt employees.

Permanent and Temporary Employees in Europe

In many European nations, as well as in Russia, employees can be classified as either permanent or temporary. Permanent employees are typically given an employment agreement that details the specific performance requirements of the job. A permanent employee is entitled to all the benefits that the employer provides, as well as being authorized to receive any government-mandated privileges and/or requirements (e.g., maternity leave duration, vacation time duration, holidays, social taxes, etc.). In some nations, such as Russia and Spain, an employee with permanent status has government-mandated rights that make it extremely difficult for the employer to remove that person from that individual's position.

An employee classified as temporary, on the other hand, has limited employment rights, and can be removed from the employee's position with limited-to-no notice. Furthermore, temporary employees in many European nations are not entitled to many of the benefits received by permanent employees. It is common for businesses in both European nations and in Russia to make use of temporary contracts whenever possible, because doing so can reduce their labor costs and makes it easier to reengineer their organization, if needed.

The Position Players in Health/Fitness Clubs

The health/fitness club industry requires a diverse array of talent to deliver the experiences that members desire, expect, need, and deserve. As such, clubs must have employees who have an appropriate blend of social/relationship skills and technical expertise. Because the services that clubs provide cover such a broad spectrum of experiences, a vast pool of talent with expertise in a broad range of services is required. Figures 15-3 to 15-5 detail the key positions in the industry and offer a brief synopsis of the responsibilities of each of those positions.

Exempt Employee	Non-Exempt Employee
Must supervise two or more employees.	Usually no supervisory responsibility or less than two.
Must allocate at least 50% of job responsibilities to supervision.	Supervision is less than 50% of the job responsibilities.
A commissioned employee can be exempt if a significant portion of their earnings is commission-based.	More dependent upon a fixed hourly rate of pay for compensation.
Examples: Manager, sales manager, sales person, fitness director, tennis director	Examples: Fitness instructor, program director, front desk staff, massage therapist, accountant

Figure 15-2. Selected differences between exempt and non-exempt employees

As Figures 15-3 to 15-5 illustrate, the health/fitness club industry involves a multiplicity of positions. While the various positions in these figures are detailed in general terms and responsibilities, club operators can decide for themselves whether to develop positions that are consistent with the aforementioned descriptions or make adjustments in the various job specifications and define the positions in slightly different ways.

Position	Description
General manager	Oversees the entire operations of a club, with responsibility for all aspects of the club including membership, accounting, and all operational departments.
Operations manager	Usually found in large club operations. Supervises the operating departments (front desk, house maintenance, pro shop, pools, etc.).
Sales manager	Usually found in larger clubs. Responsible for managing the sales staff and the sales efforts.
Fitness director	Oversees the employees and activities of the fitness department, which includes personal training, fitness floor, and group exercise.
Tennis director	Oversees the employees and activities of the tennis department, often including programming, pro shop, and related tennis activities.
Maintenance director	Found in most clubs. Oversees both maintenance and housekeeping employees and activities. In some clubs, also has responsibility for locker rooms and grounds.
Food and beverage director	In clubs with an F&B function, oversees all aspects of the food and beverage operation, including the employees and activities of the kitchen and dining areas.

Figure 15-3. Selected examples of typical exempt positions in the health/fitness club industry

Position	Description
Activity/program director	Found in larger clubs. Responsible for coordinating all club activities and programs and the employees involved in those endeavors.
Youth director	In clubs with extensive youth programming. Oversees the employees and activities involved in the youth department.
Personal-training director	A mainstay of clubs with large personal-training programs. Oversees the personal trainers and personal-training program.
Group-exercise director	Normally a part-time position, but in large clubs is often a full-time position. Oversees the group-exercise instructors and programs.
Aquatics director	In clubs with a large aquatic program. Oversees the pool and aquatic employees and the aquatic programs and activities.
Controller	In clubs with large accounting departments. Oversees the accounting department employees and the activities of the accounting department.

Figure 15-4. Selected examples of club positions that could be either exempt or non-exempt employees in the health/fitness club industry, depending on the state and federal laws and regulations involving wage and hour requirements for employees in a particular geographic area

Position	Description
Aquatic/swim instructor	Provides swimming instruction for members and guests on individual and group basis.
Personal trainer	Provides fitness instruction and coaching to members for a fee.
Fitness instructor	Provides supervision of the fitness floor, general orientation of members to the fitness centers' equipment and programs, and some personal instruction.
Group-exercise instructor	Teaches group-oriented exercise and fitness programs for members and guests.
Front-desk staff	Works the front desk. Greets members, monitors usage, answers phones, disseminates club information, and schedules appointments for club services.
Accountant/bookkeeper	Handles the basic accounting functions at clubs, including payroll, billing, accounts payable, and accounts receivable.
Maintenance/housecleaning	Provides cleaning, housekeeping, and general maintenance for the club. In many clubs, also handles the basic laundry functions as well.
Locker room	In clubs with large locker rooms, provides the general care and housekeeping of the locker rooms, but also greets members and delivers services, such as shoe shines, laundry, etc.
Child care/nursery	Provides supervision of the youth areas, including the nursery activities, but not licensed day care.
Tennis professional/instructor	Provides individual and group tennis instruction to members and guests. Also supervises leagues, mixers, camps, etc.
Activity instructors	Specialized professionals who provide individual or group instruction/coaching in their respective areas, including the martial arts, gymnastics, squash, racquetball, etc.
Massage therapists	Are professionals who are licensed by the state to provide massage therapy. Can also provide other spa services covered by their training and licensing.
Estheticians	Are professionals who are licensed to provide spa services such as manicures, pedicures, and facials.
Food-and-beverage service staff/waiters	Provide service to members and guests in the food-and-beverage area. May include waiters and bartenders.
Kitchen staff/cooks	Provide the cooking services.
Pilates/yoga instructor	Specialized instructors with advanced certifications to instruct Pilates and yoga on either an individual or group basis.
Lifeguard	Provides supervision of the pool and aquatic areas. Responsible for member/guest safety. May also have basic pool operational responsibilities.

Figure 15-5. Selected examples of non-exempt positions in the health/fitness club industry

Offsite Position Employees in Multiple-Club Operations

With the continued growth of the health/fitness club industry, multiple-club operators represent close to 50 percent of the industry at the present time. The positions of accountability in these multiple-club operations are somewhat similar to those that exist in independent clubs at the club level. On the other hand, when the offsite support of these clubs is considered, the dynamics of employee accountability differ considerably. For example, most multiple-club operations usually allocate between three and eight percent of their total revenues, although in some instances it may amount to as much as 10 percent of total revenues, to non-club or offsite overhead positions. Figure 15-6, while not inclusive, presents an overview of the offsite positions that most commonly exist in multiple-club operations.

Position	Description
Chief Executive Officer (CEO)	The CEO is the leader of the company and responsible for establishing the strategic direction of the company, serving as the public face of the company, involved with the company board, and often actively engaged in the new business development of the company. The CFO, CDO, CIO, and possibly one other position will report to the CEO.
Chief Operating Officer (COO)	The COO position and the position of president are often one in the same. The president/COO takes responsibility for overseeing all aspects of the day-to-day operations of the business, with direct leadership over the levels of management supporting the clubs.
Chief Financial Officer (CFO)	The CFO is responsible for the financial aspects of the business, including cash management, budgeting, financing, financial reporting, etc. The CFO also works closely with the financial stockholders of the business.
Director of Marketing and Sales (Vice President or higher position)	The majority of multiple-club operations have an individual who oversees the marketing and sales efforts of the company. This individual will normally provide strategic direction to the company's marketing and sales efforts and guide the systems used in marketing and sales.
Director of Human Resources (Vice President or higher position)	This individual will normally oversee all aspects of the company's human capital, including employee recruitment and selection, employee development and training, employee benefits, employee resources, etc.
Chief Information Officer (CIO) (Senior Vice President or higher position)	The CIO is responsible for the technology systems and support in the company. This position is involved in both the strategic direction of the company as it relates to technology, but also the oversight of all the employees who support the technology needs of the business.
Chief Development Officer (CDO) (Senior Vice President or higher position)	The CDO is responsible for all aspects of new business development. In many multiple-club operations, this position oversees new business, acquisitions, leasing, and construction.
Regional Operations Director or Vice President of Operations	Multiple-club operations that have a large number of clubs typically assign a freestanding manager who has direct responsibility for the operations of a set group of clubs. Normally, the regional position will oversee between six and 12 clubs, with the mangers of the clubs reporting directly to that position.
Regional Membership Sales Director	The regional membership sales person usually reports directly to the vice president of operations (the regional operations director) and indirectly to the director or vice president of marketing and sales. This position is responsible for sales management for a designated group of clubs, including supporting all corporate initiatives, as well as assisting in the recruiting and training of club sales staff.
Regional Controllers	The regional controller normally reports to either the CFO or the vice president of operations. These individuals are responsible for supporting the club's accounting and bookkeeping staff, as well as assisting in financial reporting for the respective regions of clubs.

Figure 15-6. Selected examples of exempt offsite positions in multiple-club operations

Compensation for Various Positions in the Health/Fitness Club Industry

The degree to which a club can attract and retain great employees is, in large part, dependent upon the package of compensation and benefits it provides. Figures 15-7 to 15-9 illustrate the median compensation levels for both exempt and non-exempt positions in health/fitness clubs over the past few years.

Figure 15-7. Median total compensation for senior managers

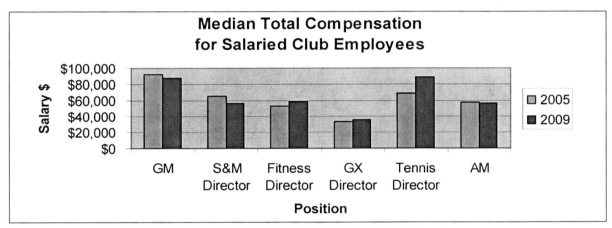

Figure 15-8. Median total compensation for salaried club employees

Figure 15-9. Median hourly rate for club level hourly employees

With regard to exempt club employees, most of these individuals are paid a base salary and receive variable incentive compensation. The variable incentive portion of the compensation tends to be position-specific. For example, in instances involving personal trainers, sales staff, tennis instructors, and spa therapists, compensation can often be composed entirely of commission (i.e., a percentage of the revenues that they generate) or involve an incentive-driven bonus (i.e., a fixed amount for achieving a designated performance target), while those individuals who are serving in exempt-level positions (e.g., managers, fitness directors, spa directors, etc.) are likely to experience a variable-based compensation package that encompasses 10 percent to 50 percent of their total compensation, based on their achieving designated performance metrics. The variable incentive portion normally consists of either a commission-based incentive (e.g., often used for such employees as the sales representatives, tennis directors, fitness directors, etc.) or a bonus, based on achieving predetermined performance targets (e.g., normally targeting individuals such as the CEO, manager, front desk manager, controller, etc.). Ideally, all exempt employees should have a compensation package that includes both a base salary and variable incentive compensation. Those exempt employees who are in sales-related positions, such as individuals working in the membership, tennis, or fitness areas of the club, should have a variable incentive compensation that is tied to their sales performance.

With regard to non-exempt employees, most of these employees are paid an hourly wage, with very few being eligible for variable incentive compensation. Three categories of non-exempt employees in the industry are typically paid on a commission structure: personal trainers, massage therapists/estheticians, and racquet/tennis professionals. These positions are considered commissioned, because the services provided directly drive incremental revenue, which, in turn, is directly impacted by the sales performance of the individual employee. Figure 15-10, based on data from the *IHRSA 2010 Industry Compensation and Benefits Survey*, details the average commissions for personal trainers and sales staff in the health/fitness club industry.

Although IHRSA did not collect data on the compensation level for either massage therapists or estheticians, the International Spa Association (ISPA), in its *2009 U.S. Spa Compensation Survey* reported the following information concerning the compensation of these particular positions:

- On average, 71 percent of the massage therapists earn between $20,000 and $50,000 annually, with 38 percent earning between $30,000 and $50,000. These earnings are based on the therapists working full time. It should be noted that the average massage therapist earns a commission equal to 40 percent to 60 percent of the massage fee.

Position	Basis of Commission		Amount of Commission	
	% Revenue	*Set Fee*	*%*	*Fixed*
Personal trainer	54%	17%	50%	$25
Sales staff	36%	38%	22%	$37

Figure 15-10. Average commissions in the health/fitness club industry for personal trainers and sales staff (2009)

- On average, 64 percent of the estheticians earn $20,000 to $50,000, while the earnings of 40 percent range from $30,000 to $50,000. Estheticians are paid a commission that is similar to that earned by massage therapists.

As a rule, the compensation package that a club offers its employees is based upon a number of factors, including the club's geographic location, its market position, and, most importantly, the level of education and experience it expects its employees to have.

Benefits Provided in the Health/Fitness Club Industry

As discussed previously, benefits are second only to wages in terms of their ability to attract top-performing employees. The primary benefits offered by most club operators include: medical, life insurance, dental, vision, short-term disability, long-term disability, Section 125 plan, employee discounts for services, paid vacations, and educational reimbursement. Some clubs also include additional benefits in the benefits package for their employees, such as domestic-partner insurance and child-care assistance. Figures 15-11 and 15-12 detail several of the major benefits that are offered to both exempt and non-exempt employees in the health/fitness club industry.

Benefit	Fully Paid	Partially Paid	Not Provided
Medical – employee	11%	80%	9%
Medical – family	5%	64%	31%
Life insurance	39%	20%	41%
Dental insurance – employee	15%	58%	27%
Educational assistance	5%	54%	42%
Employee discounts	33%	57%	10%
Section 125 plan	5%	30%	65%

Figure 15-11. Average benefits for exempt employees

Benefit	Fully Paid	Partially Paid	Not Provided
Medical – employee	5%	60%	36%
Medical – family	0%	49%	51%
Life insurance	23%	13%	64%
Dental insurance – employee	5%	44%	52%
Educational assistance	0%	45%	55%
Employee discounts	28%	51%	21%
Section 125 plan	2%	25%	74%

Figure 15-12. Average benefits for non-exempt employees

As a rule, the health/fitness club industry is not as generous with benefits as other industries are, either at the management level or the hourly, non-exempt employee level. As Figure 15-11 illustrates, at the management level, life insurance, medical benefits, and employee discounts are the most commonly offered fully paid benefits in the club industry, while dental benefits and educational assistance are next in line. For non-exempt, hourly employees, Figure 15-12 shows that the most significant, fully-paid benefits that the industry provides to this particular group of employees are medical insurance and employee discounts.

Education and Skill Competency Required of Health/Fitness Club Professionals

The health/fitness club industry is a somewhat unique business when it comes to the required educational and experience competencies of its employees. Some of the positions in the industry that were described earlier in this chapter require a relatively high level of academic qualifications (manager, accountant, fitness director), while others place more focus on the more non-traditional forms of education, such as certification and licensure (personal trainer, group exercise instructor, massage therapist). Still other positions involve a greater emphasis on work experience. The degree to which health/fitness club operators establish high academic/certification or experience standards will determine, to a large extent, their position in both the marketplace and the mindset of the customers that they are attempting to serve. Figures 15-13 and 15-14 provide an overview of the average level of education possessed by specific positions in the industry.

Position	High School	Associate's	Bachelor's	Master's	PhD
Manager	8%	6%	65%	19%	0%
Sales manager	26%	13%	58%	3%	0%
Fitness director	15%	3%	59%	6%	0%
Group exercise director	20%	17%	30%	3%	0%
Tennis director	14%	7%	50%	0%	0%

Figure 15-13. Average level of education in the health/fitness club industry – exempt positions (2009)

Position	Bachelor's	Certifications			
		ACSM	*ACE*	*NASM*	*NSCA*
Personal trainer	40%	49%	60%	46%	40%
Fitness instructor	16%	18%	25%	14%	13%
Group exercise instructor*	16%	16%	52%	8%	8%
*46% of group exercise instructors have AFAA certification					

Figure 15-14. Average level of education in the U.S. health/fitness club industry – professional non-exempt positions (2009)

It is evident that, for most exempt positions, the health/fitness club industry places a relatively high degree of importance on having at least a four-year college degree. As Figure 15-13 illustrates, at least 50 percent to 70 percent of club level exempt professionals (e.g., manager, sales manager, fitness director, assistant manager, etc.) have either a four-year degree or higher. The highest level of education in the industry is possessed by those employees who serve as either managers (19 percent have masters degree or higher) or fitness directors (six percent have masters degree or higher). On the other hand, with regard to the non-exempt professional positions that provide members with instruction in fitness, recreation, or sports-related activities, the existence of a college degree in these employees falls dramatically. Less than 20 percent of fitness instructors and approximately 40 percent of personal trainers in the U.S. have attained a four-year degree. It should be noted that in many European and South American nations, instructors and trainers are required to have a four-year college degree.

❑ *Certification and Education for Fitness Instructors, Group-Exercise Instructors, and Personal Trainers.* Personal trainers, fitness instructors, and group-exercise instructors are the positions within the health/fitness club industry that provide members and guests with instruction, counsel, and advice in fitness- and health-related issues. As such, these non-exempt professionals typically are required to have a basic understanding of exercise physiology, human movement, healthy lifestyle, behavioral change, and nutrition. While the knowledge base that these professionals need is relatively high, the actual practices of the industry often fall way short of requiring these professionals to truly demonstrate that they possess the education and training attendant to such knowledge. As shown in Figure 15-14, 40 percent of personal trainers, 16 percent of fitness instructors, and 16 percent of group-exercise instructors in the U.S. have any four-year college degree, let alone a four-year college degree in an area of study related to either fitness or exercise science. In contrast, it is interesting to note that in some foreign countries, such as Brazil, Portugal, and Russia, an undergraduate degree is, in fact, required for any individual who is providing fitness instruction.

To compensate for the U.S. industry's less-than-emphatic emphasis on these professionals having a college education, the industry has moved toward a certification-based model of competency. In the certification model of competency, fitness professionals are required to demonstrate their overall level of competency by successfully passing the certification requirements for one or more of the various fitness-professional domains (e.g., group-exercise instructor, personal trainer, lifestyle, and weight-management counselor, etc.). As of 2010, over 100 certifications for personal trainers and close to as many certifications for various types of group-exercise instructors existed. In most instances, these certification programs require prospective fitness professionals to sit for either a written exam only or both a written exam and practical exam. As a rule, most of these programs accord certification on those candidates who achieve a score greater than 70 percent on the required examinations. Once certification is achieved, most programs require that the professionals maintain their level of certification by annually earning a predetermined number of continuing education credits.

As of 2010, over 100 certifications for personal trainers and close to as many certifications for various types of group-exercise instructors existed.

In 2003, the International Health, Racquet, and Sportsclub Association (IHRSA) set a benchmark, a much-needed standard for the certification of health/fitness professionals by proclaiming that, effective January 1, 2006, it would only recognize certifications that had third-party accreditation (for example, the National Organization for Competency Assurance [NOCA] and its accreditation arm, the National Commission for Certifying Agencies [NCCA]). A direct link must be demonstrated between the certification offered and the competency requirements of a particular fitness position. As of 2010, many certifying organizations, including such prominent organizations as ACE, ACSM, NASM, and NSCA, have all earned NCCA accreditation for their base certification programs. IHRSA's actions were a necessary first step in bringing greater credibility to these fitness professional positions. Concurrent with IHRSA's position, a number of state legislatures began to push for either licensure or registration of personal trainers. As of January 2011, approximately eight states had initiated legislative action concerning the licensure or registration of personal trainers, a trend that can be expected to continue until the industry establishes criteria that the public and government feels are acceptable. Eventually (hopefully), the combined efforts of IHRSA, the certifying organizations, and state governments should bring about a greater level of demonstrable competency in each of the basic fitness professional positions in the industry. It should be noted that in Europe, the European Health and Fitness Association has established clear standards regarding the competencies that need to be demonstrated by both fitness instructors (private or group instruction) and personal trainers.

As previously discussed, the health/fitness industry currently has more than 100 certification programs for fitness professionals. Figure 15-15 presents an overview of six of the most successful and well-known certification groups for professionals in the health/fitness club industry.

> It is the responsibility of club operators to determine what educational and certification expectations and minimal standards they want to establish for the professionals in their club.

It is important to note that it is the responsibility of club operators to determine what educational and certification expectations and minimal standards they want to establish for the professionals in their club. Whatever levels they establish should be based on a clear understanding of the market's requirements in this regard and the standard of care demonstrated by the industry both as a whole and in their particular area.

Organizational Alignment and Structure in Individual Health/Fitness Clubs

It is important that independent club operators utilize and understand the various types of organizational structures that can effectively sustain accountability throughout the organization. The organizational structure a club chooses to employ is critical to establishing the flow of accountability and information that is essential if it is to achieve and maintain the desired level of profitability. Toward that end, an appropriate organizational structure helps to clarify the role of each employee, both in terms of personal and team responsibility.

Certifying Group	Sampling of Certifications	Description
American College of Sports Medicine (ACSM)	Health/Fitness Instructor Exercise Specialist Personal Trainer Clinical Exercise Physiologist	ACSM certifications have been in existence for over 30 years. Its certifications are developed by physiologists, health-care specialists, and physicians who are active members of the college. It offers both preventative tract and clinical tract certifications. As a rule, the certifications tend not to be for entry-level fitness professionals.
American Council on Exercise (ACE)	Group Fitness Instructor Personal Trainer Lifestyle and Weight Management Consultant Clinical Exercise Specialist Advanced Personal Trainer	ACE certifications have been in existence for over 20 years. ACE certifies more professionals than any other agency in the fitness industry. ACE is an industry leader in promoting exercise. Its certifications are targeted for entry-level fitness professionals.
Aerobics and Fitness Association of America (AFAA)	Primary Group Exercise Personal Fitness Trainer Fitness Practitioner	AFAA certifications have been in existence for over 25 years. AFAA currently certifies more group-exercise professionals than any other organization. Its offerings represent a front-line certification for entry-level fitness professionals.
National Academy of Sports Medicine (NASM)	Group Trainer Personal Trainer Performance Enhancement Specialist Sports Fitness Specialist	NASM has been in existence for over 10 years. Its certification program has a physical therapy/athletic trainer focus that places more emphasis on the instruction of modalities for flexibility and muscular strength and endurance. Its certifications are geared for both entry-level professionals and higher levels.
National Strength and Conditioning Association (NSCA)	Certified Strength and Conditioning Specialist (CSCS) Certified Personal Trainer (CPT)	NSCA's first certification was awarded over 20 years ago. NSCA's initial certification efforts focused on resistance training and conditioning for athletes. By the early 1990s, it created the personal trainer certification, which focused on the skills of prescriptive resistance training for average people.
Cooper Clinic	Physical Fitness Specialist Specialty Certifications for Biomechanics of Resistance Training, Optimal Performance Training, and Pre/Post Natal Fitness Instructor	The Cooper Clinic and Aerobic Activity Center, founded by Dr. Kenneth Cooper in the 1970s, has been offering a variety of professional certifications since its inception. The certifications range from fitness instructor to specialty certifications in such areas as back care, resistance training, weight management, etc.

Figure 15-15. Examples of certifying agencies in the health/fitness club industry

Figures 15-16 and 15-17 illustrate two different organizational structures that an individual club could utilize. Figure 15-16 depicts an organizational structure for a purely fitness club, while Figure 15-17 portrays a structure for a multipurpose club that offers racquet sports and aquatics.

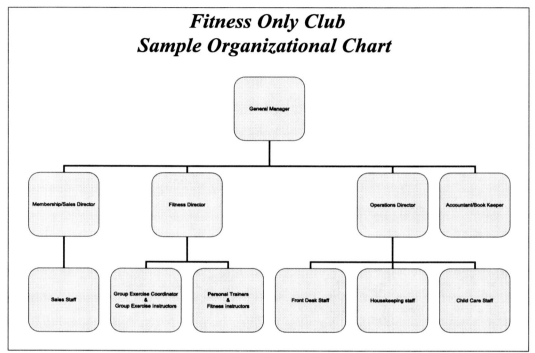

Figure 15-16. A sample fitness-club organization chart

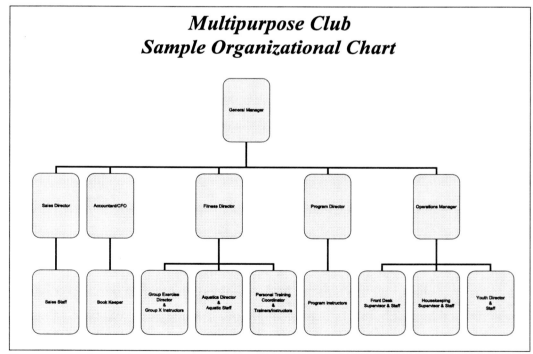

Figure 15-17. A sample multipurpose-club organization chart

The examples in Figures 15-16 and 15-17 are representative of the most common organizational structures that are utilized by individual health/fitness clubs. It is important to consider the following three critical success factors when designing a club's organizational structure:

❑ *Drive Accountability Close to the Member by Maintaining a Flat Organizational Structure.* In other words, the number of organizational layers between the member and the manager should be kept at a minimum. In the two aforementioned organizational structures, there are instances when the customer is only two layers away from the manager (sales) and other instances where the member is three layers away (personal trainers). All factors considered, the flatter the club's organizational chart, the closer the club brings accountability to the member. To achieve this objective, the club's employees need to be fully empowered.

❑ *Limit Direct Reports for any Supervisor.* Research in organizational management has determined that supervisors can be most effective if they have no more than six to eight direct reports and preferably less. If the club has a structure that requires leaders/supervisors to have too many direct reports, then it will find that these leaders/supervisors are far less effective in creating a high-performing, empowered environment for their direct reports.

❑ *Don't Create Titles; Create Accountabilities.* All too often, club management creates organizational positions to provide reward and recognition for employees. While this practice might seem like a good idea, an organizational structure should be built around the roles and the accountabilities needed to drive the club's success. As a result, all factors considered, it is often better to create fewer positions rather than more.

All factors considered, it is often better to create fewer positions rather than more.

If club operators take the aforementioned three factors into consideration, they will find it easier to create an organizational structure that supports their business objectives, without placing excessive financial and communicative strain on the organization.

Organizational Alignment and Structure in a Multiple-Club Operation

For multiple-club operations, the alignment of organizational accountabilities and positions is a sensitive issue. Since the cost of offsite overhead in a multiple-club operation can place a significant strain on club earnings (between three and eight percent of revenues), a need exists to create an organizational structure that brings accountability as close to the club employees as possible and at the lowest possible cost, while also providing the logistical and strategic resources that are essential to support the operations of each club. The three critical success factors previously detailed for establishing the organizational structure for a single club also apply to the organizational structure of a multiple-club operation. Figure 15-18 provides an example of a multiple-club organization chart. This sample organizational chart is representative of a typical multiple-club operation, with only the number of direct reports varying, depending upon the size of the company. A multiple-club operator, such as Western Athletic

Clubs, that has 10 clubs, will have a smaller and flatter organizational chart than either a company, like Lifetime Fitness, that has over 90 clubs, or a much larger company, like 24 Hour Fitness, that has over 375 clubs. It is important to note that as the number of clubs within the organization grows, the greater the number of organizational layers that tend to appear. Accordingly, while the Western Athletic Clubs may only have one or two regional operational managers, 24 Hour Fitness might need as many as 15 to 20.

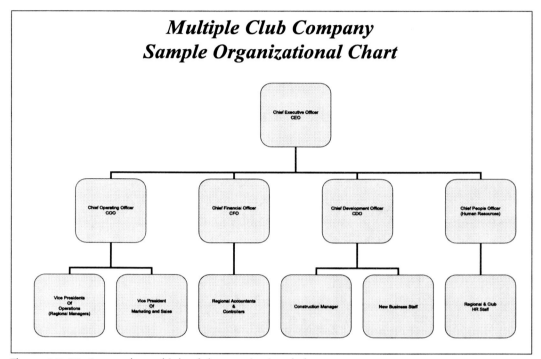

Figure 15-18. A sample multiple-club organizational chart

16

Building and Leading a Successful Health/Fitness Club Team

Chapter Objectives

According to the article, the "Service Profit Chain," written by Leonard Schlessinger, profit is driven by great service to the customer, which, in turn, is driven by a great employee team that is the recipient of great internal service from management. In that regard, this chapter examines the process of creating an exceptional health/fitness club team. Initially, the four "E's" of developing an extraordinary team are discussed. Next, the role of recruiting and selecting team players is reviewed. Then, the underlying principles and concepts attendant to effective leadership are detailed. Finally, the chapter addresses two very important issues: determining job descriptions and developing compensation agreements that provide an incentive for high-performing team players.

The Four "E's" of Building a Great Team

The process of building a great employee team is one of the most important responsibilities that management has. The process of team development is neither an easy undertaking nor a short one. Rather, it is a task that requires an understanding of the critical stepping-stones that need to be laid in order to build a strong team foundation and provide the basic roots that are needed for a continual evolution and empowerment of the team. The four "E's" are a relatively easy-to-remember tool that outlines four key steps in the team-building process. In order to be better prepared to build a great team, it is essential for club managers to be aware of and sensitive to the key factors attendant to the four "E's": expectations, equipping, encouragement, and evaluation.

❏ *Expectations—Setting the Course for the Team.* The club's first step in building its team of employees is to establish clear expectations for both individual and team performance. Without clear expectations, individuals and teams will not have the direction that they need to be successful. Among the components that are essential for creating clear expectations in that regard are the following:

> In order to be better prepared to build a great team, it is essential for club managers to be aware of and sensitive to the key factors attendant to the four "E's": expectations, equipping, encouragement, and evaluation.

All employees should be given a copy of their personal performance goals that are updated on at least a six-month cycle.

- *Provide each team member with an introduction to the club's core values and philosophies.* These values and philosophies serve as the core foundation of the decision-making process. Families, relationships, cultures, and businesses should have a set of common values that each member respects and lives by. If the club wants its team to be strong, it must ensure that the team is values-oriented.

- *Provide each team member with a job model, a copy of the club's organizational chart, and a listing of each individual's personal annual performance goals.* The job model should detail the specific accountabilities of the employee's position, as well as the manner in which that position interacts with the other members of the team. In addition, all employees should be given a copy of their personal performance goals that are updated on at least a six-month cycle. Collectively, these documents should help eliminate any confusion or misunderstandings concerning each person's accountabilities as either an individual or a team member. The organization chart should help clarify each team player's role and how the team members should interact with each other and work as a single, functioning unit.

- *Have a clear set of employee policies and rules.* While policies and rules can be relatively brief in scope, they play an essential role as a means of helping communicate the expectations of the business concerning employee and team behavior. Together with the club's core values, they set the framework for the behavior of the team.

- *Provide each employee with a personal development plan.* The personal development plan is a relatively simple tool that helps an employee to establish a path for professional development. By helping each employee set a course for such growth, the club is facilitating the team's overall development and, at the same time, creating a succession plan that will have team members ready to take on new roles when and if needed.

- *Have regular meetings of the team.* Team meetings are critical to setting and supporting the club's expectations. These meetings should be viewed as an opportunity to reinforce expectations, share achievements, and create new directions. They are also a time to build team trust.

- *Develop new tools to share the club's expectations with the team.* Newsletters, videos, weekly line-ups, and web pages for employees are all methods that can be employed to share the expectations and the performance achievements of a team with its members.

❑ *Equipping the Team Through Education and Growth.* The second step in building a great team is to provide an environment that equips the members of the team to successfully undertake and fulfill the club's expectations. Too many businesses mistakenly assume that once their expectations have been defined, their employees will proceed to successfully achieve them. In reality, the process is not automatic. Rather, club owners and operators should provide the members of their teams with the resources that they need to meet both theirs and the team's expectations. This process is commonly referred to as "equipping the team" and includes the following:

- *Institute an internal formal-education system for all employees.* In this instance, a formal educational program refers to a standardized program that educates all of a club's employees on its values, philosophies, policies, traditions, and basic operating systems. Every new employee and even the tenured employees should go through a formal education system that constantly updates the employee's knowledge of the club's business and expectations. At ClubCorp, this system was called Star Education. All employees were expected to complete the Star Education Program and become certified in their assigned specific area of responsibility. At the Russian Fitness Group, the company has a training director who assists the company and various department supervisors in developing and implementing educational programs that can help facilitate the professional development of the employees.

- *Establish an external continuing-education program for the enhancement of each team member's technical, sales, and people skills.* Beyond its own education system, the club should develop and implement a system that affords its employees the opportunity to pursue continuing education that can help them advance their technical skills, sales skills, and people skills. For fitness employees, this process could involve several measures, such as bringing in outside speakers to discuss technical topics, offering scholarships or shared funds that would enable the fitness professional to attend industry-sponsored workshops, etc. For employees in other areas of interest, this undertaking could involve such steps as bringing in sales trainers or individuals to speak on customer service. The key point to note in this regard is that educational efforts, such as these, can play an important role in developing a strong team.

- *Provide the tools that employees need to do their jobs.* One of the biggest mistakes that club operators can make is to set expectations for their team and then not provide the tools that their employees need to get the job done. In this instance, tools refer to the assets/resources that are essential to completing a particular task. For example, if a piece of equipment is needed to do a job, that resource is provided. By the same token, if a job requires access to certain information, then that information is made available. All factors considered, the most powerful and valuable tool that a team can have is information. Accordingly, the club should ensure that its employees are able to access the information that they need to be able to do their job.

- *Open the communication lines.* Club management should make sure that the club has an open communication process that allows its employees to ask questions of management and share comments with management. The process should also make it relatively easy for management to share ideas, results, and feedback with its employees. As a rule, the greater the degree to which these lines of communication are opened up, the better the flow of information and resources will be between the team and management.

- *Walk the talk.* The axiom that leaders should act in a manner that is consistent with what they espouse has been around for a long time.

One of the biggest mistakes that club operators can make is to set expectations for their team and then not provide the tools that their employees need to get the job done.

Many club employees feel that one of the most important tools that the club has to equip them to perform their duties is to know that management is willing to perform those same responsibilities.

❏ *Encouragement—The Fuel of Champions.* The next step in building a great team is to create an environment that encourages employees to take ownership in their own and their team's performance. Such an environment should also reward the club's employees when certain process and outcome goals are achieved. Encouragement is normally a blend of strategies, including:

- *Have a formal employee-recognition program.* Formal recognition programs are an effective method for fostering an environment of reward and encouragement. The focus of a formal employee-recognition program should be to reward employees for performing in a manner that is consistent with the club's core values and delivering upon the team's expectations. At ClubCorp, this program was called Star Recognition, and they rewarded employees on the basis of how well they delivered on the company's values and philosophies. At the Russian Fitness Group, they had several awards that recognize employees, including the "Legends" award to recognize those employees whose efforts over the long haul had a significant impact on the success and reputation of the organization. Other clubs undertake efforts that attempt to provide a similar level of recognition, for example employee-of-the-month programs, employee-of-the-week programs, etc. Some key elements of an employee-recognition program include:
  ✓ The program should focus on objective measures so that it is consistent from one employee to the other.
  ✓ The program should be designed to encourage employees to deliver on the values and standards of the business.
  ✓ The program should have employee ownership, such as an employee committee that oversees its conduct.
  ✓ The rewards provided by the program should be relevant to the employees, not merely what management feels that the employees would value.
  ✓ The delivery of the program should be consistent.

- *Leaders must be cheerleaders.* According to Ken Blanchard, in his best-selling book, *The One-Minute Manager*, management should catch employees doing things right. As a rule, the best encouragement that employees can receive is the personal recognition that comes from a leader recognizing their efforts and providing them with a thank you and job well done. When employees talk about encouraging environments, they often speak about the personal recognition that they receive from their managers/leaders. In the 80s and 90s at ClubCorp, Robert Dedman, Sr., the company founder and chairman, made a habit of writing personal notes to company employees, thanking them for their efforts. These notes were treasured by those employees who received them. Accordingly, leaders should make it a habit to walk the club, looking for employees who are doing great things and then letting those

> The focus of a formal employee-recognition program should be to reward employees for performing in a manner that is consistent with the club's core values and delivering upon the team's expectations.

employees know how much their efforts are appreciated. Another key factor is to make sure that other employees see the encouragement provided by management.

- *Have recognition meetings.* Another valuable tool that the club can utilize to provide encouragement is to hold open meetings with its employees, during which the results of the club's performance are shared and discussed. At the Russian Fitness Group, quarterly meetings are held at which the employees whose contributions made a difference in the attainment of company goals are recognized and honored. Sharing the results in an open setting and letting the employees know how much the club values their efforts creates an open and honest team environment, which is a critical factor in encouraging employees to do their best.

- *Avoid finger pointing.* One of the easiest approaches to creating an environment of encouragement is to foster a workplace that does not condone finger pointing and blaming. Instead, it fosters a workplace focus on solutions. In that regard, leadership should cultivate an environment where employees are not afraid to make mistakes. Rather, employees should be willing to take risks and should have a sense of ownership toward addressing key issues, because they realize that no blame will be placed as long as they act in a professional manner.

❑ *Evaluate the Expected.* The final step in the four "E's" is evaluation. If the club wants its employees to succeed both individually and collectively, it needs to establish an evaluation system that measures what is expected of its employees and provides constructive feedback for their continuous growth. Among the key evaluation tools that a club should consider in this regard are the following:

- *Create objective performance evaluations for each employee.* Each employee should have a performance evaluation that is tailored to the specific performance goals set forth in their job model. The evaluation tool should be specific to each employee and include the measurement of both the personal goals and team goals in which the individual employee has a role.

- *Evaluate at least twice a year.* Performance evaluations are most effective if they are done at least twice annually. The longer the club waits between performance evaluations, the less likely it will be able to create a link in the employee's mind between what the club expects and what feedback is being provided to each employee.

- *Make it a habit to evaluate daily.* Leaders need to actively engage in the evaluation process by walking around the club. If they observe behavior that warrants their feedback, the best time to provide comments of any kind is to do so immediately.

- *Create a business scorecard.* To help facilitate the team's performance, leaders should develop a club business scorecard that every employee can understand. This scorecard should be to help assess team performance, as well as communicate recognition and education. The scorecard can be incorporated as part of every meeting to either recognize the team or educate it. The scorecard should be more than

If the club wants its employees to succeed both individually and collectively, it needs to establish an evaluation system that measures what is expected of its employees and provides constructive feedback for their continuous growth.

One of the biggest challenges in any business, and in particular the club industry, is building a great team.

a financial tool. Rather, it should help evaluate the performance of the club's employees against the core values and standards of operation of the business.

- *Never let performance go without recognition, education, and follow-up.* If the club's managerial staff sees good performance, they should make sure that the individual or team is recognized and rewarded. By the same token, if they see performance that falls below their expectations, they should acknowledge the performance misstep, educate the employee involved about how to improve it, and then follow-up to make sure that the individual's performance has changed appropriately.

Recruiting and Selecting the Club's Team

One of the biggest challenges in any business, and in particular the club industry, is building a great team. Before the aforementioned four steps to building a great team can be undertaken, however, the club needs to have the right people as employees. The easiest way to build a great team is to hire great employees, a practice approach that requires a systematic approach to recruiting and selecting the best available employees to serve on the team. In this regard, the following factors apply:

Recruitment

❑ *Develop a Hiring Model and Posting for Each Position.* The first step in recruiting is to create a model of what the employee profile should be. A hiring model is a shortened version of the job model that identifies the values, attitudes, and skills expected for each position.

❑ *Place the Postings/Models in the Appropriate Areas.* When the club is ready to recruit, the club should make sure that it places its hiring models/posting with the right lead sources, including:

- Local two-year and four-year colleges can be excellent sources of employees. If the club is looking for fitness staff, it should contact the college's kinesiology department. On the other hand, if it is looking to hire swim instructors, it should get in touch with the coach of the college's swim team.
- The ad seeking new employees should be posted on the appropriate career-center websites for the respective specialty areas. For example, when the club is seeking to hire fitness staff, the websites of ACSM, ACE, NSCA, and IHRSA would be excellent sources. If massage and spa employees were wanted, the club should contact any institution/entity that might be aware of individuals who would accommodate the club's needs, such as the local massage schools, the American Massage Therapy Association, etc.
- The club should consider creating a career center on its website. Companies, such as 24 Hour Fitness, ClubCorp, Equinox, Fitness First, Lifetime Fitness, and Virgin Active, have developed their own recruitment sites, as have some independent clubs, such as the Eastbank Club in Chicago, and Gainesville Health and Fitness in Gainesville, Florida.

❑ *Develop Internship Programs With Colleges*. Possibly the best recruiting tool is to develop an internship program with local colleges and high schools. By creating internships, the club can provide learning opportunities for those students who have an interest in fitness and health and, at the same time, give the club a chance to evaluate each intern's potential as a future employee. In fact, many of the top club companies in the industry offer internships. These companies report finding that their best employees often are those individuals who have previously served in internships. IHRSA has developed an internship manual that clubs can utilize to help implement a successful internship program.

❑ *Recruit From Other Service Industries*. If a club is seeking people who have a servant's heart and understand how to work within a hospitality/service business, it should consider recruiting from similar businesses. The recruiter should carry business cards and, if and when they observe a worker whose performance aligns with the club's culture, hand the worker a card and invite that individual to visit the club. Over the years, I have personally made it a habit to leave my business card with those employees of other organizations whom I feel represent the type of employee we wanted in our company.

Selection

❑ *Compare Applications and Resumes to the Hiring Model*. The first step that a club should take when deciding whom to hire is to compare every application and resume, via a checklist, with its hiring model. Clubs can subsequently rank the applications and resumes by how closely they align with the hiring model. Performing this step allows the club to limit the number of candidates it takes to the next step of the selection process. Clubs can employ this method to identify those applicants who most closely reflect their hiring model.

> The first step that a club should take when deciding whom to hire is to compare every application and resume, via a checklist, with its hiring model.

❑ *Use Multiple Interviews*. Every candidate under consideration should go through a series of interviews. The first interview should be conducted by the immediate supervisor and should focus on uncovering the basic values, beliefs, attitudes, and skills of the applicant. This first interview can be conducted using a structured interview format and checklist. The goal of the interview should be to evaluate the candidate against a specific model. While most initial interviews are conducted in person, a growing trend is to conduct the first interview over the phone, over Skype, or even in a virtual environment, such as Second Life. If the candidate meets the expectations of the first interview, then a second interview should be conducted with multiple members of the team, using a structured format. The second interview should be more detailed than the first and should focus on role-play situations, based on predetermined questions that are designed to be value indicators of success in the club business. If the candidate gets through the second interview successfully, then the third interview should be conducted in a team format with several members of the team present. This interview can be more free-flowing than the other two, because its primary focus is to determine if an appropriate fit exists between the team and the applicant.

❑ *Consider an Industry Profile.* Many club operators employ personality and job-profile surveys that are designed to help compare the candidate's personal profile against the known attitudes and attributes of a successful employee. These profiles, typically used with senior-level employees, are usually available through human-resource organizations and private companies that are focused on profiling new employees. As a rule, these profiles measure such key attributes as leadership, communication, teamwork, work ethic, relationship skills, etc. By comparing the profile of a candidate with the standardized profile of a top-performing employee, the club can obtain a better reading of the candidate's potential for success.

❑ *Only Hire From the Top of the List.* After completing all of the aforementioned steps, the club should develop a list of potential candidates, with the best candidate placed at the top and the others ranked in a priority order. Leaders should make an effort to let their team help compile the rankings. Once the rankings are completed, they should initiate the selection process by contacting the candidate at the top of the list.

Leadership

> Over the years, teachers, scholars, and philosophers have attempted to provide a variety of definitions for leadership and have put forth a seemingly endless abundance of theories on what it takes to be an effective leader.

Leadership has been a topic of discussion for decades. In both large business organizations and small businesses, one of the most common concerns is their perception that they don't have enough good leadership. In fact, this issue is often ranked as the number one perceived weakness in most organizations. Over the years, teachers, scholars, and philosophers have attempted to provide a variety of definitions for leadership and have put forth a seemingly endless abundance of theories on what it takes to be an effective leader. One factor that seems to be a common thread among all the definitions and theories on leadership is that organizations that want to be successful need leaders at all levels of the organization. This section is not intended to provide a detailed description of leadership or any particular style of leadership. Rather, its primary goal is to present an overview of what leadership is, how leadership impacts the club business, and how every employee of a club, from fitness instructors to managers, can develop the basic attributes of leadership.

❑ *The Role of Leaders.* The primary responsibility of leaders is to determine the culture and goals of the business and help establish an environment in which every employee takes ownership in living the culture and achieving the goals. Realistically, an effective leader might be defined as an individual who is able to influence the passion, vision, and commitment of others in order to channel the efforts and talents of individuals who are going separate directions into a cohesive team of employees who are functioning as a single unit. Among the roles that leaders most often assume in an organization, such as a health/fitness club, are the following:

• To establish a compelling vision and culture for the business. This role is most often assumed by the primary club leader (e.g., owner or manager). The vision and the culture serve as the foundation for the success that the business achieves.

• To communicate the culture and vision of the club every day. This role should not just involve the club's top leader, but also every employee who interacts with and has responsibility for the behavior of another employee.

- To develop a team of employees who will take ownership in a common vision and goal by seeing how working together benefits both the individual and the team.
- To demonstrate trust in their team and, in return, gain the respect and trust of their team.
- To build consensus when appropriate, but also to make tough decisions when they are needed.
- To see themselves as servants for their team by providing a vision, the support, and the resources that their team needs to achieve the club's vision and goals.
- To set the course, provide guidance along the way, remove barriers, build bridges, leverage talent, recognize the need for change, and hold people and teams accountable for their actions.
- Challenge the status quo by seeking to identify and execute business strategies that can enhance the efficiency and quality of their business.

Within every club, these roles should be assumed by those employees who are entrusted to work with other employees.

❑ *The Qualities of Leaders.* Great leaders who can take on the aforementioned roles and successfully execute them often exhibit certain basic qualities, including:

- *Dare to be different.* Daring to be different involves capitalizing on whatever is unique about the individual in such a way that it positively impacts the business. Having attributes (e.g., passion, creativity, vision, imagination, etc.) that can be leveraged to the advantage of the business are an important trait of all leaders.
- *Emotional intelligence.* Great leaders have the ability to sense what is occurring in the business environment around them. This instinct does not emanate from the ability to analyze the impact of relevant numbers on the situation. Rather, it involves having the ability to sense the soft data and the emotions of the people and then being able to interpret that information to the benefit of the organization. Leaders with emotional intelligence are sensitive to the emotions of their staff members and are able to openly discuss these emotions with these individuals as they relate to the work environment. Emotional intelligence also requires the ability to listen without prejudice, to hear what is actually being communicated.
- *Empathy with strength.* Great leaders have the ability to communicate through their actions to their employees that they care about them. Empathetic leaders demonstrate genuine care about the members of the team and are legitimately interested in the work that their employees do. This empathy evolves not only from respect and trust, but also from the ability to deal with each employee in an honest and ethical manner.
- *Reveal their weaknesses.* Great leaders realize that all other factors being equal, they can enhance the level of trust in the organization by being

> Great leaders have the ability to communicate through their actions to their employees that they care about them.

Leaders understand that people manage themselves. Leaders understand that their job is to create and support systems that enable people not only to manage themselves, but also to achieve the expectations set forth for them by the business.

willing to show their weaknesses to other individuals in the organization. Revealing weakness involves the ability to let their team know that they are willing to take accountability for their actions and behaviors, rather than hiding them. Exposing their own personal limitations also enables leaders to surround themselves with people whose strengths can counterbalance the weaknesses exhibited by the leaders. In other words, leaders who are willing to lay bare their weaknesses are not threatened by the strengths of others. Instead, they are able and prefer to utilize the strengths of others to strengthen the team.

- *Manage systems, not people.* Leaders understand that people manage themselves. Leaders understand that their job is to create and support systems that enable people not only to manage themselves, but also to achieve the expectations set forth for them by the business. A leader ensures that systems are in place that will allow the goals of the business to be accomplished and then empowers employees to leverage those systems for the benefit of the organization.

- *Let the people lead.* Leaders understand that if, figuratively, they get out of the way and let the members of the team lead, then everyone will be successful. In other words, effective leaders are able to get everyone to take ownership of the business. They are also able to establish a work environment that enables the individual skill-sets of each employee to link together. In essence, each employee becomes a leader of the team's other employees, with each person headed in the same direction. As such, the process involves creating leadership disciples.

❑ *Characteristics of Great Managers.* Great managers build great teams and produce great results. As a rule, great managers in the health/fitness club industry possess the following characteristics:

- *They plan for success.* One attribute that all great managers have is that they have a plan for success at their club. In other words, they develop a comprehensive plan that identifies specific objectives for their business, including quantitative benchmarks for such areas as membership growth, revenue growth, expense control, people development, marketing, community development, and facility enhancement. Each objective is stated in relatively simple terms with clearly definable, measurable targets and is subsequently communicated to all members of that person's team. The plan includes a detailed financial budget that delineates specific financial targets for each aspect of the business. As such, great managers leave nothing to chance.

- *They know their numbers.* Great managers always seem to know their facility's numbers. In other words, they know what the budgeted targets are for every possible area of importance in their club and are aware of how well their facility is doing with regard to these key parameters on a daily, weekly, and monthly basis. Want to know what their club's membership retention level is—just ask them. Want to know what their facility's payroll percentage is—just ask them.

- *They are coaches and educators.* One of the most notable characteristics of great managers is how much time that they spend with their "people." The employees of great managers tend to speak very highly of them, particularly how they have helped them grow both professionally and personally. These manager-coaches make sure that all of their employees know the club's business plan, ensure that employees know they care about them, and expend substantial time teaching and counseling their employees. Great managers educate, motivate, and inspire their employees.

- *They get their hands dirty.* Great managers are someone who will do any job in the club, whether it is working the front desk, teaching a class, or cleaning the locker room. They do not see themselves as being above the fray. Whatever the situation, they are willing to "get their hands dirty." It is not that they spend a lot of time performing a particular task; rather it's that they do the job when it is needed, the way it should be done. In the process, they set the perfect example for their staff.

- *They have great relationships with the members.* When members stop by the manager's office or approach that person on the floor to converse, that manager probably has a positive relationship with the club's members. Great managers tend to make it a practice of getting close to the membership and building trust between the club's management and its members. In that regard, they try to learn (and remember) the members' names and get somewhat knowledgeable about the members' families. They express sincere interest in the members—particularly how each member is doing in the club, how well the facility is treating the person, etc.

- *They have an open door.* Individuals who want to know if the club has a great manager should just go to the manager's office. Great managers have an open-door policy in which they maintain an environment that encourages employees and members alike to approach them about their concerns—good or bad. Those managers who try to hide behind their office door have neither the courage nor the wisdom to fulfill their assigned role. Confident, successful managers, on the other hand, do not set such barriers. Rather, they make every effort to ensure that their club's members and employees know that they are there to support them and assist them.

- *They are sponges for learning.* Great managers make it a habit to continually expand their horizons. They are aware of the need for lifelong learning. They make a commitment to establish an organization with a suitable environment for group learning. They accept the value of critical thinking. They understand that learning is reciprocal. They exhibit a number of characteristics, including a thirst for relevant knowledge concerning the industry and their organization, a desire to learn, and a willingness to be teachable.

- *They are sales people.* Great managers seem to have an affinity for selling—not the hard-core approach to selling, but rather the understanding that every relationship is an opportunity for selling. These managers build upon their relationships with other people to identify opportunities to make their members aware of the fact that the facility has offerings (services, programs, and products) that they may need. Managers who are sales people are able to create an environment that

Great managers seem to have an affinity for selling— not the hard-core approach to selling, but rather the understanding that every relationship is an opportunity for selling.

encourages every employee to see themselves as a "sales person." Great managers emphasize the point that sales is about identifying the needs of the members and then providing a service that fulfills that need.

- *They are passionate.* Anything worth doing is seldom achieved without passion. In that regard, great managers are incredibly passionate about the health/fitness club business. In a very real sense, passion is the lubricant of their success. They have the ability to exercise sound judgment, control their emotions, be passionate about what they do, and be aware of the tremendous value of a physically active lifestyle.

- *They know the competitors.* Great managers know their competition. They know everything about them, from their facilities to the way that they program their clubs. They subscribe to one of the basic principles highlighted in Sun Tzu's Art of War, which essentially states, "Keep your allies close and your enemies even closer." A tendency exists among some managers to criticize and belittle their competitors. Rather, they should learn from them and take advantage of their good ideas.

A tendency exists among some managers to criticize and belittle their competitors. Rather, they should learn from them and take advantage of their good ideas.

❑ *The Situational Leadership Model.* For the first-time supervisor or manager, the responsibility of leadership can be overwhelming. While the attributes detailed in the previous sections are essential to great leadership, a person who is new to the obligations that leadership entails cannot develop and refine all of those qualities overnight. For those novice leaders, the model of situation leadership, as presented in Ken Blanchard's best-selling book, *The One Minute Manager and Leadership*, can be an excellent tool. Blanchard's model of leadership reviews the following four styles of leadership and details how they can be applied with different employee populations:

- *Directive leadership.* This style of leadership is most effective when undertaken with new employees, as well as with other employees whose knowledge of the job (i.e., skill level/technical expertise of job) and its expectations are relatively low and their desire to achieve is high. The leader needs to provide direction to these individuals concerning how the job should be performed. This direction might be presented in several formats, including checklists, regular meetings, teaching, goal setting, etc.

- *Coaching leadership.* This style of leadership is most effective when utilized with those employees who have garnered a relatively strong understanding of the job and whose level of desire or passion may have waned slightly. As a rule, these individuals are usually more tenured employees who have yet to achieve an empowered status, as an outgrowth of their skill, passion, and understanding of the job. With these employees, the leader should listen to the employee, be supportive of the employee's efforts, and if needed, provide the direction or goals for the job to get done.

- *Supportive leadership.* This style of leadership is usually employed with employees and teams of employees who have the knowledge, experience, and an understanding of what needs to occur in the workplace. With these employees, the leader must listen, support, and facilitate change. This style is not about giving direction; rather, it involves facilitating interaction and supporting the employees, and only stepping in if needed.

- *Delegating leadership*. This style of leadership is appropriate for use with employees and teams who are knowledgeable, experienced, focused, and passionate. With these employees, the leader is focused on providing an environment of trust and handing over the reigns of leadership. This type of leadership involves fully empowering employees and letting them lead.

It is important to understand that each style of leadership is applicable to every employee. While it might appear that the needs of each employee would dictate that a specific style of leadership be utilized, it is far more likely that each employee will require each of these styles at different times over the course of their employment. Occasions will arise when an employee or team needs to be directed, while at other times, those same individuals will need to be coached, supported, or delegated. It is the role of the leader to know which style to use and when to use it. This responsibility can involve several factors, including emotional intelligence, empathy, and being open to and in touch with the work environment.

Developing Job Descriptions and Compensation Agreements for Employees

As previously discussed, one of the keys to building a team is providing each employee with a job description (model) and a compensation agreement. These two documents are two of the most critical tools in establishing expectations, offering encouragement, and providing evaluation. In reality, the job description and compensation agreement are not documents, as much as they are living roadmaps for the employee.

> The job model is a roadmap for the employee, because it points out the expectations that the club has for a particular job (position) and details how that job interacts with the other members of the team.

❑ *Building the Job Model*. The job model is a roadmap for the employee, because it points out the expectations that the club has for a particular job (position) and details how that job interacts with the other members of the team. Building a job model involves the following steps:
- *Begin with the job overview*. The first part of the job model is a simple paragraph that summarizes the primary responsibilities and accountabilities of the job. This narration should be clear and direct.
- *Identify whether the position is exempt or non-exempt*. The job model should detail how the various positions in the club are to be categorized. For example, a fitness director would be an exempt position, while a personal trainer would be a non-exempt position.
- *List the essential accountabilities of the job*. The essential accountabilities of the position involve the top five behaviors/areas for which the employee will be held accountable. Collectively, these factors should reflect the big picture. For example, employees might be held accountable for their department achieving its annual budget target for revenues.
- *List the secondary accountabilities*. Secondary accountabilities involve those areas/behaviors over and beyond the aforementioned essential

accountabilities for which the club will hold the employee accountable. These areas are not tasks; rather, they are areas of accountability. For example, employees might be held accountable for completing their work schedule each week.

- *Identify the reporting lines*. This factor involves clarifying whom employees report directly to, whom the employees have indirect reporting responsibility to, and whom they supervise (if anyone). For example, an employee might report to the operations manager, but is expected to work with the fitness director when needed, and is responsible for the personal trainers.

- *Identify the physical requirements of the job*. This stipulation is an OSHA requirement. It involves identifying the specific physical tasks, such as lifting, walking, etc., that a particular job requires.

- *Identify the educational expectations for the position*. This measure refers to the fact that the club should provide a listing of any educational requirements for the position, such as certifications, licenses, etc.

Several examples of job models that are employed in the health/fitness club industry, which can help illustrate what a completed job model might look like, are included in the appendix of this book.

> **Every employee should receive a written compensation agreement, in addition to a copy of the job model for the position.**

❑ *Building the Compensation Agreement*. Every employee should receive a written compensation agreement, in addition to a copy of the job model for the position. A compensation agreement is a non-binding understanding of the compensation that will be provided for performing the duties expected of a specific position, rather than a contract for employment. On the other hand, it should be noted that in many European countries, the compensation agreement is actually a contract of employment. The compensation agreement should be consistent with the accountabilities of the job and spell out in detail for the employees exactly how they derive their personal earnings. Building a compensation agreement can involve several critical elements, including:

- *Non-exempt hourly employees*:
  - ✓ Identify their hourly wage and share with them the changes in that rate for overtime and holiday work.
  - ✓ Identify what benefits they are eligible for as a non-exempt employee.
  - ✓ If employees are being paid by commission only, make sure that the commission structure is completely outlined and provide a sample template so that they can see how the compensation process works for them.
  - ✓ For employees who are paid by commission, also include a second hourly rate that can be applied for holidays and vacations.

- *Exempt employees*:
  - ✓ Identify their base salary. This step should be communicated in terms of the club's standard pay period and also be outlined in an annualized amount. For example, the employee will receive a base salary of $2,000 every two weeks equal to $52,000 annually.
  - ✓ Identify any incentive or variable pay, based on performance. Make sure that employees understand clearly how their variable or incentive pay will be given. For example, employees have the potential to earn $10,000 each at year-end if they achieve 100 percent of their revenue goal. Furthermore, they will receive a percentage of the $10,000 that is proportional to the percentage of the revenue goal they achieve (e.g., $5,000 for reaching 50 percent of the assigned goal, etc.).
  - ✓ Identify all benefits provided, including vacation, education allowances, medical, profit-sharing, etc.

(Note: To help visualize what a compensation agreement might look like, several sample compensation templates are provided in the appendix of this book.)

Employees must understand clearly how their variable or incentive pay will be given.

FACILITIES AND EQUIPMENT IN THE HEALTH/FITNESS CLUB INDUSTRY

Part Six

Essenza Architecture, Boulder, CO

17

Health/Fitness Club Facilities

Chapter Objectives

The health/fitness club industry is heavily dependent upon its facilities for driving business profitability. This chapter presents an overview of the facilities that make up the majority of health/fitness clubs. The chapter initially reviews the various types of facilities. The chapter then discusses the areas that typically are found in these types of facilities. The chapter continues by examining the design and construction process for health/fitness club facilities, including providing examples of cost guidelines for construction. Finally, the chapter provides several examples of various facility designs.

Types of Health/Fitness Club Facilities

The International Health, Racquet & Sportsclub Association in its 2010 industry data survey, the *IHRSA Profiles of Success*, separates facilities into two generic categories: fitness-only and multipurpose. While these categories enable the various kinds of facilities to be grouped into two primary types of facilities, each of these major categories can be separated into even greater detail, based on the actual business operated in the facility:

❑ *Fitness-Only Facilities (Gym-Only in Europe)*. Fitness-only facilities are defined as those clubs that have facilities that provide space specifically for the pursuit of fitness activities. These facilities typically consist of activity-specific areas for cardiovascular equipment, resistance-circuit equipment, free-weight equipment, and group-exercise studios, as well as common areas, such as locker rooms and reception areas. Fitness-only facilities typically range in size from 3,000 square feet (280 meters) to as large as 40,000 square feet (2,800 meters), depending upon whether they include group-exercise studios, and how large the local market is. Based on the average membership for a fitness-only club, as reflected in IHRSA's 2010 research, these fitness-only facilities provide approximately 10 square feet per member. In fact, several of the leading operators in the fitness-only segment actually provide as few as 2.5 to 3 square feet per member.

> Fitness-only facilities typically range in size from 3,000 square feet (280 meters) to as large as 40,000 square feet (2,800 meters), depending upon whether they include group-exercise studios, and how large the local market is.

Some of the leading global industry players whose focus is providing fitness-only facilities include:

- *Planet Fitness, U.S.* Planet Fitness is one of the leading global gym operators in the high-volume, low-priced business segment (dues under $20 a month). The Planet Fitness model is a pure fitness-only operation, with relatively small locker rooms, a reception area, and expansive equipment areas. A Planet Fitness facility will typically range in size from 10,000 to 20,000 square feet.

- *24 Hour Fitness, U.S.* 24 Hour Fitness began as a fitness-only company and, over the past decade, has expanded its product offering to include a range of multipurpose facilities (Sport, Super Sport, and Ultra Sport). A significant number of its existing facilities are still fitness-only operations (Express, Active, and Fit Lite). These facilities are typically less than 30,000 square feet and offer both a gym and group-exercise studios.

- *Anytime Fitness, global franchise.* Anytime's typical franchise model is a 3,000 to 4,000 square foot, fitness-only facility.

- *McFit, Germany.* McFit, which like Planet Fitness operates in the high-volume, low-price (budget) segment of the fitness industry, offers a fitness-only facility. McFit facilities are typically fitted out at around 12,000 to 25,000 square feet and do not include group exercise.

- *Fitness First, UK.* Fitness First got its start in the 1990s by building out 12,000 to 20,000 square foot, fitness-only facilities. Originally, these facilities typically had one studio, small locker rooms, and a large gym area. In recent years, the company has branched out into multipurpose facilities under the Fitness First Platinum and Black Label brands.

Fitness-only facilities are commonly found in strip malls, office buildings, residential buildings, and corporate wellness and fitness programs.

Fitness-only facilities can be further broken down into more specialized units with sub-categories, such as exercise studios, free-weight gyms, personal-training studios, and express facilities, such as Curves for Women. Fitness-only facilities are commonly found in strip malls, office buildings, residential buildings, and corporate wellness and fitness programs. The various types of specialized fitness-only facilities range in both scope and popularity:

- Exercise studios normally have one or two group-exercise studios, a reception area, and locker rooms. Examples of exercise studios include:

  ✓ Yoga studios. The majority of yoga studios are independent studios, such as Pure Yoga in New York. Recently, this segment of the exercise-studio community has experienced growth in the number of multi-location yoga studios, such as YogaWorks, a chain of approximately 25 yoga studios operated in California and the Northeast corridor of the U.S.

  ✓ Pilate studios. Private Pilate studios dominate the landscape, and only a few actually offer more than one location.

  ✓ Cycling studios. Over the past few years, studios dedicated purely to cycling have evolved, such as the ever-popular SoulCycle in New York.

- Free-weight gyms usually provide a relatively large free-weight area, a reception area, and locker rooms. Free-weight gyms have become less prevalent over the past few decades, as they have evolved into offering other forms of exercise equipment.

- Personal-training studios are composed primarily of resistance, cardiovascular, and stretching areas. Some might have reception desks and locker rooms or changing rooms. Personal training studios have evolved significantly over the past five years and now represent a growing segment of the fitness industry.

- Express facilities, such as Curves for Women and Ms. Sporty in Germany, typically have a small open area for equipment, a small reception area, and in some cases, changing facilities. These smaller fitness-only facilities tend to occupy less than 3,000 square feet of space, with many express clubs being less than 1,000 square feet.

❏ *Multipurpose Facilities.* Multipurpose facilities are defined as clubs that offer fitness facilities and one or more recreational spaces, such as racquet courts, pools, gymnasiums, spas, and outdoor recreational areas. The typical multi-purpose facility will range in size from 45,000 square feet to 60,000 square feet. Based on data reported in the publication, the *IHRSA 2010 Profiles of Success*, the average multipurpose club provides approximately 14 square feet per membership, approximately 40 percent more space per membership than offered by fitness-only clubs. Similar to what occurs in the fitness-only market, some multipurpose clubs, such as those operated by Lifetime Fitness or LA Fitness, provide as little as 5 to 10 square feet per membership. The largest single multipurpose club in the U.S. is the member-owned Multnomah Athletic Club, located outside Portland, Oregon, at over 550,000 square feet. Just behind Multnomah in terms of size is the Eastbank Club in Chicago at 450,000 square feet. Some of the other massive multipurpose clubs in the U.S. include the Michigan Athletic Club in East Lansing, Michigan at over 250,000 square feet; the Rochester Athletic Club in Rochester, Minnesota at over 200,000 square feet; and Red's in Lafayette, Louisiana at over 185,000 square feet. Some of the leading global industry players that focus on providing multipurpose facilities include:

- *Millennium Partners Sports Clubs.* Millennium Partners operates six luxury multipurpose clubs in several major urban markets (e.g., New York, Boston, San Francisco, Washington, DC, and Miami), under the Reebok Sports Club and Sports Club/LA brands.

- *Western Athletic Clubs (WAC).* WAC operates nine premium and luxury multipurpose clubs throughout California, including the Pacific Athletic Club in Redwood City; the Pacific Athletic Club in San Diego; and the Courtside Club in Los Gatos.

- *David Lloyd Leisure Clubs.* David Lloyd operates 89 clubs throughout Europe, most of which are large-scale multipurpose clubs, with gyms, spas, racquet courts, and pools.

- *Lifetime Fitness.* Lifetime Fitness is the biggest operator of large multipurpose clubs in the U.S., and one of the largest globally. The

Personal training studios have evolved significantly over the past five years and now represent a growing segment of the fitness industry.

typical Lifetime Fitness facility ranges in size from 100,000 to 120,000 square feet.

- *Companhia Athletica.* Companhia Athletica operates 13 premium multipurpose clubs in Sao Paulo, Brazil, most of which are over 40,000 square feet.

Several sub-categories of multipurpose clubs exist, including racquet courts only, pools only, gymnasiums only, clubs with tennis courts, and clubs with a blend of each type of activity area. The majority of multipurpose clubs have fitness facilities, racquet courts, gymnasiums (sometimes referred to as sport courts), pools, and in some instances, tennis courts. Some multipurpose facilities also have outdoor facilities, such as outdoor pools, ball fields, and even team-building venues. The largest multipurpose clubs tend to be those with tennis facilities, gymnasiums, and outdoor facilities.

Multipurpose facilities are typically located in suburban settings, due to their space demands and the lower cost of land. Since late 2010, 24 Hour Fitness and Bally have established a standardized multipurpose club model of 45,000 square feet, which closely approximates the size of a standard LA Fitness facility, a company that has suburban multipurpose clubs that tend to range in size from 45,000 to 65,000 square feet.

The Spaces Within a Health/Fitness Club Facility

This section presents a brief overview of the most common spaces found in health/fitness clubs (fitness-only and multipurpose). A description is provided of each area's function, space requirements, and any critical design or construction requirements. For ease and clarity of understanding, the discussion of the areas is separated into physical-activity areas and service areas.

Primary Physical-Activity Areas

❑ *Aquatic Areas.* The aquatic areas of a facility can serve multiple functions, ranging from lap swimming and exercise classes to full-scale aquatic entertainment and recreation centers. A number of aquatic spaces are commonly found in clubs, including lap pools, therapy pools, and recreational pools:

- *Lap pools.* Lap pools are designed primarily for individuals who want to swim laps, but can also be used for other activities, such as water-exercise classes and swim lessons. The typical lap pool in clubs will be 25 yards long (75 feet) and 15 yards wide (45 feet and six lanes) and will be four to five feet deep at its deepest. Lap pools that are going to be used for swim meets must have both a depth of at least seven feet at one end of the pool to accommodate surface diving and lane widths of seven feet (2.15 meters). In fact, many of the lap pools that were built before 1980 have depths of 10 to 12 feet and can be used for board diving. The current trend in lap pools is to build them between 60 and 75 feet in length and provide only three or four lanes for lap swimming. The larger multipurpose clubs often install regulation

The aquatic areas of a facility can serve multiple functions, ranging from lap swimming and exercise classes to full-scale aquatic entertainment and recreation centers.

short-course competitive pools in their facilities that are either 25 meters (international) or 25 yards (domestic) in length and have eight lanes of 2.15 meters width. Most lap pools are built with gunite or stainless steel, though fiberglass structures also exist. The surface of these pools is plaster, stainless steel, or tile. Most clubs keep the water temperature in their pools between 78 degrees and 86 degrees Fahrenheit. Starting in March 2012, pools that have over 300 linear feet of edge will be required to provide two ADA accessible entries to the pool, rather than the single one that is now required.

- *Therapy pools.* Therapy pools are designed primarily for group classes and therapeutic exercise. These pools may be as small as 20-feet wide by 20-feet long or as large as 40-feet wide by 60-feet long. The average size of therapy pools in the club industry is approximately 1,500 square feet. With a depth that typically ranges from 2.5 to 5 feet, these pools are designed to be handicap accessible. The materials used to construct these pools are similar to those employed with lap pools. The water temperature in most therapy pools is kept between 84 degrees and 92 degrees Fahrenheit.

> **Recreational pools are the newest trend for indoor multipurpose facilities.**

- *Recreational pools.* Recreational pools are the newest trend for indoor multipurpose facilities. These pools are designed to accommodate various types of recreational activities (wading, swimming, sliding, splashing, etc.). The most common features of recreational pools are zero-depth entry (sloping from deck level to the desired depth), water slides, splash pads (sprays, fountains, and similar), lazy-river features, and non-traditional shapes. These pools can have two to three times the area of a typical lap pool. Lifetime Fitness offers both indoor and outdoor recreational pools in many of its facilities, each of which is composed of areas for water slides, splash pads, and general recreational aquatic activity. In fact, a few clubs in the industry have recreational pools that occupy as much as 5,000 square feet of pool surface area and an additional 5,000 square feet of deck surface. Most of these pools have starting depths of zero feet and normally go no deeper than four feet, unless the pool has water slides, in which case, additional depth levels are usually required by local codes. The water temperature in most recreational pools is kept between 82 degrees and 86 degrees Fahrenheit.

Many of the newer multipurpose facilities, such as those of Lifetime Fitness, headquartered in Minnesota, the Michigan Athletic Club in East Lansing, Michigan, and the Maryland Athletic Club in Timonium, Maryland, have aquatic environments that include two or more of these aquatic spaces.

❑ *Fitness Areas (Gym Areas in Europe).* The fitness areas in most clubs include four primary spaces to house the fitness and exercise equipment of the club. The typical gym space may range in size from 1,500 square feet (e.g., Anytime Fitness, Snap, etc.) to over 10,000 square feet (e.g., Eastbank Club, Lifetime Fitness, etc.) and include as many as 400 to 500 pieces of equipment. As a rule, these spaces involve the cardiovascular area, the resistance-circuit area, the free-weight area, and the stretching area:

Cardiovascular areas normally allocate between 50 and 60 square feet of space per piece of exercise equipment.

- *Cardiovascular area.* The cardiovascular area houses the club's cardiovascular equipment, including treadmills, elliptical machines, mechanical stairclimbers, and stationary bicycles. Cardiovascular areas normally allocate between 50 and 60 square feet of space per piece of exercise equipment (the typical manufacturer space recommendation for a piece of equipment). On average, the club's cardiovascular area occupies between 1,000 and 5,000 square feet, These areas are typically located in relatively open spaces, with fluorescent lighting and durable floor surfaces. Usually, the floor surface in this area is either carpet or rubber (e.g., Everlast, Mondo, or Softpave). In Europe, many clubs have wood flooring in the cardiovascular area. Many of the clubs provide an entertainment system as part of their cardiovascular area, such as the systems manufactured by Broadcast Vision or Cardio Theater. One of the newest industry trends in this regard is to provide individual viewing screens for each piece of cardiovascular equipment, a practice that many manufacturers currently follow. As a rule, the club's cardiovascular areas require sufficient airflow (measured in cubic feet a minute—CFMs) to maintain a temperature range of 68 to 72 degrees Fahrenheit and a relative humidity level of under 50 percent, based on the expected head load.

- *Resistance-circuit area.* The resistance-circuit area in a club normally holds the selectorized-resistance machines, such as those manufactured by companies such as Cybex, Free Motion, Life Fitness, Precor, and Technogym. As a rule, these areas allocate between 40 and 60 square feet of space per machine, based on the manufacturer's requirements. The average health/fitness club has one or two resistance circuits, each of which has 10 to 12 machines per circuit and occupies approximately 800 to 1,000 square feet per circuit. It is a common practice in the industry for a club to have one circuit dedicated to those members who wish to follow a dedicated circuit and another circuit that is devoted to the serious weight-training members. Some of the larger clubs, such as the Gainesville Health and Fitness Center, located in Gainesville, Florida, and Lifetime Fitness, provide several circuits of resistance equipment.

  Most resistance-training areas are commonly located in wide-open spaces, with a rubberized floor surface. A few club operators use carpet or wood, instead of a rubber surface. Most of the newer facilities also provide some form of audiovisual entertainment in this area. Most resistance circuit areas also have at least one wall with mirrors so that members can check on their posture and mechanics while exercising. These areas require sufficient air circulation (CFMs) to maintain a temperature range of 68 to 72 degrees and a relative humidity level of under 50 percent.

- *Free-weight area.* This area of the club houses the free weights and the plate-loaded weight machines. The free-weight area is similar to the resistance-circuit area, in that it requires 40 to 60 square feet per piece of equipment and a rubber floor surface. The size of this area varies from club to club, depending upon the amount of equipment provided. Some clubs only devote a few hundred square feet to this area, while others allocate over 5,000 square feet of space to it (e.g., LA Fitness,

Sports Club/LA, Red's, East Bank Club, etc.). It is a common industry practice for the free-weight areas to have one or more mirrored walls so that members can monitor their mechanics and posture while training. These areas require sufficient CFMs to maintain a temperature range of 68 to 72 degrees and a relative humidity level of under 50 percent.

- *Stretching area*. Over the past decade, a number of clubs have made stretching areas an integral part of their physical-activity space. While no specific design parameters currently exist for stretching areas, it is a common practice for facilities to allocate between 200 and 800 square feet to these areas. The stretching area is usually a quiet area that utilizes exercise mats for a floor surface. The temperature for this area is normally the same as for the other fitness spaces, although in an ideal environment, it should be slightly warmer to facilitate the dynamics of stretching.

While the aforementioned four spaces are typical of most fitness areas, since 2000, a growing trend has existed in the club industry to include an additional space for functional-fitness training, featuring accessory equipment, such as medicine balls, tubes, balance boards, exercise balls, steps, cones, and plyometric implements. With regard to air circulation and floor surface, these spaces are similar to the other fitness areas in the club. Some clubs dedicate a specific room for these functional fitness areas, while others devote an open area in the gym for the same purpose.

A recent trend in the design of fitness areas involves the creation of specific zones, separated by low walls or other partitions, so that instead of massing all the equipment together, facility operators can offer smaller, less intimidating zones that include no more than 15 to 20 pieces of equipment. Life Fitness, a leading manufacturer of exercise equipment, has developed what it calls the Journey system, which is a concept that provides club operators with a custom-designed floor plan that separates a gym floor into distinct zones of equipment, that are often based either on the equipment in the zone or the interests of the members.

❑ *Group-Exercise Studios*. The group-exercise area is a space designed to provide a suitable environment for offering group-exercise and fitness activities (note: these areas were formerly called aerobic-exercise studios). The group-exercise space in a club can be as small as one multipurpose studio or as extensive as four or five studios with dedicated functions. The most common group-exercise studio spaces are multipurpose, group cycling, Pilates, and yoga:

> The group-exercise space in a club can be as small as one multipurpose studio or as extensive as four or five studios with dedicated functions.

- *Multipurpose studio*. The multipurpose studio provides space to offer the majority of group-exercise activities, such as step classes, sculpt classes, resistance classes, stretch classes, yoga, and group cycling. Because such studios serve multiple activities, their design must accommodate the variety of activities performed in the allotted space. As a rule of thumb, these studios should allocate between 40 and 60 square feet of space per user, with an average of 50 square feet per user being the norm. Typically, multipurpose studios in clubs range in size from 1,000 to 4,000 square feet. These rooms most commonly have a cushioned wood floor (i.e., a floor with a shock-absorbing sub-layer, plywood underlayment, and solid wood surface). Two of the leading manufacturers of these floors are Conner Flooring and Robbins Sports Surfaces.

Another typical requirement for a multipurpose studio is to have mirrors on at least two adjacent walls. The multipurpose studio should also have its own thermostat to control airflow and temperature, with the temperature range during class set between 68 and 72 degrees and a relative humidity of less than 50 percent. When these classes are not in session, these rooms may seem cold. The multipurpose room should also have lighting as standard equipment that can be adjusted to different levels, depending upon the needs of the class.

- *Group-cycling studio.* The group-cycling studio is designed for the specific demands of group cycling. As a rule, this room requires 50 square feet per cycle, although some clubs offer far less space. The ideal floor surface for this studio is either wood or rubber, with rubber floors being the most common. Some clubs carpet the area, but this practice is not recommended because of the high level of perspiration that is generated in these studios. These studios should have at least one wall with a mirror, normally the wall behind the instructor. These studios should also have adjustable lighting as well, since many instructors like to vary the lighting levels to establish certain mood states during class. Recently, many clubs have begun to theme their group-exercise studios, similar to what Fitness First did in Australia with its Cosmic Cycling studios. The group cycling studio should have its own thermostat to control airflow and temperature, with the temperature range during class set between 68 and 72 degrees and a relative humidity of less than 50 percent. When classes are not in session, these rooms may sometimes seem cold. The industry trend in the past few years has been to combine the group-cycling studio with the multipurpose studio, rather than devoting a separate space to this activity.

- *Pilates studio.* The Pilates studio, a relatively new addition to the group-exercise area of most clubs, should be designed to accommodate the unique requirements of group and private Pilates training. This room requires approximately 60 to 80 square feet per user, primarily due to the equipment that is used. These rooms may have a wood, rubber, cork, or even carpeted floor surface. Instructors like to have a studio with at least two mirrored walls. Like the other group-exercise studios, this room requires adjustable lighting and a separate thermostat for temperature control. The Pilates room normally has a higher temperature range than either the group-cycling or the multipurpose studio. As a rule, most Pilates exercisers prefer to work out in rooms in which the temperature is over 70 degrees. Normally, the temperature is set in most Pilates studios between 72 and 76 degrees Fahrenheit.

Yoga, along with Pilates, has been one of the two fastest growing forms of group exercise over the past decade.

- *Yoga studio.* Yoga, along with Pilates, has been one of the two fastest growing forms of group exercise over the past decade. In some clubs, yoga comprises over 50 percent of all class offerings. Because of the unusual space demands of yoga, a separate studio is often required. Many of the newest club facilities in the industry have standard yoga studios. The yoga studio requires between 50 and 75 square feet per user. The floor surface for the yoga studio can be wood, rubber, or carpet, with wood floors being the most common. Regardless of what material is used for the floor of the yoga studio, the surface must be firm and level to accommodate the postures and movements of yoga. Most yoga studios require adjustable lighting, similar to the other studios. Like the other studios, at least one wall should be mirrored. The yoga room normally has a higher temperature range than the other studios, with most users preferring temperatures over 70 degrees. Typically, the temperature in most yoga studios is somewhere between 72 and 80 degrees Fahrenheit. The practitioners of Bikram style yoga or hot yoga often turn the temperature in the studio as high as 105 degrees Fahrenheit (note: all factors considered, this is not a healthy environment for exercise). Some yoga studios also have special built-in wall units and ceiling mounted features that allow selected exercises to be performed either against the walls or hanging from the ceiling (e.g., antigravity yoga).

❑ *Racquet Courts.* Racquet courts are as varied in their design and function as are the games that are played on them. The types of racquet courts that are most frequently found in health/fitness clubs are racquetball courts, squash courts, and tennis courts. In addition to these court areas, some clubs also have some of the less-commonly used court areas, such as court tennis, paddle tennis, badminton, and platform tennis.

Racquet courts are as varied in their design and function as are the games that are played on them.

• *Racquetball courts.* In the past two decades, racquetball has been far less popular than it was when it achieved its pinnacle of participation in the 1970s and early 1980s. A racquetball court is typically used for racquetball, although it can also be utilized for activities such as handball and walleyball. A regulation racquetball court is 20-feet wide by 40-feet long (800 square feet) and 20-feet high.

Racquetball courts usually have a suspended wood floor and walls composed of panels of a compressed wood material, unlike the courts that were built in the early days of the sport's infancy, which were often constructed with plaster walls or wood-panel walls. The typical racquetball court floor should be refinished on a regular basis. Most racquetball courts have a back wall that is composed of glass, although some clubs have courts that are fully enclosed by compressed panels or plaster, with only a rear door providing visibility within. Racquetball courts require separate air circulation control due to the volume of the space and the temperature and humidity requirements for that space. Under normal conditions, the court temperature should be between 60 and 68 degrees Fahrenheit. One common mistake that is often made in the construction of racquetball courts is failing to allow the wood-floor materials to acclimate to the indoor environment before laying them (e.g., a 7 to 10 day acclimation period is recommended). The lighting of a racquetball court should allow for at least 40 to 50 foot candles at floor level.

- *Squash courts.* Over the past 10 to 15 years, squash has grown in popularity to the point it has overtaken racquetball as an indoor racquet activity in many clubs. Squash courts originally could be grouped into two categories—North American courts and International courts. The North American courts were the primary playing surface in the United States, while the International courts were the primary playing surface throughout the rest of the world. Since the early 1990s, the International game has been adopted as the accepted version of squash. As a result, the North American courts are no longer built.

  The International court is 21-feet wide by 32-feet long (672 square feet), with a ceiling height of 20 feet. The court surface in an International court is unfinished hardwood. The walls and ceilings can be a compressed-wood panel system, plaster, wood, or a sand-filled, panel wall system. At the present time, most courts developed in recent years employ the compressed-wood panel system, although the sand-filled panel system is the surface of choice for serious squash players. Squash courts are similar to racquetball courts in their lighting and air circulation requirements. In that regard, they need a temperature range of 60 to 68 degrees and lighting levels of at least 40-foot candles.

  While the International court is the preferred court area for squash, many clubs still have either North American courts or converted racquetball courts as their squash-court area. The North American court, which is 18.5-feet wide and 32-feet long, requires a completely different game and ball and offers a somewhat less-than-satisfactory-playing space for the game of squash.

Tennis is the most popular court sport in the U.S., with over 23 million participants.

- *Tennis courts.* Tennis is the most popular court sport in the U.S., with over 23 million participants. Tennis is somewhat different than the other racquet-court games, because it offers players multiple playing surface options, as well as variable playing environments—ranging from outdoors to indoor-climate controlled to somewhere in between. A regulation tennis court requires a total square footage of 7,200 square feet, with the court area being 120 feet long by 60 feet wide. The actual court area (where the ball is in play) is 36 feet wide (doubles area) and 78 feet long, with a court surface that extends 12 feet to either side of the playing area and 21 feet to either end of the playing surface (note: a singles court is only 27 feet wide). If the playing area is an indoor court, it requires a ceiling height of at least 24 feet, preferably 30 feet high.

  A tennis court surface can be grass, clay, or hard-court. Grass is predominately an outdoor playing surface and is not very common in North America. Grass surfaces require considerable care and produce a relatively faster game of tennis. Clay is also a predominately outdoor playing surface, although it can be used on indoor courts. The Mayfair Racquet and Fitness Clubs in Toronto, Canada, for example, have indoor clay surfaces. A clay surface can be red clay or green clay. The brand name of the most common type of clay is Har Tru. Clay courts require constant care, including watering, raking, taping, and resurfacing. Clay courts offer an outstanding playing surface for older adults because they tend to place less physical strain on the player's joints and slow the game down. Hard-court is the most common playing surface in the United States and is best suited for indoor courts. Hard courts can be either blacktop or a synthetic surface that has been laid over a concrete foundation, which is the most common type of hard court. Tennis courts can also have surfaces that use either carpet or artificial turf. In reality, neither material is utilized as a court surface, as a rule, in North America, although many indoor courts in Europe (primarily in England) employ such coverings.

The ideal lighting environment for tennis is to provide at least 50-foot candles of light at the net surface (for competitive play, 75- to 100-foot candles is preferred), using one of the following light sources: metal halide, halogen, or even fluorescent. If the courts are indoors in a climate-controlled environment (i.e., heating and cooling provided), then the air temperature of the area should be maintained between 60 and 68 degrees Fahrenheit.

❑ *Gymnasiums (Sport Courts)*. The gymnasium is a multipurpose area in which a host of recreational sports can be conducted. The most common activities offered in the gymnasium are basketball, volleyball, badminton, group-exercise classes, and youth-oriented activities. Depending upon the club and the market in which it is located, a variety of less common activities can also be programmed in the gymnasium, including such activities as roller hockey, roller skating, and indoor soccer. Since the primary function of a gymnasium is normally for basketball, most facilities design and build their gymnasiums to accommodate the space requirements of basketball, which has parameters that are more than sufficient for activities, such as volleyball and badminton.

The standard practice for clubs that desire to offer a full array of activities in the gymnasium is to build the space in accordance with the American collegiate-sized court, which is 94-feet long and 50-feet wide, with a recommended 10-foot perimeter around the playing area of the court (7,980 square feet). Another option is to build the gymnasium to North American high-school dimensions, which are 84-feet long by 50-feet wide, with a 10-foot perimeter around the playing area of the court (7,280 square feet). On the other hand, because of the aforementioned relatively large space requirements, some clubs develop courts that are comparatively smaller, usually 60-feet long by 40-feet wide, with a minimum perimeter distance of three feet (3,036 square feet). These smaller courts are primarily used for basketball and volleyball.

The gymnasium typically has a suspended wood floor that is comprised of a cushioned or suspended sub-floor structure, with a hard-wood floor surface (maple, beech, etc.) Clubs also have the option of installing a rubber-floor surface on the floor of the gymnasium court, which is less expensive than wood-floor systems.

Since the primary function of a gymnasium is normally for basketball, most facilities design and build their gymnasiums to accommodate the space requirements of basketball, which has parameters that are more than sufficient for activities, such as volleyball and badminton.

When a gymnasium is built, the standard practice is to mark the floor surface for basketball and volleyball, and sometimes for badminton. Most gymnasiums have six basketball hoops, so that games can be played either full-court or half-court. The recommended lighting levels in the basketball area are similar to indoor tennis courts, with somewhere in the neighborhood of 40- to 50-foot candles at the floor surface.

Service Areas

While the main spaces found in health/fitness clubs are physical-activity areas, service areas are also essential. Service areas are those physical spaces that are used by members for non-physical activity. It is critical that a club provides an appropriate number, as well as a mix, of service areas. The most common types of service spaces in a club are locker rooms, child-care areas, day spa/ massage areas, and reception-and-greeting areas.

> **It is estimated that on average, members may spend as much as 30 to 50 percent of their time in the locker rooms.**

❑ *Locker Rooms.* The most heavily used area in most facilities, locker rooms are provided in over 90 percent of health/fitness clubs. It is estimated that on average, members may spend as much as 30 to 50 percent of their time in the locker rooms. Locker rooms can serve several purposes, including providing an area for members to relax, network, and change their clothes before and after working out. Most clubs offer lockers, wet areas, rest-room facilities, and relaxation amenities in this area.

• *Lockers.* In the health/fitness club industry, two distinct approaches exist concerning providing locker facilities. Some clubs have day-use lockers that members can access at no charge; others offer lockers that can only be rented, and finally, some clubs offer a blend of both alternatives. The most common scenario for a club is to provide day-use lockers. The most desirable feature of this practice involves the fact that the club only needs to provide a sufficient number of lockers to accommodate the expected number of users during any given time period. For example, a club might have 4,000 members, and might expect that approximately 1,000 members a day (25 percent of its membership) will utilize the facility. In all likelihood, no more than 10 percent of the membership will be present in the club during any given two-hour time period. In other words, because no more than 400 members would need lockers, the club would only require 400 day-use lockers in the facility. Most high-volume, low-priced clubs, economy clubs, and middle-market clubs prefer this approach. Clubs operated by companies, such as 24 Hour Fitness, LA Fitness, and Town Sports International, utilize this approach for providing lockers.

Renting lockers is a practice that higher-priced clubs (i.e., premium and luxury clubs), serving a more affluent member base, employ. These clubs build lockers and offer members the opportunity to rent the lockers on a monthly, semi-annual, or annual basis. As a rule, this scenario involves having the club provide enough lockers to accommodate at least 70 percent of the expected membership. For example, if the club has 2,000 members, it needs to provide approximately 1,400 lockers.

The Houstonian in Houston, Texas, the Reebok Club in New York, and the ClubCorp sports clubs are examples of health/fitness companies that utilize this particular approach to providing lockers. On the other hand, some facilities offer both day-use locker areas and rentable locker areas. The recent trend is to create "executive-locker areas," which are separate areas in the club with full-size rentable lockers (e.g., Reebok Club, N.Y.; Sports Club/LA, Boston; Eastbank Club, Chicago; and Pacific Athletic Club, CA).

The actual lockers are offered in a variety of sizes. The most common size for day-use lockers is 36 to 42 inches tall, 12 to 15 inches wide, and 20-inches deep, while the size of rentable lockers can vary from simple 12 inches-by-12 inches-by-20-inches locker spaces to full-size 72 inches-by-15 inches-by-21-inches lockers. The dimensions of lockers are influenced by cost, the space available, and the type of market being served. Most lockers are composed of solid wood, wood laminate, or a polyvinyl material.

- *Wet areas.* The wet areas encompass both the showers and the wet-amenity spaces, such as the sauna, the steam room, and whirlpools. The number of showers that a club needs depends on the number of users that it expects to have. Some clubs have as few as one shower per locker room, while other clubs have several dozen per locker room. While no standard quantitative measure exists for determining the number of showers that a club should have, a basic guideline is to provide one shower in each locker room for every 250 to 500 members of the facility. For example, if a club has 2,000 members, it should have at least four to eight showers per locker room. The typical shower is at least nine square feet and is constructed with a surface of tile or other solid material (e.g., granite, stone).

> While no standard quantitative measure exists for determining the number of showers that a club should have, a basic guideline is to provide one shower in each locker room for every 250 to 500 members of the facility.

The amenities normally offered in the wet area include a sauna (60 percent of clubs offer), a steam room (37 percent of clubs offer), and whirlpools (41 percent of clubs offer). The sauna is the most favored feature because of its popularity among both men and women and its relatively low installation cost. The typical sauna occupies approximately 80 to 150 square feet and is constructed of wood. A recent trend is the development of wet saunas that are a blend of sauna and steam. A steam room, on the other hand, is more popular among men than women. A standard steam room takes up between 80 and 150 square feet and is built similar to a shower. The whirlpool requires considerable space and dollars to install, which are the primary reasons for whirlpools not being located in more clubs. As a rule, whirlpools are constructed of fiberglass, stainless steel, or concrete.

It is important to note that both men and women prefer the aforementioned wet amenities only in their own locker rooms, although a number of international clubs (e.g., Germany, England) offer these amenities in a common wet area. Industry-compiled data from the U.S. indicate that individuals do not like or use coed wet-amenity spaces very

The quantity of restrooms in a particular area or club is normally determined by the existing building codes and the occupancy levels expected in the space.

often. In some international clubs, wet areas will also integrate unique water-therapy amenities, such as Turkish baths, snow rooms, and stone therapy pools.

• *Relaxation areas.* A number of health/fitness facilities include relaxation areas as part of their locker-room offerings. Among the more popular relaxation areas are lounges, nap rooms, and massage rooms. Lounges are usually found in locker rooms that provide rental lockers, because they serve as an area in which members can relax before heading out. Nap rooms exist in many of the higher-end club facilities that cater to an affluent member demographic. Massage rooms are the most common relaxation-area amenity, since most clubs do not have separate spa facilities.

• *Restroom facilities.* Every locker room has restroom facilities. As a rule, the quantity of restrooms in a particular area or club is normally determined by the existing building codes and the occupancy levels expected in the space.

❏ *Child-Care and Children's-Service Areas (Creche in Europe).* Traditionally, facilities that offered nurseries and dedicated children's centers were not the norm. At the present time, however, such spaces are becoming an integral part of many clubs. A nursery is an area that is dedicated space for providing basic children sitting or care—not licensed day care. In most states, specific guidelines exist for these spaces. In that regard, two of the most common regulatory stipulations are children cannot be left in these areas for more than a couple of hours and their parents/guardians must be on the club's premises. These rooms may be as small as 80 square feet or as large as 5,000 square feet. In most instances, these spaces include a small area for cribs and playpens, an area for games and activities, and an area for television. In some clubs, these spaces are separated by age group, in an effort to provide dedicated space to specific age categories.

A dedicated children's area is a space in which services and activities (beyond simply offering nursery services) are provided, such as arts and crafts, recreational games, nap-and-rest areas, and even birthday parties. The Pacific Athletic Club in Redwood City, CA, for example, has over 10,000 square feet in its children's area, including a small gymnasium, an arts and crafts area, a game area, and a nursery area. Lifetime Fitness has over 15,000 square feet in many of its clubs that are set aside specifically for a children's area. The Belair Athletic Club, in Belair, Maryland, operated by Wellbridge of Denver, Colorado, has a separate building just for children's services, while the Boston Sports Club in Wellesley, Massachusetts has a dedicated children's area of over 5,000 square feet. In all of these facilities, the focus is on providing a space that is safe for young people. As a rule, these spaces typically have rubber flooring, no edges, no mirrors, and no breakable materials that could otherwise harm a child. Finally, most state laws require a separate children's restroom that is handicap accessible.

❏ *Spa and Massage Facilities.* Massage has grown increasing popular over the past decade, as have day spas, in the health/fitness club environment.

The space allocated to either massage or spa services ranges drastically in the health/fitness club industry. Some clubs offer one room for massage, while other clubs, such as the Houstonian in Houston, Texas or the Village Health Club and Spa at Gainey Ranch, which is operated by DMB Sports in Phoenix, Arizona, have full-blown spas that encompass over 15,000 square feet. Many of the larger premium and luxury club chains, such as Sports Club/LA and Lifetime Fitness (e.g., LifeSpa), offer a branded spa facility in each of their clubs. The most common spaces in a day spa include:

- *Massage rooms*. The standard massage room is at least 90 square feet, preferably 100 to 110 square feet. A massage room will normally have a wood floor or other floor surface that is both attractive and easily cleaned (a carpet is not a good choice). These rooms typically have indirect lighting on dimmer switches to control the light levels and are constructed with soundproofing to reduce noise from entering the room. As a rule, most massage rooms also have both a sink and a storage space.

- *Facial rooms*. Typically, the facial room (a room for providing facial and basic skin care services) shares space with the massage room, since both involve the same basic design and construction. Facial rooms can often be as large as 150 square feet in order to accommodate the space required for a separate shower.

- *Wet-treatment rooms*. Wet-treatment rooms are areas that are normally used for body scrubs and body wraps. As such, these activities involve considerable moisture. The room should be at least 150 square feet, have floors and walls that are impervious to water, and have a shower and sink. On occasion, these rooms are utilized for Vichy showers, hydrotherapy treatments, and related water treatments, all of which require additional plumbing.

- *Pedicure space*. The typical pedicure space requires an operational area of between 50 and 60 square feet. This area should have a floor that is impervious to water (e.g., be constructed of tile or a similar material) and have drainage that accommodates the small footbaths that commonly are a part of the newest pedicure stations.

- *Manicure space*. The manicure space requires an operational area of between 25 and 50 square feet. This space should be open, rather than enclosed, like the other treatment rooms. Preferably, the floors of this room should be either wood or another hard surface that is easily cleaned.

In addition to the aforementioned facility spaces in a spa area, the spa facilities in many clubs also include a relaxation area that allows customers to sit and relax before and after receiving a treatment. In fact, many of the larger spas also offer reception areas and have separate relaxation areas for men and women. Ideally, a club-based day spa should be designed to be between 1,400 and 2,000 square feet—collectively, a space that would accommodate a relaxation area, four to eight treatment rooms, two to three manicure and pedicure stations, and a small retail area.

Ideally, a club-based day spa should be designed to be between 1,400 and 2,000 square feet—collectively, a space that would accommodate a relaxation area, four to eight treatment rooms, two to three manicure and pedicure stations, and a small retail area.

❑ *Reception-and-Greeting Areas.* The reception-and-greeting area is one of the most important spaces in the club. This area is the first internal space in the club that members see when they arrive and the last space that they see when they leave. Accordingly, this space should be designed and constructed to provide a positive impression and to facilitate the immediate needs of the members and guests who are entering and leaving the facility. In most clubs, the reception area (i.e., the front-desk area) serves as the entry point for the club and is designed to accommodate such essential functions as security, member greeting, appointment scheduling, phone answering, and information dissemination. Some larger clubs often have a separate area that is dedicated to scheduling appointments and answering the phones. The reception area normally occupies 400 to 2,000 square feet and includes a desk and a small lounge space. As a rule, this area often has some of the most aesthetically pleasing features in the club, including stone or wood floors, wood or solid surface desks, and attractive low lighting.

Other Facility Areas

Besides activity and service areas, most clubs also have operational spaces that are used to support the operational and administrative functions of the business. Examples of such spaces include offices for the key staff, the laundry room, and storage area(s). In most clubs, the amount of space allocated to offices is 80 to 100 square feet per office, with the typical facility providing offices for accounting, membership sales people, the manager of a club, and the key department heads. In most facilities, the total space that is allocated to offices does not exceed 1,000 to 1,500 square feet. The typical laundry (two washers, two dryers, and circulation space) ranges in size from 150 to 200 square feet. Storage space is often the area that receives the least amount of attention in the design phase of developing the club, and yet is the most needed area when the facility finally opens. Since the typical club design allocates 10 to15 percent of the facility's total space to circulation, at least 25 percent of that area should be allocated to storage.

> Storage space is often the area that receives the least amount of attention in the design phase of developing the club, and yet is the most needed area when the facility finally opens.

The Design and Construction Process

Whether the endeavor involves building a new health/fitness facility, expanding an existing facility, or just renovating some space, it is important to understand the basics of the design and construction process. Understanding this process can help club owners/operators avoid many of the pitfalls and expenses that often occur during these processes.

❑ *The Design Process.* The design process occurs in several stages, which if carried out in their proper sequence, will help ensure that the facility is properly designed. One of the first steps that every club operator should take is to hire a licensed architect to design any facility additions, expansions, or renovations. In most cases, an architectural firm will charge a fee, ranging from as low as six percent to as high as 12 percent of the total construction costs for the design work. The average rate is seven to nine percent. With small jobs, some architectural firms will charge their clients a higher rate than normal, simply because certain services are required on all jobs. It is recommended that owners enter into one of the standard agreement forms between an architect and owner, as provided by the Architectural Institute of America (AIA). As a rule, the design process involves several phases, including:

- *Programming phase.* The programming phase is primarily an internal process in which the club team identifies its specific program and activity needs for the spaces they want in the facility. Most architects will ask to meet with the team and conduct a review of the club's program plan so that they have a clear understanding of what the team believes is needed in the space that will be designed. This phase is usually part of the schematic-design phase for architects. The key for the club team is to be as specific as possible concerning what their needs will be with regard to facility space.

- *Schematic-design phase.* This phase of the design process involves the architect taking the programming information and combining it with the field work of the architect that has been undertaken to that point to identify a preliminary floor plan and "appearance" for the facility space. During this phase, the architect normally takes pictures of existing spaces, performs field measurements, asks for existing plans, and meets with local authorities about special regulations and zoning issues. The architect uses this information to prepare a preliminary floor plan and some sections (vertical representations) of the design that are then shared with the club team. This process normally can take from two to six weeks, depending upon the size of the project. The cost for this phase normally ranges from 10 to15 percent of the overall architectural fee.

- *Design-development stage.* During this stage, the architect, using feedback from the club team on the schematic design, prepares a more complete set of plans. During this phase, the architect utilizes the services of structural, electrical, and mechanical engineers, as well as those of soil engineers and surveyors, if needed. The goal of this stage is to provide the owner with a set of plans that offers substantial detail on each space, including the basic electrical, plumbing, mechanical, and structural work. During this stage, the architect also provides the owner with additional details on the space dimensions and elevations of the facility. Upon the completion of this stage, it is essential that the club owner/operator reviews the plans and provides input. Once this stage has been concluded, many architects then obtain initial cost estimates for the work that is to be performed so that they can get an initial estimate of the approximate cost of the planned project. The cost of this phase can range from 15 to25 percent of the overall architectural fee.

- *Construction-document stage.* During this stage, the architect takes the design development plans and the feedback that has been received from the club and local authorities to prepare a full set of construction documents. Most top architectural firms usually meet at least once during this phase with the owner to give the club owner an additional opportunity to review the plans, which are usually at 90 percent of completion at that point. During this phase, the architect completes a

The programming phase is primarily an internal process in which the club team identifies its specific program and activity needs for the spaces they want in the facility.

full set of construction documents, which contain details on all aspects of the project. The architect also works closely with the local authorities at this point in the process to address all use and permit requirements so that finished plans can be submitted for building permits. At the completion of this stage, the architect and club owner normally meet one final time to make sure all plans are correct. At the end of this stage, the architect, at the owner's direction, then forwards the design plans to at least three general contractors for bidding documents. The bidding process normally takes approximately 30 to 45 days to complete, at which time, the owner should receive three cost estimates (bids) from the general contractors. The cost for this phase is the balance of the architectural fees already paid subtracted from 85 percent of the total estimated design cost.

- *Construction-administration stage.* This phase includes the architect's involvement in the bidding process and the selection of the general contractor (which is typically undertaken with the club owner), as well as the architect's efforts during the construction process. During construction, the architect reviews and approves all general contractor submittals for work, approves all changes recommended by the contractor, reviews pay applications, and checks the progress of work through inspections at each phase of construction. Subsequently, in concert with the owner, the architect completes the final punch list and approves the final conditions of the construction. The cost for this phase of services is normally 15 percent of the overall design work.

❑ *The Construction Process.* The construction process begins once a general contractor has been selected and hired. The selection of the contractor should be based on several factors, including bid price, references, and experience with similar projects. It is important to note that accepting the lowest contractor's bid does not always lead to the best work or even the lowest price once the project has been completed. Once the decision has been made to hire a particular contractor, the club owner should consider and be sensitive to the following factors, all of which can impact the job:

- *Be aware of the fact that contractors have a fudge factor in their price.* General contractors base their submitted bid on cost estimates that they have received from sub-contractors. Most sub-contractors double their costs in order to arrive at their bid price. In turn, the general contractor applies a 20 to 100 percent profit margin to each sub's bid price. Furthermore, the general contractor includes a line item for general conditions in their bid, which consists of their cost to supervise the job, along with another line item for profit and overhead that normally runs from 5 to 15 percent of the total cost from all bids. In other words, the final bid price that the club owner receives from the contractor usually has another 15 to 25 percent of wiggle room for price negotiation.

- *Get a contract.* Club owners should utilize one of the standard agreements from the American Institute of Architects (AIA), such as a lump-sum agreement, with the contractor. These agreements provide considerable protection for the owner. Such an agreement should address all details

It is important to note that accepting the lowest contractor's bid does not always lead to the best work or even the lowest price once the project has been completed.

of the project, including the payment schedule, change orders, pay applications, liability insurance, performance criteria, etc. The owner should consider including deadlines and penalties in the agreement to cover situations in which the contractor fails to finish a particular part of the project on time, as well as for cost overruns. It is critical that the contract stipulate that between 5 and 10 percent of the contract price is held out of each payment (referred to as a contingency), until after the final punch-list work is completed. The contract should also require the contractor to provide evidence of liability insurance (it is important that the owner is listed on the contractor's insurance as co-insured) and, if the contractor is from a relatively small company, evidence of bonding.

- *Limit change orders.* Change orders occur when a contractor has to perform work that is not reflected in the original construction documents. As a rule, contractors charge a premium for change orders (typically a 20 percent profit premium). Once a change order has been received, the contractor obtains a bid from a sub-contractor for the work involved in the change order and adds a premium of at least 10 percent to the bid (note: the degree of mark-up that is permissible can be specified in the contract). Change orders occur most often because owners want to make changes during the construction phase or the architect and owner have not clarified the plan documents. As a result, it is critical that the plans are reviewed by all parties involved so that no misunderstandings exist and that the owner is aware of the fact that any changes to the plan once construction begins will involve additional costs. Finally, all change orders should be submitted to the architect for approval before any work mandated by the change order can begin or be paid for.

- *Review all pay applications in detail.* Contractors submit a pay application for work performed each month. The pay application provides a detailed listing of all divisions of work and the percentage of work completed for each category. The amount to be paid is based on the work completed. On each application, the contractor lists the contract price, the amount paid to date, the balance, the amount due, and the retainage held out. The pay application should be reviewed and approved by the architect first and then by the owner to ensure that the work that has actually been completed corresponds with the figures shown on the pay application and that no extra costs are included.

- *Conduct regular meetings with the contractor.* The owner and architect should meet regularly with the contractor during the course of construction. In most cases, these meetings are held once a month, while on smaller jobs, they might be scheduled once a week. These meetings should focus on a review of all work, change orders, and pay applications. These meetings should also include an inspection of the job site.

> **The owner and architect should meet regularly with the contractor during the course of construction.**

- *Get partial and full lien waivers.* A lien waiver is a form that says that the contractor has received payment for the work completed and that all subcontractors and parties have been paid for their work. When a contractor submits a pay application, lien waivers should be turned in at the same time that correspond to the amount of work completed and the amount of the work paid for by the club owner. This process ensures that a lien is not placed on the business if a sub-contractor claims that they have not been paid for work that they performed. The final lien waiver should be submitted when all of the work has been completed.

- *Conduct a punch list.* After the contractor completes the job, the owner, architect, and contractor should walk through the job and complete a punch list. The punch list identifies any work that either has been performed in an unsatisfactory manner or work that still needs to be done. The punch list ensures that the work is completed to the satisfaction of the owner. Once the punch list is completed, the contractor is paid the retainage fees that have been held out during the course of each pay application.

- *Obtain the warranties and owner's manuals.* At the completion of a construction project, the contractor is obligated to provide the owner with an operator's manual on each product that was utilized in the project (e.g., carpet, HVAC, lighting, floor surfaces, etc.). The operator's manual provides the owner with resources that might be useful with any product-related problems that might subsequently arise with the construction. The standard practice for contractors and their subcontractors is to provide a one-year guarantee on all work and products, commencing from the time the project is completed. Before making a final payment to the contractor, the owner should obtain these warranties from the contractor.

- *Be aware of the fact that under certain circumstances, the contractor can be removed from the job.* If the owner uses a standard AIA agreement, that agreement includes a section that spells out the owner's right to remove the contractor, select another contractor, and let the new contractor finish the job, using the original contractor's equipment. This stipulation can be important, because some small contractors start out relatively strong and then fade as the project moves forward.

> The standard practice for contractors and their subcontractors is to provide a one-year guarantee on all work and products, commencing from the time the project is completed.

Costs Associated With Design and Construction

Some general cost guidelines for design and construction exist that can be useful in determining the scope of a project, including:

- ❑ *Design Costs.* As discussed previously, an architect's costs can run from as low as six percent to as high as 12 percent of total construction costs. The fees of structural engineers, mechanical engineers, and electrical engineers are all included in this expense. Among the items that are not included in the architect's fees are the costs attendant to landscape design, civil engineering, acoustical engineering, surveys, and other specialty work. Collectively, the total cost for all design work can run as high as 14 to 15 percent of the overall construction costs.

- ❑ *Construction Costs.* Most construction is priced on a unit basis, either in linear feet, square feet, or some other basic unit of measurement.

- *Overall construction costs.* The cost per square foot can vary considerably, depending on the facility's level of finish. The average cost for building a shell (i.e., site work, foundations, bringing in utilities, and building a frame) normally runs approximately $75 to $125 a square foot, depending on the region of the country. The national average would be in the neighborhood of $75 to $100, depending on the local conditions. The balance of construction after the shell has been completed is considered finish work (i.e., plumbing, electrical, HVAC, surfaces, etc.). The cost range for this stage varies considerably, based on finish levels, with costs as low as $50 a square foot to as high as $200 to $300 a square foot in some geographical areas. The national average for this kind of work would be in the neighborhood of $50 to $125 a square foot. For example, if a freestanding facility was being constructed in a state like Florida or Texas, it might cost from $125 to $200 a square foot, whereas the cost of that same facility in California or New York might be between $250 and $400 a square foot.

Examples of Health/Fitness Facility Designs

The schematic designs, isometrics, and renderings illustrated in this section are intended to showcase some of the unique elements discussed in the previous sections of this chapter.

Ohlson Lavoie Collaborative, Denver, CO

Schematic plan (first floor) of Stonecreek Club & Spa, Covington, LA

Schematic plan (second floor) of Stonecreek Club & Spa, Covington, LA

Schematic plan (first floor) of Fizkult Meshchera, Nizhny Novgorod, Russia

Essenza Architecture, Boulder, CO

Schematic plan (second floor) of Fizkult Meshchera, Nizhny Novgorod, Russia

Essenza Architecture, Boulder, CO

Isometric floor plan (first floor) of World Class Zhukovka, Moscow, Russia

Isometric floor plan (second floor) of World Class Zhukovka, Moscow, Russia

Isometric floor plan (third floor) of World Class Zhukovka, Moscow, Russia

Fitness area rendering, U.S.

Ohlson Lavoie Collaborative, Denver, CO

Rendering of a cycle studio, City Club, Fort Worth, TX

Essenza Architecture, Boulder, CO

Rendering of a fitness floor, World Class Four Winds, Moscow, Russia

Essenza Architecture, Boulder, CO

Rendering of a locker room, World Class Four Winds, Moscow, Russia

Essenza Architecture, Boulder, CO

Rendering of a reception desk, World Class Zhukovka, Moscow, Russia

Rendering of an aquatic zone, World Class Zhukovka, Moscow, Russia

Rendering of a mind/body zone, World Class
Zhukovka, Moscow, Russia

Examples of Health/Fitness Facility Areas From Around the World

Cafe, Virgin Active, UK

Group exercise entry, body + soul, Munich, Germany

Lobby, Pfitzenmeier Sport & Wellness, Schwetzingen, Germany

Clay tennis courts, Vilas Club, Buenos Aires, Argentina

Pilates studio, Buenos Aires, Argentina

Circular fitness floor, Ocampo Wellness, Buenos Aires, Argentina

Activity pool, Hamilton-Lowe

Ohlson Lavoie Collaborative, Denver, CO

Fitness floor, Lakeshore Athletic Club, Broomfield, CO

Ohlson Lavoie Collaborative, Denver, CO

Group exercise studio, Lakeshore Athletic Club, Broomfield, CO

Ohlson Lavoie Collaborative, Denver, CO

Entry to mind/body group exercise, Telos Fitness Center, Dallas, TX

Telos Fitness Center, Dallas, TX

Women's locker room whirlpools, Telos Fitness Center, Dallas, TX

Telos Fitness Center, Dallas, TX

Reception desk, Telos Fitness Center, Dallas, TX

Telos Fitness Center, Dallas, TX

18

Fitness Equipment for the Health/Fitness Club Industry

Chapter Objectives

The health/fitness club industry is capital-intensive, with facilities and equipment encompassing the majority of that capital outlay. According to industry research, as reflected in IHRSA's publication, *Guide to Lenders and Investors*, most newly built clubs expend approximately $15 to $25 a square foot on fitness equipment. It is not uncommon, however, for the cost of fitness equipment to typically run from $20 to $30 a square foot. This initial investment in equipment is compounded by the need for club owners to reinvest in equipment on an annual basis to stay current with equipment trends in the industry and to deal with the depreciation and wear on existing equipment. This chapter reviews the basic categories of fitness equipment in the industry, the leading equipment manufacturers, and the costs associated with the equipment, including a brief discussion of the pros and cons of purchasing versus leasing. The chapter is not intended to delve into great depth on this subject; rather, it is designed to provide a basic overview of the key factors attendant to the equipment end of the industry. As such, the information is grouped and reviewed according to the major equipment categories in the industry, including cardiovascular equipment, resistance-circuit equipment, free-weight equipment, cardiovascular-entertainment equipment, and other types of equipment that are frequently required in the health/fitness club industry.

Cardiovascular Equipment

Cardiovascular equipment exists in nearly all health/fitness clubs and is second only to free-weight equipment in terms of its availability and popularity in the industry. Although cardiovascular equipment has been around since the 1870s (when the Curtis indoor rowing machine was first introduced in clubs), it has only been since the 1970s that it has been accorded such a prominent role in the marketing and programming of clubs.

Most newly built clubs expend approximately $15 to $25 a square foot on fitness equipment.

❑ *Historical Overview.* The first pieces of cardiovascular equipment that were utilized in the club industry were stationary indoor rowing machines, the first of which was the Curtis rowing machine introduced in 1871 by William Curtis, a founding member of the New York Athletic Club. During the late 1800s and early part of the 1900s, rowing machines, such as the Curtis rowing machine, Kern's & Laflin rowing machine, and those rowing machines that were marketed and sold by A.G. Spaulding and Narragansett Machine Company, represented the primary form of indoor cardiovascular conditioning equipment in clubs. In 1932, the Exercycle, invented by Gordon Berg, became a part of the club industry. In the process, it became the second most popular indoor cardiovascular training machine (after rowing machines). The first commercial treadmill (Quinton treadmill) was a relatively large machine that was developed by Robert Bruce (who is relatively well-known in some circles for devising the Bruce protocol) and Wayne Quinton. In the 1960s, the Pacemaster treadmill, developed by Bill Staub and Kenneth Cooper, M.D., was introduced, a machine that was followed shortly thereafter by the Trotter treadmill in the early 1970s.

In 1968, the Lifecycle was invented by Keene Dimmick. Six years later, in 1974, Ray Wilson purchased the rights to the Lifecycle and, along with his first employee, Augie Nieto, introduced it to the club industry. As the first mass-produced electronic piece of cardiovascular equipment, designed specifically for the health/fitness club industry, it subsequently became the benchmark for all future developments in the industry. The Lifecycle established itself as one of those brands that become virtually synonymous with the product type. Fairly or not, all indoor exercise cycles, at one time

Life Fitness, Chicago, IL

Lifecycle 2000

or another, have been called Lifecycles. The Lifecycle subsequently gave rise to other early brands of indoor electronic cycles, such as Biocycle and Universal. During the late 70s, treadmills began to have a presence in the health/fitness club market through models built and sold by companies such as Pacemaster, Quinton, Marquette, and Trotter. Since then, treadmills have blossomed into the largest segment of cardiovascular equipment in the industry, a segment that is dominated by companies such as Cybex, Life Fitness, Precor, Star Trac, and Technogym.

The next landmark type of cardiovascular equipment to hit the industry was the development of StairMaster machines in 1984. To many industry observers, StairMaster evolved into the industry equivalent of the Lifecycle in the 80s and early 90s. The developmental evolution of cardiovascular equipment continued in the mid-1990s when in 1995, Precor introduced the first elliptical machine. Subsequently, the Precor EFX became the StairMaster of the previous decade.

During the 1970s, a number of other types of cardiovascular equipment were also popular, including the Nordic Track cross-country ski machine, the Cybex upper-body ergometer, and the Concept II Rower. The late 1980s and early 1990s also witnessed industry efforts to expand the types and features of "cardio" equipment. Some of these machines, such as the Reebok Sky Walker, had an early, but not lasting, impact on the industry. At the present time, cardiovascular equipment continues to evolve, as manufacturers incorporate new technology and improved mechanics and as the public looks for even better/newer exercise tools.

❑ *Categories.* Cardiovascular equipment can be grouped into the following major categories: elliptical machines, stairclimbers, recumbent and upright bicycles, adapted movement machines, and treadmills. In addition to these major categories, a few, less-prominent categories exist, such as rowing machines, upper-body ergometers, and cross-country ski machines.

Elliptical machines are the fastest growing category of equipment in the health/fitness club industry.

• *Elliptical machines.* Elliptical machines are the fastest growing category of equipment in the health/fitness club industry. Since their introduction by Precor in 1995, they have become the second most popular form of cardiovascular machines in clubs. Elliptical machines reflect an evolution in how the industry looks at cardiovascular exercise. These machines exert load forces on the body similar to those imposed on an individual's musculoskeletal system while walking and running, but with significantly less impact. These machines also feature technology that allows for integrated upper-body movement with lower-body movement. At the present time, elliptical machines are available both with and without upper-body movement arms. The industry leader in this type of equipment is the Precor EFX. Companies such as Life Fitness, Star Trac, Matrix, Cybex (Arc Trainer), Octane, and Technogym also manufacture well-received models of elliptical machines. Most of the elliptical machines currently available in the market offer heart-rate technology, integrated entertainment technology (e.g., touch screen LED screens and iPod compatability), and accessories for holding items, such as water bottles and reading materials. The average retail cost of a commercial-grade elliptical machine ranges from $4,000 to $6,000 per machine.

- *Stairclimbers.* Mechanical stairclimbers have lost much of their market share since the introduction of the elliptical trainers. Once the highest volume seller in the industry, stairclimbers currently rank behind treadmills, elliptical machines, and bicycles in terms of their popularity among health/fitness club users. StairMaster Sports/Medical Products, Inc. (a company that is part of the Nautilus Group), which developed and manufactured the first mechanical stairclimbing machine, remains the industry leader in this equipment category. Several other companies, such as Life Fitness, Star Trac, Precor, Technogym, and Cybex, also produce stairclimbing machines that are popular in the industry. The first model of a stairclimbing machine that Stairmaster produced (originally called the Gauntlet, but subsequently renamed as the Stepmill), which featured a series of stairs that actually rotated, is often still the piece of cardiovascular equipment of choice among those individuals who either would like to engage in a particularly intense workout or see a direct correlation between the exercise afforded by revolving stairs and a personal activity interest (e.g., outdoor climbing). The technology involved in mechanical stairclimbing has not changed all that much since these machines were first introduced. Some of the newer stairclimbing machines feature heart-rate monitor technology and entertainment technology, as well as offer soft pedals and accessories to hold water bottles and reading materials. The average retail price for a commercial-grade stairclimber ranges from $3,000 to $5,000.

- *Recumbent and upright bicycles.* Upright bicycles were the first type of cardiovascular equipment that was introduced to the club market. Within the industry, they remain popular among club users. Recumbent bicycles, the more popular of the two types of bicycles (recumbent and upright), were introduced in the industry in the late 1980s and early 1990s, to ostensibly serve an older demographic. Bicycles are third in popularity, behind treadmills and elliptical machines, among current facility users. The current trend in the technology for both types of bicycles is to provide lower starting workloads, heart-rate feedback, fully adjustable seats and pedals, self-adjusting workloads based on heart-rate response, and integrated entertainment technology. The leading manufacturers of bicycles include Life Fitness, Star Trac, Precor, and Technogym. The average retail price for either a recumbent or upright bicycle ranges from $1,500 to $4,000.

- *Treadmills.* Treadmills are the single most popular piece of cardiovascular equipment in the industry and involve the largest expenditure for cardiovascular equipment by clubs. As previously discussed, the first treadmills offered to the club industry were models developed by Quinton, Pacemaster, and Trotter, each of which was relatively large and cumbersome to use. Over the years, treadmills have become the cardiovascular modality of choice for many club members. Much of

> Treadmills are the single most popular piece of cardiovascular equipment in the industry and involve the largest expenditure for cardiovascular equipment by clubs.

their popularity can be attributed to the evolution of technology, often based on research into the mechanics of human motion, which is featured in most treadmills. For example, almost every treadmill offers some form of soft deck (shock-absorbing surface), programmable features, controllable speed that ranges from less than 1 to 15 mph (some as high as 20 mph), adjustable grades (negative-degree grade to as high as a positive 50-degree grade), contact and remote heart-rate monitoring, integrated audiovisual entertainment, accessories for holding items, such as water bottles and reading materials, and, on occasion, fans for "cooling" the individual who is using the machine. The leading manufacturers of commercial-grade treadmills are Star Trac, Life Fitness, Precor, Cybex, Technogym, and Woodway. Some smaller companies, such as True, Matrix, and Sport Art, also produce treadmills. Two of the newest innovations in treadmills are built-in fans, introduced initially by Star Trac, and LCD entertainment, introduced initially by Life Fitness. The average retail price of a quality commercial-grade treadmill ranges from $3,500 to $10,000.

> The average retail price of a quality commercial-grade treadmill ranges from $3,500 to $10,000.

- *Adaptive movement machines.* In the early part of the 21st century, several manufacturers introduced a new category of cardiovascular equipment, one of which was an offshoot of the elliptical and total-body training machines introduced in the late 1990s by companies such as Precor and Life Fitness. These new machines leveraged the popularity of the elliptical trainer by establishing adapted movements that were similar to those of an elliptical trainer, but which also provided a different modality for the user. The first adaptive movement machine was the Arc Trainer, which was introduced by Cybex. The Arc Trainer provided users with both upper- and lower-body movement that followed a semi-arched or elliptical-type movement through the lower body. One of the Arc Trainer's unique features is that it allows the user to be "suspended" in air while performing the movement. The second adaptive movement machine to hit the market with a bang was the Cardiowave from Technogym. The Cardiowave, released in 2005, simulated the movement of ice skating or uphill Nordic skiing. Interestingly, back in the 1990s, Nautilus introduced an ice skating simulator that had provided a similar movement pattern. The Cardiowave's unique design allows users to develop several physical attributes, including cardiovascular endurance, lower-body muscular endurance, and lower-body muscular strength. In 2007, Precor released a machine called the Adaptive Motion Trainer (AMT). The AMT provides users with three distinct movement patterns—stepping, elliptical training, and running. The AMT allows the user to adapt their stride length and mobility patterns to simulate one of the abovementioned movements.

Selectorized/Variable Resistance Equipment

According to the published report, the *IHRSA 2010 Profiles of Success*, selectorized/variable-resistance equipment is found in a majority of all facilities. In reality, almost all clubs offer some form of variable-resistance equipment. Variable-resistance or selectorized-resistance equipment encompasses strength-training equipment that utilizes weight stacks and pulley mechanisms to provide resistance to movement, while the user typically assumes (and maintains) a set position. The primary advantage of this type of resistance exercise is that it provides a safe and efficient strength-training modality, while reducing the level of exercise anxiety and the perceived need for demonstrable fitness prowess that some individuals experience.

❑   *Historical Overview.* Resistance-training machines, in one form or another, have been in existence for more than 150 years. The first such resistance machines, which look similar to today's modern resistance machines, were developed in the 1860s by Dr. Gustav Zander. Dr. Zander developed over 27 different mechanical machines that featured graduated levers, springs, weights, and pulleys to create resistance. His machines included a number of devices, such as the pulldown machine, the abdominal punching machine, and the torso resistance machine.

In the 1880s, another industry legend, Dudley Allan Sargent, director of the Heminway Gymnasium at Harvard, invented the first variable-resistance pulley machines. Over time, Sargent created more than 30 distinct machines, including the chest pulley system and abdominal pulley system. By the late 1880s, Sargent's pulley systems could be found in gymnasiums around the country and were being replicated by several other equipment companies, such as A.G. Spalding.

The selectorized resistance machines that currently exist in the health/fitness club industry originated in the late 1950s, as a result of the efforts of Harold Zinkin, Sr. to develop the first Universal machine. Zinkin's equipment featured a single-training unit that had multiple-exercise stations, each with

*Gustav Zander's torso
resistance machine (1903)*

its own weight stack. These early machines employed a system of levers to move the weight stack and provide resistance (Universal called it dynamic-variable resistance). As a rule, Zinkin's machines were somewhat limited by the fact that they had an uneven distribution of the resistance load at different points in the range of motion. Until the 1970s, however, Universal and Paramount were the preferred choices of the industry where it involved the purchase of resistance-training machines.

In 1970, Arthur Jones revolutionized the equipment manufacturing and club industries with the introduction of Nautilus machines. Nautilus machines featured variable resistance, made possible by the use of a cam that controlled the level of resistance afforded to the user. The cam allowed the resistance offered by the machine to vary based on the fulcrum's (mechanical movement arm) position on the cam while the machine was being used. Concurrently, the concept of "strength curves" was introduced into the mindset of many club members. According to Nautilus, one of the most desirable features of its equipment was the machine's capacity to provide resistance to the user that is applied in a manner that is consistent with the normal strength curve of the user's muscles. Another selling point for Nautilus machines was their ability to isolate specific muscle groups while exercising. Nautilus also featured mechanisms that allowed users to adjust their seat position and body position while exercising, which is designed to enhance both the mechanical efficiency and effectiveness of their exercise bout. Nautilus advocates adhered to a prescription and training concept that involved performing one set of each exercise to near muscular fatigue, doing each repetition in relatively slow motion (e.g., four to six seconds each), and placing equal or greater emphasis on the eccentric portion of the exercise movement (versus the concentric phase).

Nautilus Blue Monster

Legends of the Iron Game, Bill Pearl Enterprises

While the number of variable-resistance equipment manufacturers grew over the years, no new innovations hit the industry until 1978 with the introduction of Keiser pneumatic machines.

Eventually, Nautilus was followed by a new group of equipment manufacturers, such as Eagle (later to become Cybex), Body Masters, and Icarian, among others, who led the effort to expand the technology involved in variable-resistance machines. For example, by the early 1980s, Eagle had entered into the market for variable-resistance machines and captured much of the demand for such equipment. Cybex and many of the resistance equipment companies that followed improved on the original Nautilus design by creating lighter machines that required less space, employed airplane cable or Kevlar belts instead of chains, offered additional color options, and were aggressively marketed at a lower-price point to the industry.

While the number of variable-resistance equipment manufacturers grew over the years, no new innovations hit the industry until 1978 with the introduction of Keiser pneumatic machines. The Keiser machines involved a new, innovative concept—the use of air pressure to create resistance. This feature provided exercisers with greater flexibility in adjusting either the level of resistance or speed. Subsequently, companies, such as Hydra Fit, introduced a line of resistance-training machines that were powered by pneumatic cylinders, while others developed machines that employed water as a means to adjust the level of resistance. At the present time, Keiser is one of the few manufacturers of resistance machines that do not employ a weight stack.

The next stage in the evolution of resistance-training machines occurred in the early 1990s, when several manufacturers introduced computerized-resistance training (e.g., Powercise, Life Circuit) machines. These machines employed electromagnetic forces (controlled through computer chips) to produce resistance. The most noteworthy feature of these machines was their ability to adjust the resistance level, based on the user's strength that day, as well as memory of how the user had performed on the previous workout. This approach to resistance training did not catch on with consumers and disappeared from the industry within a few years.

At the end of the 1990s, Ground Zero, later renamed Free Motion, developed a line of functional resistance-training equipment, featuring pulleys that enable users to exercise in a variety of positions and planes. The efforts of Free Motion have since given rise to an entire manufacturing segment in the industry attempt to design and produce functional resistance-training machines.

❑ *Categories.* Variable-resistance equipment can be grouped into three distinct categories: fixed-position weight stack, functional fitness-based weight stack, and alternative resistance.

  • *Fixed-position weight stack.* This category encompasses over 80 percent of the market for variable-resistance equipment. This type of machine provides resistance through the use of cams or other pulley-based systems that are attached to weight stacks. These machines enable users to perform a specific exercise movement in a fixed position that isolates one or two muscle groups. The basic design of these machines provides a high degree of user safety since most of the postural and mechanical alignment errors that can occur in more functional exercise are eliminated. Another benefit category of variable-resistance equipment is the ability to set up circuits of the machines that allow a user to perform movements for each of the major muscle groups by exercising on 8 to12 machines that have been arranged in a circuit. Most of these machines also allow personalized position adjustments to accommodate multiple body types, as well as feature more aesthetically pleasing designs. A host of manufacturers of this type of equipment exists in the industry, including Life Fitness, Cybex, Technogym, Nautilus, Precor, Paramount, Star Trac, and Matrix The average retail price for a complete circuit of 12 machines is approximately $30,000 to $40,000, with each piece ranging from $2,500 to $5,000 in price.

- *Functional fitness-based weight stack.* This category of variable-resistance equipment has evolved from having a relatively small role in the club industry to being a major focus of variable-resistance equipment manufacturers. At the present time, all of the leading manufacturers of variable-resistance equipment offer machines in this category. This type of equipment is based on the two primary concepts. First, muscles don't contract in isolation. Rather, a synergy of contraction occurs during exercise, involving agonist, antagonist, and stabilizer muscle groups. Second, the body does not function in an isolated or a fixed position. Instead, the functional performance of movement requires both balance and posture. Accordingly, the design of these machines features pulley and cable systems that allow users to adjust their position and angle of movement, as desired. Furthermore, these machines often require that users perform the movement in a standing or similar position—where the body is not fixed in a set position, thus incorporating an element of balance in the exercise. The manufacturing leader in this area is Free Motion Fitness, although additional companies, such as Life Fitness, Cybex, Precor, Star Trac (Human Sport), and Matrix, among others, have developed their own models of this equipment. These machines range in cost of approximately $2,500 to $5,000 each, with a complete circuit of 12 machines retailing in the neighborhood of $30,000 to $40,000.

The body does not function in an isolated or a fixed position. Instead, the functional performance of movement requires both balance and posture.

- *Alternative resistance.* Alternative-resistance machines are similar to the fixed-position, weight-stack equipment, except that they utilize a resistance source other than weight stacks. These machines operate on the same basic principles as the other two basic categories of variable-resistance equipment (i.e., most of these machines provide isolated movements, with the user set in a fixed position). The leader in this category is Keiser, which manufactures a line of equipment that uses air resistance. Keiser has been able to attract a relatively strong following in some segments of the industry, based on the ability of air resistance to allow for loads light enough for the weakest individual and loads in excess of what the strongest human could lift. Keiser has also capitalized on the fact that its equipment nearly eliminates placing undue load forces on the joints, which makes it a very suitable resistance-training modality for older adults. Other manufacturers exist that use alternative forms of resistance, such as water, air, and hydraulics. On average, these machines retail for between $3,000 and $5,000 per machine and for approximately $30,000 to $40,000 for a complete 12-station circuit.

Free-Weight Equipment

Free-weight equipment has been around longer than any other form of exercise equipment. According to the publication, the *IHRSA 2010 Profiles of Success*, 83 percent of all clubs indicate that they offer free-weight equipment, thereby making it the most popular type of exercise equipment in the health/fitness club industry.

> *Free-weight equipment has been around longer than any other form of exercise equipment.*

❏ *Historical Overview.* Free-weight equipment has been around for well over two thousand years. The first piece of free weight equipment introduced to physical culturists was dumbbells (originally called halteres when they were introduced during the Greek period of 300 to 700 BC), followed shortly thereafter by the medicine ball. The kettlebell was introduced around 1700. By the mid-1800s, globe barbells and dumbbells (bells were filled with either sand or metal pellets that were loaded to the end of a bar), also became popular, along with Indian clubs.

Milo Barbell, founded by Alan Calvert in 1902, was the first company to commercially produce free-weight sets. These early free-weight sets allowed the user to easily change weights and brought free-weights into gyms and homes throughout America. During the early years of the health/fitness club industry in the late 1940s, most free-weight equipment consisted of barbells, dumbbells, and benches built by individuals for their gyms. The free-weight equipment industry underwent its first major thrust in popularity with the introduction of the York barbell in the late 1930s. Developed by the legendary Bob Hoffman, the York Company purchased the assets of Milo Barbell and proceeded to create an entire market for barbells, dumbbells, and free-weight benches. In fact, until the late 1980s, York was one of only a few companies that made free-weight equipment,.

The popularity of free-weight equipment received a substantial boost in popularity in the late 1980s and early 1990s, when research began to document and reinforce the enumerable benefits of strength training for all segments of the population. As a result of the impetus for resistance training that was provided by this research, companies began to expand into the free-weight market. Among the manufacturing companies that were at the forefront of this effort were Cybex, Icarian, and Body Master. By the turn of the 21st century, nearly every major exercise equipment manufacturer offered full lines of free-weight plates, benches, and accessories.

One of the biggest developments in the history of the free-weight industry occurred in 1989, when Hammer introduced plate-loaded resistance equipment. Hammer machines featured the functional advantages of free-weight movements, combined with the advantages of variable-resistance, weight-stack equipment. Initially, Hammer developed a significant following in both colleges and professional sports, before gaining in popularity in the club industry. Hammer's prime engineer was none other than Gary Jones, son of Arthur Jones, the creator of Nautilus.

The most recent attempt at innovation in free-weight technology has been the introduction of weight plates with holes for easier grasping. Free-weight equipment has evolved from an exercise tool primarily targeted at bodybuilders to the resistance-training modality of choice for many average consumers.

❑ *Categories.* Free-weight equipment can be grouped into three primary categories: barbells and dumbbells, benches and support machines, and plate-loaded equipment.

- *Barbells and dumbbells.* Barbells and dumbbells have evolved very little since they were first introduced. At the present time, most barbells involve Olympic-style bars and plates that have ball-bearing sleeves that allow the weights to revolve around the end of the bar. The most innovative change in barbells in recent years has been the introduction of plates (technology first introduced by Iron Grip) that have holes that allow the user to more easily grasp the plates.

  Dumbbells have also not evolved all that much over the last century. Two changes that have occurred in dumbbells, however, are the use of rubber-plate coatings that have been put on the plates to protect them and the presence of more ergonomic handles that have been developed. Another change has been the use of kettlebells, which have become quite popular in the past few years. First used in the early 1700s by Russian strongmen, kettlebells are large metal balls with a fixed handle on top. The leading manufacturers of barbells and dumbbells are Ivanko and Iron Grip. The retail cost of barbells varies, with most commercial grade bars retailing for between $150 and $500 dollars, while plates cost between $.30 and $1.00 per pound. The cost of solid dumbbells ranges from less than $.30 a pound to over $1.00 a pound, depending on the actual weight (e.g., heavy dumbbells cost less per pound).

- *Benches and support machines.* Benches and support machines comprise the largest segment of the free-weight product line. These products range from simple Olympic style flat benches for performing bench presses to power racks and Smith machines. Each bench and accessory is designed to be used with barbells and dumbbells. The variety of products in this category is substantial and includes such items as adjustable incline benches, flat benches, decline benches, leg- press machines, Smith machines, power racks, cable-crossover machines, curling benches, T-bar rowing machines, calf machines, 45-degree back benches, and abdominal benches. The leading manufacturers of this product segment include Life Fitness, Cybex, Technogym, Precor, Star Trac, Matrix, and Gym 80. These benches and machines have wide-ranging retail prices. For example, most benches retail for between $400 and $900 each, while larger machines, such as power racks and Smith machines, cost in the range of $1,000 and $4,000 each.

Free-weight equipment has evolved from an exercise tool primarily targeted at bodybuilders to the resistance-training modality of choice for many average consumers.

- *Plate-loaded machines.* Plate-loaded equipment is the most recently developed type of free-weight equipment, having only been around since1989. Plate-loaded machines involve a hybrid piece of equipment that allows the average health/fitness club user to experience some of the benefits of free weights, while simultaneously receiving the advantages that variable-resistance equipment can provide, such as enhanced safety and the ability to exercise isolated muscles. Plate-loaded equipment enables users to perform a variety of fixed-position (isolated exercise movements) and functional based movements (exercises that involve closed-chain movements). The leading manufacturer of this type of free-weight equipment is Hammer (owned by Life Fitness), although other companies, such as Cybex, Precor, Nautilus, and Star Trac, also offer plate-loaded machines. The majority of plate-loaded machines retail for between $1,000 and $2,000, with only a few pieces ever exceeding $2,000 in cost.

Cardiovascular Entertainment Equipment

Cardiovascular entertainment equipment involves a system of apparatus that is employed in concert with cardiovascular-exercise equipment (e.g., indoor cycles, treadmills, elliptical machines, stairclimbers, etc.) that allows individuals to watch televised images while they work out. Such a system can accomplish several goals, including: enable individuals to disassociate from the perceived effort to exercise, help mask general feelings of fatigue, enliven the workout, make the exercise bout more interesting, etc.

> **Cardiovascular entertainment equipment involves a system of apparatus that is employed in concert with cardiovascular-exercise equipment (e.g., indoor cycles, treadmills, elliptical machines, stairclimbers, etc.) that allows individuals to watch televised images while they work out.**

❑ *Historical Overview.* Assumptions concerning how to "entertain" individuals while they are exercising changed substantially when Tony DeLeede introduced Cardio Theater to the health/fitness club industry in 1991. Before Cardio Theater, the entertainment efforts of most clubs were strictly limited to background music systems that played soundtracks from either licensed programs, such as Musak, or from radio stations. Prior to Cardio Theater, a few clubs set up televisions in their cardiovascular areas and tuned them to established stations so that members could watch and listen to television while they trained. The constraints of these various efforts became quite apparent when Cardio Theater developed a system that allowed users to tune into the television or music station of their choice through a special control that is mounted on the equipment on which the individual is exercising. The popularity of Cardio Theater led to the development of other audiovisual entertainment systems, including one produced by Broadcast Vision. The effort was further advanced when two companies, E Zone and Net Pulse, developed personal viewing systems that were attached to each piece of equipment. Net Pulse created individual kiosks for each piece of equipment that allowed users to surf the net or tune into their favorite television station. E Zone established a system, featuring small viewing screens that could be mounted in front of each piece of equipment and allowed users to view television stations, listen to CDs, or listen to music stations. E Zone also introduced personal headsets that enabled users to navigate throughout the club and continue listening to the station to which they were tuned. By the beginning of the 21st century, both E Zone and Net Pulse experienced problems with their business models and basically disappeared from the cardio-entertainment industry. Subsequently, both Broadcast Vision and Cardio Theater developed personal viewing systems that have been incorporated into their offerings. Starting in 2005, many equipment manufacturers began integrating personal viewing systems (PVS) into their equipment design. The first to leverage this approach was Life Fitness. The development of integrated personal viewing systems continues to evolve and currently includes systems that offer touch-screen technology, HD LED screens, MP3 compatibility, and streaming from the Internet.

❑ *Categories*. Cardio-entertainment systems are offered in three distinct categories: personal viewing systems, interconnected audiovisual systems, and personal tuner audiovisual systems.

• *Personal viewing systems (PVS)*. Personal viewing systems involve individual LCD screens (13 inches to 15 inches) that are either mounted in front of each piece of equipment and are connected to an integrated audiovisual network or integrated into the control panel of the equipment. Each user is able to tune into the station to which they want to watch or listen, using either a control module that is mounted on the equipment or through touch-screen technology that is integrated into the control panel of the equipment. As a result, users have their own personal entertainment system while exercising. As of 2010, most manufacturers of cardiovascular equipment offer models that include fully integrated entertainment systems that are compatible with the newest media devices, such as iPhones, iPads, etc. The price of PVS ranges between $1,000 and $1,300 per unit.

> Personal viewing systems involve individual LCD screens (13 inches to 15 inches) that are either mounted in front of each piece of equipment and are connected to an integrated audiovisual network or integrated into the control panel of the equipment.

• *Interconnected audiovisual entertainment systems.* These systems integrate wall/ceiling-mounted televisions with audio and video channels that are connected through a transmitter and equipment-mounted control boxes. Users can utilize the control box to select a channel that corresponds to either a television station or an audio channel. These systems have a varied number of channels (e.g., 4, 8, or 16) that allow users to select from a variety of audiovisual options. These systems feature headsets that users connect to the equipment-mounted control boxes. Most of the systems are wireless, but a few clubs employ hard-wired systems. The leading manufacturers of these systems are Broadcast Vision and Cardio Theater. The cost of these systems varies, based on the number of televisions, the number of channels on the system receiver, the number of control boxes needed, whether a DVD or video deck is provided, and whether wiring is needed. The control boxes retail for between $140 and $175 each, while an 8-channel receiver ranges in price between $1,300 and $1,500. A club that has 50 pieces of cardiovascular equipment might expect to spend in the range of $20,000 to $30,000 for a full system. One of the biggest challenges facing clubs that have these systems is the ongoing need to replace headphone jacks that are damaged through the constant placement and removal of user headsets.

- *Personal tuner audiovisual systems.* These systems are similar to the aforementioned integrated systems, except that they do not involve having control boxes on the equipment. These systems require that all televisions are set to specific, unused FM frequencies. This feature enables users to bring their own personal audio machine to their workout and tune into the frequency that corresponds to the television station they want to watch. Users can also tune into their favorite radio station. Many clubs prefer these systems, given that they involve less upfront expense and do not cost as much to operate, because they don't include equipment-mounted control boxes.

Other Frequently Required Equipment for the Health/Fitness Club Industry

As discussed previously, the health/fitness club industry is a capital-intensive business, especially from an equipment perspective. The majority of the capital spent on equipment is expended in one of the aforementioned four categories. Nonetheless, some relatively smaller categories also exist that can play an important role in the delivery of the health/fitness club experience, including:

❏ *Whole Body Vibration Machines (WBV).* Whole-body vibration training, sometimes referred to as acceleration training, was initially introduced to the club industry in 2001 by Power Plate, a European-based company. Whole-body vibration training equipment involves the transfer of an alternating mechanical wave from a vibrating platform to the tissues of the body. The transfer of these alternating mechanical waves from the machine platform to the body's tissues results in the creation of physical and neural overloads, which then lead to muscular and soft-tissue adaptation. The advocates of this style of training promote its ability to create improvements in muscular tone and conditioning in relatively brief bouts of activity. Although WBV equipment is popular in Europe and South America, as of 2010, it has not established traction in the U.S. market. The two leading brands of WBV equipment are the Power Plate and the iTonic, distributed by Free Motion. It should be noted that many exercise scientists remain somewhat skeptical of this particular form of training.

The majority of Pilates equipment purchased by clubs falls into the category of personal reformers (e.g., a single-user reformer that can be used in an individual or group setting), which is the primary piece of equipment employed in both personal-Pilates training and group-Pilates training.

❏ *Pilates Equipment.* Pilates equipment has slowly evolved into a significant equipment category with the expansive growth of Pilates programs. Pilates equipment consists of reformers, trapezes, ladder barrels, towers, Wunda chairs, combo chairs, and step barrels and arcs, as well as some additional pieces of accessory equipment. The majority of Pilates equipment purchased by clubs falls into the category of personal reformers (e.g., a single-user reformer that can be used in an individual or group setting), which is the primary piece of equipment employed in both personal-Pilates training and group-Pilates training. The leading manufacturers of Pilates equipment are Balanced Body, Peak, and Stott. The cost of Pilates equipment varies from item to item, brand to brand, and model to model. For example, the average retail price for studio reformers ranges between $3,000 and $4,500 each, with the classroom-designed reformers, such as Balanced Body's "Allegro Reformer," retailing for around $2,400. Another popular piece of Pilates equipment, the Cadillac (which is also referred to as the "Trapeze") ranges in price from $5,000 to $6,000, depending on the accessories purchased with it. (Note: The Cadillac is a Pilates table with a series of attached overhead implements.)

❑ *Spa Equipment.* As day spas have evolved into a noteworthy profit center for many clubs in the health/fitness club industry, the market for the equipment utilized in day spas has grown substantially. An incredible variety of equipment is needed to operate a successful spa, including:

- *Massage tables.* Massage tables range from fixed tables to adjustable tables, including hydraulic-driven adjustable tables. The price of a massage table ranges from $800 to $1,200 if it is self-adjusting and closer to $2,200 to $3,000 if it is hydraulic.

- *Facial tables.* Facial tables are similar to massage tables, except that they also have armrests and backs that enable users to be elevated so that they can be placed in a partially seated position. The cost of these tables ranges from $1,200 to $4,000, depending on the features desired.

- *Manicure tables.* The typical manicure table includes all the storage that is needed for the manicure products. A high-quality manicure table retails for between $900 and $1,500.

- *Pedicure stations.* The most popular pedicure stations include a number of features, such as a custom chair with armrests and a separate footbath/whirlpool. These stations retail for between $4,000 and $6,000. Some pedicure stations are also available that employ portable footbaths and chairs, rather than the more first-rate features. These stations cost approximately $2,000 less than the more upscale models.

- *Facial Stations.* A facial station encompasses a variety of devices necessary for performing basic facials, such as a magnifying light and rotary brush. A quality facial-station system retails for around $2,500 to $3,500.

Examples of other equipment that is often employed in spas include hot wax units, paraffin baths, thermal heaters for hot packs, Vichy shower units, hydrotherapy tubs, scotch hoses, massage chairs, wet tables, and aromatherapy diffusers. Purchasing spa equipment can be a somewhat difficult task, since no single manufacturer makes all of the items needed to operate a day spa. Some companies, such as Living Earth Crafts and Golden Ratio, provide a variety of tables and accessories, but not the full line of spa equipment. A few companies, such as Universal and Takara Belmont, distribute spa equipment from a variety of different suppliers.

Because the equipment industry is an ever-changing, fast-evolving enterprise, health/fitness club professionals need to stay abreast of the changes that occur if they want to be knowledgeable about essential equipment-related factors. IHRSA annually produces a publication, *FIT* (Fitness Industry Technology), that provides an overview of the various equipment categories and a listing of the various equipment suppliers. Several industry-related magazines, including *Athletic Business, Club Industry,* and *Recreation Management,* also publish editions that detail the equipment that is utilized in the health/fitness club

IHRSA annually produces a publication, *FIT* (Fitness Industry Technology), that provides an overview of the various equipment categories and a listing of the various equipment suppliers.

industry. (Note: A list of the leading manufacturers of health/fitness equipment in the industry is included in the appendices of this book.) One of the best ways to stay abreast of changes in equipment is to attend one of the major industry tradeshows, such as Club Industry (typically held in October), Athletic Business (held in December), IHRSA (usually held in March), and FIBO (held in Germany every April).

Purchase or Lease Equipment

Many of the most successful club operators choose to lease their equipment rather than purchase it, which enables them to save the initial investment that would be required if they had purchased it.

As previously stated, outfitting a health/fitness club with new equipment can range from $15 to $30 a square foot. As a result, a typical health/fitness facility might have to spend between $300,000 and $1,000,000 on exercise equipment. Because this expense can often represent a significant financial hurdle for owners, leasing becomes a viable alternative to acquisition and later depreciation. Many of the most successful club operators (e.g., LA Fitness, 24 Hour Fitness, etc.) choose to lease their equipment rather than purchase it, which enables them to save the initial investment that would be required if they had purchased it. The following list provides a brief overview of the pros and cons associated with either leasing or purchasing equipment.

❑ Purchasing Equipment
  • Pro:
    ✓ Outright ownership of the equipment
    ✓ Able to depreciate the equipment on financial statements
    ✓ Not at the mercy of leasing companies
    ✓ Causes club owners to have a greater "stake" in the business and a resultant commitment to making the business work (they cannot walk away as easily from the business)
  • Con:
    ✓ Initial up-front investment can be overwhelming and consume a significant amount of start-up funds
    ✓ Equipment depreciates in value as an asset (loss in asset value)
    ✓ Clubs are often less likely to invest in new equipment in coming years

❑ Leasing Equipment
  • Pro:
    ✓ Eliminates up-front investment
    ✓ Allows cost of equipment to be spread over several years
    ✓ Provides opportunity to upgrade equipment more readily and remain current with industry equipment trends
    ✓ Owners can step away from leases in the event of financial challenges
  • Con:
    ✓ Increases the cost of equipment due to interest payments to leasing company
    ✓ May require club to have leases with more than one company

OPERATIONAL PRACTICES IN THE HEALTH/FITNESS CLUB INDUSTRY

Part Seven

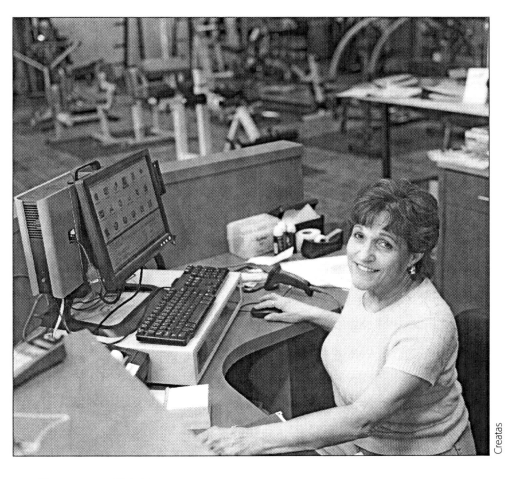

Creatas

19

Risk Management

Chapter Objectives

Risk management refers to the practices and systems that businesses put in place to help reduce and/or eliminate their exposure to liability and financial loss due to unsafe operating practices. In the health/fitness club industry, risk management refers to the practices, procedures, and systems by which the club reduces its risk of an employee or member experiencing an event that could result in harm to the individual (employee or customer) or the business itself. This chapter reviews the most critical risk-management practices and factors that clubs should address in order to provide an environment that presents the lowest possible risk to the employees, members, and business.

Risk Management Practices to Reduce Employee and Business Risk

Clubs should consider a number of key practices, policies, and systems when managing their business risk as it applies to their employees, and ultimately to their members, including:

❑ *Background Checks for Specific Employee Populations.* Most of the employees in the health/fitness club industry are actively involved in providing personalized experiences that can expose not only themselves, but also the club, to considerable risk. Numerous club personnel, such as personal trainers, massage therapists, fitness instructors, and swim instructors, among others, typically work closely with members in a one-on-one environment, where the chance of a risk-related situation occurring exists. Some club employees, such as child-care workers, swim instructors, summer camp instructors, tennis instructors, etc., are in even more potentially risk-vulnerable positions, because they work closely with young adults and children. The key point that should be emphasized is that clubs should seriously consider doing criminal background checks on every employee who comes into personal contact with the members to ensure that each individual member of the staff has no prior record of unsavory behavior that

> Clubs should seriously consider doing criminal background checks on every employee who comes into personal contact with the members to ensure that each individual member of the staff has no prior record of unsavory behavior that might expose other employees, members, or guests to harm.

might expose other employees, members, or guests to harm. For example, a simple criminal background check can be performed by an outside agency to determine whether an employee has a past criminal record. In addition to those individuals who work closely with people, any employee who is responsible for handling money on a regular basis should also be a serious candidate for a background screening.

As such, numerous businesses, including many in the health/fitness club industry, conduct annual background checks of those employee populations who present the greatest risk, such as those who meet the aforementioned criteria. It is important that if a club performs background checks, it should make its employees aware of its practices, policies, and procedures in this regard.

❏ *Drug and Alcohol Pre-Employment Testing.* The use of alcohol or drugs can impair an employee's judgment, which, in turn, could ultimately expose other employees or members to harm. Accordingly, drug and alcohol pre-employment testing is recommended for individuals employed in certain positions, such as those that require the handling of dangerous equipment, working with minors, or dispensing of alcohol. Such testing can help reduce the risk of an employee being impaired while acting on behalf of the club. Clubs should also consider testing other employees, such as bartenders, servers, housekeepers, engineering staff, locker-room attendants, and even fitness instructors. By law, drug, and alcohol pre-employment screening cannot be conducted without the permission of the individual who will be tested. As such, clubs must give their employees (actual and prospective) the option of whether to participate in the testing program. Fair or not, many businesses will view the refusal of an individual to undergo testing as a negative factor with regard to that person's worthiness as an employee.

> **Drug and alcohol pre-employment testing is recommended for individuals employed in certain positions, such as those that require the handling of dangerous equipment, working with minors, or dispensing of alcohol.**

❏ *Ensure That Employees Have the Right Credentials to Perform Their Job.* The health/fitness club industry has numerous positions that require specific licensing, registration, or certification. In that regard, clubs can limit their risk by ensuring both at the time of an individual's employment and during the course of employment that each employee's credentials are valid and current. If a person who holds a particular position that requires special education, training, registration, or licensure is found to be lacking, that club may be exposing itself to considerable financial risk. Among the positions in a club where an individual's credentials should be checked at the time of employment or contract signing and thereafter on an ongoing basis are the following:

 • *Massage therapists.* In the majority of states, massage therapists must be either licensed or registered to practice. Accordingly, clubs should ask all of their massage therapists for a copy of their license or registration documents (as appropriate) at the time of their employment and ensure that these are maintained.

 • *Estheticians.* Estheticians are employees/contractors who provide selected spa services, such as manicures, pedicures, facials, and hair styling. Because these employees must be licensed, similar to massage therapists, clubs should obtain evidence of licensure upon employment.

- *Dieticians/nutritionists.* Many clubs offer nutritional counseling and related dietary advice. A registered dietician is a professionally trained individual who is recognized as having the education and qualifications needed to counsel and prescribe a nutritional plan. If the employee or contractor is not a registered dietician, then the club is exposing itself to an increased risk of liability.

- *Personal trainers and instructors.* At the present time, no established national standard or law exists concerning the required qualifications for a personal trainer. Both the American College of Sports Medicine, in its highly regarded text, *ACSM's Health/Fitness Facility Standards and Guidelines*, and IHRSA, in its book, *Standards Facilitation Guide: Health and Safety, Legal, and Ethical Standards for U.S. IHRSA Clubs as of 1998*, indicate that it is essential that personal trainers and other exercise instructors have the appropriate level of education and credentials. In fact, IHRSA (since January 1, 2006) only recognizes those professional certifications with third-party accreditation from a nationally recognized certifying agency [e.g., National Commission of Certifying Agencies (NCCA)]. Accordingly, personal trainers should be certified by a nationally recognized certification program, such as those offered by ACE, ACSM, NSCA, and NASM. As of 2011, eight state legislatures have introduced legislation to compel personal trainers to be either registered or licensed. If a personal trainer does not have the appropriate certification, the club is exposing itself to greater risk.

- *Lifeguards.* In all states, lifeguards are required to have advanced lifesaving and water safety certification. Employing lifeguards without those credentials would expose a club to a substantial risk in the event of an accident.

Besides ensuring that their employees/contract labor possess the appropriate credentials, clubs should be aware of exactly what actions these individuals are legally permitted/qualified to perform. For example, a personal trainer is not qualified or legally recognized as someone who can prescribe either supplements or rehabilitative exercises. Likewise, a personal trainer cannot diagnose a member's health status. Similarly, massage therapists are not legally qualified to perform therapeutic treatments using massage, unless they have the appropriate credentials. Clubs can avoid these issues by making sure that their job descriptions and employee policies clearly clarify such matters.

❏ *Handling Hazardous Chemicals and Materials.* The health/fitness club industry is a field in which many of its employees are exposed to materials that the Occupational Safety and Health Administration (OSHA) considers dangerous. Club positions, such as housecleaners, lifeguards, locker-room attendants, maintenance staff, and fitness staff, among others, are occasionally exposed to hazardous chemicals and materials. These chemicals and materials include items such as cleaning agents, paints, and lubricants. For example, employees who work in closed areas where air circulation is inadequate, particularly in locations where sanding, drilling, or similar activities are occurring, can suffer undue exposure to particle matters. To comply with OSHA guidelines and reduce the level of risk involving the

Besides ensuring that their employees/ contract labor possess the appropriate credentials, clubs should be aware of exactly what actions these individuals are legally permitted/ qualified to perform.

handling of hazardous chemicals and materials to their employees, clubs should undertake the following actions:

- Ensure that the material data sheets (MDS) for every chemical and agent used in the club are posted in a visible location for all employees to view.
- Provide an MDS binder for all employees/contractors to review. Confirm that these individuals have viewed the information and understand the issues, usually by having them sign a designated sheet.
- Store all chemicals and agents in secure locations. Make sure that these materials are stored off the floor and in an area that is off-limits to the members. These storage areas should have locks in order to prevent their access by unauthorized individuals. In addition, only those staff who receive training in the handling of these agents should be allowed access to these secured storage areas.
- Provide regular training in the proper handling of hazardous chemicals and materials.
- Make sure to provide employees with the proper protective apparel, e.g., protective gloves, aprons, face masks, respirators, etc.

❏ *Handling Body Fluids.* The health/fitness club industry is a field that exposes its members and employees to various bodily fluids. In fact, almost every individual who works in the industry can come into contact with bodily fluids, thereby being exposed to the resultant risk of blood-borne pathogens. Too many club operators fail to realize that even the handling of towels involves an increased risk of exposure for employees and members to the problems that can arise from handling bodily fluids. As a result, an increased risk to the business itself exists in such circumstances. Among the key steps that every club can take to minimize their risk in this area are the following:

- Provide training for employees. Make sure that employees are taught how to handle bodily fluids. In this regard, OSHA provides training materials, as do many other organizations.
- Provide literature for employees on the handling of bodily fluids.
- Make sure employees who are handling towels, cleaning, or picking up papers wear gloves (surgical-style gloves). Employees who have to handle bar soap or razors should be provided with latex or similar type of gloves.
- Have a system within the club for the disposal of items that contain bodily fluids. If the club provides razors for members' use, it should have a biowaste container for their disposal. If the club washes the towels that are utilized in the facility, it should use bleach, which will help kill most of the pathogens that are carried in bodily fluids.
- If blood is visible, clean it immediately with bleach or similar agent, and do not let employees or contractors handle it without the proper protective apparel.

❏ *Have an Employee Safety Program.* Clubs that want to reduce their level of risk involving their practices, policies, and procedures and the costs associated with those factors need to provide worker safety programs that

> **Too many club operators fail to realize that even the handling of towels involves an increased risk of exposure for employees and members to the problems that can arise from handling bodily fluids.**

address the key safety issues inherent in each job. Many of the costs and liabilities incurred by clubs result from not having a safety program in place that provides the proper education to employees about the risks of each job and how to prevent them. For example, massage therapists, tennis instructors, and group-exercise instructors experience more work-related injuries than any other positions in the health/fitness club industry. The key point that should be emphasized in this regard is that a club must establish clear guidelines concerning certain positions and job responsibilities, for example, setting limits on the time a therapist can perform massage during a given schedule or placing strict boundaries on the number of classes that instructors are allowed to teach. A sound employee-safety program addresses several factors, including:

- Making sure that every job description identifies the tasks and activities of that job that may expose an employee to an increased risk of being injured (e.g., fitness instructors can be exposed to lifting and moving heavy objects, while massage therapists can be open to incurring chronic repetitive motion injuries). Having the employee sign-off that they are aware of these job-related parameters and risks is important.
- Providing ongoing educational programs on worker safety.
- Establishing a reward program for safety that recognizes actions that increase the safety level of the work environment.
- Making sure that all accidents or incidents are immediately reported and documented and that appropriate action is taken to deal with the incident.

❑ *Have the Appropriate Insurance Policies.* Clubs should maintain the appropriate types and the proper amounts of insurance in order to minimize their level of risk in the work environment and help protect both the physical and intellectual assets of their business. In this regard, club operators should carry the following types of insurance:

- *General liability insurance.* Every club should have a general liability insurance package that provides at least one million dollars in coverage per occurrence and up to three million dollars of total coverage. General liability insurance covers most incidences of negligence or accidents.
- *Professional liability insurance.* Professional liability insurance is one key type of insurance that many clubs fail to provide. Certain positions in a club, such as personal trainers, group-exercise instructors, and massage therapists, should be covered by professional liability insurance. This insurance covers issues involving professional competency. Although most clubs do not have this type of insurance, they should. Several of the professional associations in the industry (e.g., ACE, ACSM, NSCA, etc.) offer professional liability insurance-coverage packages, which members of those associations can obtain.
- *Worker's compensation insurance.* Clubs should consider establishing a worker's compensation program for their employees, especially if they have individuals who are performing jobs that expose them to injury and loss of work. In many states (e.g., California), such a program is required.

Many of the costs and liabilities incurred by clubs result from not having a safety program in place that provides the proper education to employees about the risks of each job and how to prevent them.

- *Property insurance.* Although property insurance covers the physical assets of a business, this type of insurance can be another key element in managing a club's risk, particularly its risk of financial loss if something happens (damage or loss) to its property or other physical assets.

- *Business interruption insurance.* Business interruption insurance provides clubs with insurance against revenue loss due to unforeseen circumstances. For example, if a club has to close for a month due to fire damage, this insurance would protect their revenue stream during the time they are closed.

Risk Management Practices to Reduce Member/User and Business Risk

Effectively managing the level of risk to which members are exposed is important to clubs for at least two reasons. First, having sound member risk-management practices can help provide a safer environment in the club for the members and help reduce their chances of being injured or suffering other health-related problems. Second, properly managing the risks that members encounter in a club's facility can help reduce the likelihood of litigation directed to the club that can drain the financial health of the business. In that regard, several policies, practices, and systems exist that clubs can utilize to reduce the level of risk for their members.

❑ *Pre-Activity Screening.* The first basic step in increasing member safety and reducing risk is to make sure every member and club user has completed a pre-activity screening. According to both the most recent editions of the two most highly regarded texts on the subject, IHRSA's *Standards Facilitation Guide* and *ACSM's Health/Fitness Facility Standards and Guidelines*, a club must provide pre-activity screening for its users. Pre-activity screening should involve, at the minimum, screening for certain basic health risks, particularly, coronary-risk factors. In that regard, proven tools, such as the Par-Q or a simple medical history questionnaire (samples of which are included in the Appendices), can be extremely useful.

> The first basic step in increasing member safety and reducing risk is to make sure every member and club user has completed a pre-activity screening.

❑ *Medical Clearance.* Clubs that utilize pre-activity screening tools should also have a system by which those individuals who are identified as having an increased risk due to their health profile either are referred to a physician for physician clearance before engaging in physical activity or if they refuse to obtain a physician's release (for whatever reason), are required to sign a waiver or other legally drawn up form, indicating that they have decided not to obtain clearance from a physician and, as a result, are releasing the club from any liability associated with their participation in any physical-activity offering of the club.

The medical release can be as simple as a one-page document that is forwarded by the club to the member's physician or provided to the member to personally take to their physician. The medical-release form should clearly indicate that the member has been identified as being at an increased risk of incurring an injury or health-related problem if the individual participates in a physical-activity program and that by completing and signing the form, the physician is clearing the member to participate in physical activity. The release should allow physicians to provide any recommendations they may have concerning the individual's participation in physical activity. An example of a medical-release form is included in the Appendices.

❑ *Waiver of Liability.* A waiver is a legal document that members/users sign, indicating that they are aware of the risks associated with their participation in a physical-activity program that involves the club's facilities, programs, and services and that they knowingly accept full responsibility for their decision to participate in such offerings and are releasing the club from any and all responsibility for their participation. A waiver should be prepared by an attorney and should address the following:

   • The facilities, programs, and services that the member has access to and might use to pursue a program of physical activity
   • The risks involved in engaging in physical activity, including and up to the risk of a cardiac event or even death
   • A statement that the member is aware of the risks involved, that the club has explained those risks thoroughly, and that the member is willing to accept those risks
   • The member's willingness to accept all responsibility for their participation in light of the information they have been provided and that they are accepting complete responsibility for their actions and releasing the club from any and all liability associated with their decision

   The use of a waiver should be standard practice for every club in legal jurisdictions that allow the use of a waiver. Ideally, all members/users should complete and sign a waiver form upon joining a club. Both *ACSM's Health/ Fitness Facility Standards and Guidelines* and IHRSA's *Standard Facilitation Guide* indicate that waivers should be a standard practice for health/fitness club operators. (Note: Some recent court rulings have upheld a plaintiff's right to legal action even when a waiver has been signed.)

❑ *Emergency-Response System.* Having an appropriate emergency-response system is an essential factor in the effort to establish a safe environment for members and employees, as well as a sound risk-management practice. In that regard, health/fitness clubs must develop emergency response systems that help ensure that their members have the highest reasonable level of safety. An emergency-response system should encompass several key elements, including:

   • Local healthcare and/or medical personnel should be solicited to help develop the emergency-response system that the club utilizes. Most emergency-medical services are willing to assist a club in developing an emergency-response program. Clubs can also pay for the services of a qualified person, such as a physician, registered nurse, or certified emergency-medical technician, to help guide the development of their program.

Having an appropriate emergency-response system is an essential factor in the effort to establish a safe environment for members and employees, as well as a sound risk-management practice.

- The club's emergency-response system should address the major medical emergency situations that might occur, such as heart attacks, strokes, orthopedic-related injuries, accidents, etc., as well as non-medical emergencies, such as fires and natural disasters.

- The club's emergency-response system should detail explicit steps or directions concerning how each emergency situation should be handled, including the roles that should be played by first, second, and third responders to an emergency. In addition, the emergency-response system should specify the locations of all emergency equipment and all emergency exists.

- The emergency-response system should be fully documented and kept in an area that can be easily accessed by the club's staff. In addition, the emergency-response system should be reviewed with each employee on a regular basis.

- The emergency-response system should be physically rehearsed by everyone involved at least once annually and preferably once every quarter.

- The emergency-response system should incorporate the use of an automated external defibrillator (AED) and cardiopulmonary resuscitation equipment (both of which are covered in greater detail in a later section of this chapter).

- The emergency-response system should address the availability and location of first-aid kits within the club.

- The emergency-response system should identify an on-site coordinator for the program (the employee who is responsible for the club's overall emergency readiness).

❑ *Signage.* Clubs can reduce their level of business risk and, at the same time, help create a safer physical activity environment for their members by developing signage that is then posted in appropriate locations that communicates to its members those areas of the club that involve a potentially substantial risk to an individual's health and safety. This signage should indicate the risks involved and include information that can lessen the member's risk if they respond appropriately to the information provided to them. Detailed information on developing proper signage for the health/fitness club industry is available from the American Society for Testing and Materials (ASTM) in its *Standard Specification of Fitness Equipment and Fitness Facility Signage and Labels (F 1749-96).*The key areas of a health/fitness facility that should have signage include:

- *Sauna, steam room, and whirlpool.* Due to exposure to high heat and humidity, these areas present an elevated risk to both apparently healthy and at-risk users. As a result, clubs should post signage that provides users with the basic warnings and information concerning these areas that can help them make a more-informed decision about whether to utilize these facilities. Signage in each of these areas should include:

  ✓ Information about the temperature range to which the user will be exposed

Clubs can reduce their level of business risk and, at the same time, help create a safer physical activity environment for their members by developing signage that is then posted in appropriate locations that communicates to its members those areas of the club that involve a potentially substantial risk to an individual's health and safety.

✓ A warning about the increased risk of hyperthermia if too much time is spent in any of these facilities

✓ A warning about specific populations that should avoid exposure to these areas unless they have their physician's approval, such as those individuals with either high blood pressure or coronary artery disease, women who are pregnant, members on vasodilator medications, etc.

✓ A warning to cool down after exercise before entering these areas

✓ Guidelines on what constitutes a reasonably safe time period for individuals to utilize these areas

✓ A warning about not entering the pool if the individual has an open wound

- *Aquatic areas.* Most state and local health departments require certain signage be posted in the pool areas. These signage requirements are designed to protect users from exposure to risky behavior. Among the key elements that are normally indicated in pool signage are the following:

  ✓ A warning about not running or playing on the pool deck

  ✓ A warning about deck surfaces being slippery when wet

  ✓ A warning about no diving

  ✓ Information about food not being allowed around the pool

  ✓ Information that no supervision or lifeguard is present (if the pool is not required by law to have lifeguards)

  ✓ Information about not entering the pool immediately after eating

  ✓ Information about showering before entering the pool

  ✓ A warning about not entering the pool if the individual has an open wound

  With regard to signage for aquatic areas, club operators should be familiar with the local laws and regulations to ensure that their facilities are in full compliance with all the legally required signage expectations.

- *Enclosed racquet courts (e.g., handball, racquetball, and squash).* Clubs should provide signage that indicates that individuals should wear appropriate eye protection when using the courts.

- *Fitness areas.* Certain risks exist in the fitness areas of a club with which many users might not be familiar. In those circumstances, the use of relatively simple signage can help rectify the situation. Examples of signage in these areas might include:

  ✓ Recommendation to have a spotter when performing certain free-weight exercises (free-weight area)

  ✓ Recommendation to get instruction or guidance from a professional before embarking on a fitness program

  ✓ Recommendation to stop exercising if the individual experiences dizziness, pain, or unusual discomfort

  ✓ Instructional signage that helps enhance the safety level of a particular piece of equipment

  ✓ Signage indicating that a piece of equipment is out of order

Certain risks exist in the fitness areas of a club with which many users might not be familiar. In those circumstances, the use of relatively simple signage can help rectify the situation.

✓ Recommendation to read the labels and operational instructions provided on all equipment prior to using it

In addition to signage in the fitness areas that focuses on the aforementioned information and warnings, clubs should also provide either perceived-exertion charts or target heart-rate charts so that members/users can monitor their level of exertion while exercising.

- *Hazardous conditions signage.* Hazardous conditions signage is general signage that warns members/users of any unusual risk attendant to a particular physical condition or practice at the club. For example, these signs should be used in situations such as:

  ✓ When equipment is out of order, and the club wants to make its members aware that the equipment is out of use

  ✓ When floors are being wet, and the club wants to make its members/users aware of slippery conditions

  ✓ When a condition exists, such as damaged walking surfaces, loose impediment, or a related condition that would increase the risk to the club's members/users exists

  ✓ When repairs or construction are being performed and the club wants to warn its members/users of specific dangers or locations to avoid

❏ *Preventative Maintenance Schedules and Audits.* One of the best practices that clubs can adopt for increasing member/user safety and reducing their business risk is to implement preventative maintenance procedures that are audited on a daily or weekly basis. The majority of accidents in the health/fitness club environment occur because club operators fail to execute basic preventative maintenance procedures and provide the necessary inspection of these procedures. Among the core practices that a club can execute in this regard are the following:

- Employ cleaning and preventative maintenance checklists for all fitness equipment. Clubs should ensure that its equipment is maintained on a daily, weekly, and monthly basis. This endeavor should include checking all bolts, checking all cables, checking for loose parts, cleaning surfaces, etc.

- Adhere to daily, weekly, and monthly schedules for cleaning all areas of the club.

- Utilize checklists for performing preventative maintenance of lights, plumbing, and HVAC.

- Make sure to follow the manufacturer's guidelines concerning the care of equipment. In that regard, clubs should have operator manuals for each piece of equipment in the facility.

The most critical factor is to have a system in place to verify compliance with the aforementioned, prescribed checklists. Many club operators employ supervisors to conduct regular audits of their maintenance procedures and practices. When audits are conducted, it is important to make sure the audit is documented, and the results are kept on file.

> One of the best practices that clubs can adopt for increasing member/user safety and reducing their business risk is to implement preventative maintenance procedures that are audited on a daily or weekly basis.

❏ *Incident Reports.* Incident reports are standard forms that a business completes whenever an accident or incident occurs on its property. For health/fitness clubs, it should be standard practice to complete an incident report each time an accident or safety-related event occurs at the club. The purpose of the incident report is to obtain the necessary information attendant to a particular event, such as the nature of the event, time of the event, witnesses, extent of any injury resulting from the event, response of the club to the incident, etc. This information can be extremely important for situations involving insurance, litigation, and responding medical agencies.

For health/fitness clubs, it should be standard practice to complete an incident report each time an accident or safety-related event occurs at the club.

Automated External Defibrillators (AEDs)

❏ *Overview.* AEDs are sophisticated, computerized machines that are simple to operate and enable a layperson, with minimal training, to administer a potentially lifesaving intervention to individuals who experience cardiac arrest. AEDs are devices that can be employed in an emergency situation to detect a life-threatening cardiac arrhythmia and then to administer an electrical shock that can help restore the normal sinus rhythm. AEDs represent the third step in the American Heart Association's (AHA's) renowned "chain of survival"—after calling 911 and administering CPR.

The AHA reports that research shows that the delivery speed of defibrillation, as provided by an AED, is the major determinant of success in resuscitative attempts for ventricular fibrillation (VF) cardiac arrest (the most common type of cardiac arrest). Survival rates after VF decrease 7 to 10 percent with every minute delay in defibrillation. A survival rate as high as 90 percent has been reported when defibrillation is administered within the first minute of collapse, but decreases to 50 percent at five minutes, 30 percent at seven minutes, 10 percent at 9 to 11 minutes and two to five percent after 12 minutes.

Those communities that have incorporated AEDs into their emergency systems have achieved significant improvements in the survival rates for those individuals who have experienced cardiac events. In the state of Washington, for example, the survival rate increased from 7 to 26 percent, whereas, in Iowa, the survival rate increased from 3 to19 percent. Some public programs have reported survival rates as high as 49 percent with prompt administration of an AED. The American Heart Association is a strong proponent of having AEDs as accessible to the public as possible. The use and application of AEDs in a public setting is detailed in the American Heart Association's book, *Guidelines for Emergency Cardiac Care.* A revised version of the *Guidelines* was released in 2010.

As of January 2010, 11 states had passed AED legislation, as it pertains to health/fitness facilities (Arkansas, California, Illinois, Indiana, Louisiana, Michigan, Massachusetts, New Jersey, New York, Oregon, and Rhode Island). In addition to these states, several local districts—Suffolk County, NY; Weston, Florida; and Montgomery Country, Maryland—have passed legislation requiring health/fitness facilities to have AEDs. Similar legislation requiring clubs to have AEDs is also pending in Wisconsin. Only four states have legislation that accommodates unstaffed fitness facilities.

The movement toward requiring an AED in health/fitness facilities received strong support in 2007, when the American College of Sports Medicine, in the 3rd edition of *ACSM's Standards and Guidelines for Health/ Fitness Facilities*, indicated that an AED must be a part of every health/ fitness facility's emergency response plan. Among the U.S. health/fitness club companies that have adopted that standard are ClubCorp, Dallas, Texas; Fitcorp, Boston, MA; Sport and Health, Washington, DC; Tennis Corporation of America, Chicago, Illinois; Townsports International, New York, New York; Wellbridge, Denver, Colorado; and Western Athletic Clubs, San Francisco, California.

❑ *Guidelines for Implementing an AED Program in a Health/Fitness Club:*

- Every site with an AED should make an effort to get the response time from collapse to defibrillation to three minutes.

Every site with an AED should make an effort to get the response time from collapse to defibrillation to three minutes.

- AEDs that are located in the club facility should ideally be within a 1.5-minute walk of a potential collapse site. A responder should be able to reach an AED within a 1.5-minute walk time.
- The FDA requires that a physician must prescribe an AED before it can be purchased. The AHA strongly recommends that a physician, licensed to practice medicine in the community, should provide the oversight of the facility's emergency system and the role of AEDs in that system. In most cases, the company from which the AED is purchased will assist the club with identifying a physician to provide these services, or will include those services with the purchase an AED. Physician oversight refers to:
  ✓ Prescribing the AED
  ✓ Reviewing and signing off on the emergency plan
  ✓ Witnessing at least one rehearsal of and providing a written report of such events
  ✓ Providing standing orders for the use of the AED
  ✓ Reviewing documentation of any instances when the emergency plan is initiated and the AED is used
- A club's emergency plan and AED plan should be coordinated with the local emergency medical services (EMS) provider (the product provider normally does this step). Coordinating with the local EMS provider refers to:
  ✓ Informing its local EMS provider that the club has an one or more AEDs
  ✓ Informing its local EMS provider of the location of each AED in the club's facility
  ✓ Working with the local EMS provider in providing ongoing training of the club's staff in the use of the AED
  ✓ Working with the local EMS provider to provide monitoring and review of AED events

- The AHA's Emergency Cardiac Care Committee, as well as numerous international experts, encourages a skills review and practice sessions with the AED at least every six months. Regular practice drills every three to six months are recommended.

- The AED should be monitored and maintained to the manufacturer's specifications on a daily, weekly, and monthly basis. All results from those efforts should be recorded. AEDs currently on the market provide this capability through an automated process.

- All incidences involving the administration of an AED must be recorded and then reported to the physician who is providing oversight. It should be noted that the HIPPA (Health Insurance Portability and Protection Act) does not allow medically sensitive information to be released to anyone other than the medical director.

- Each club should have an AED program coordinator who is responsible for all aspects of the facility's emergency-response plan and the use of the AED, as outlined in *ACSM's Health/Fitness Facility Standards and Guidelines, 4th Edition.*

- All employees who are likely to be involved in a situation in which they might have to administer an AED should complete a program in basic life support (BLS) and AED usage from an accredited training organization. The two most recognized organizations in this regard are the American Heart Association (AHA), which offers its Heart Saver CPR/AED training and certification, and the American Red Cross, which offers separate courses in CPR, AED, and First Aid training. Numerous local and national organizations, including the American Council on Exercise (ACE), facilitate either AHA or ARC courses in the administration of an AED and CPR. These programs involve a minimum of four hours of direct-contact training. Because certification in these areas lasts for two years, employees should be required to complete such training on an every-other-year basis.

- A club should have at least one employee on duty at all times who is currently trained and certified in CPR/AED administration. Ideally, more than one such trained and certified employee should be on duty at all times.

- Four special situations exist involving the use and application of an AED that the club should be familiar with and which should be reviewed during the initial AED training of the club's employees:

  ✓ AEDs should not be used in or around water. Because electricity takes the path of least resistance, it should not be used in or near puddles of water (e.g., shower, steam room, whirlpool, etc.) or in the rain. If necessary, the patient should be moved and dried off before attaching the AED.

  ✓ The American Heart Association, in its 2005 *Guidelines* that include references to emergency cardiac care, and the Pediatric Life Support Task Force (PALS) of the International Liaison Committee on Resuscitation, in its 2002 position paper, both indicate that an AED can be used on children under eight years of age when no sign of

All employees who are likely to be involved in a situation in which they might have to administer an AED should complete a program in basic life support (BLS) and AED usage from an accredited training organization.

circulation exists. In these instances, the electrical shock should be delivered in a pediatric dose.

✓ External factors, such as clothing, jewelry, medication patches, and too much hair on the chest, could interfere with the AED effectiveness, and as a result, these items should be removed. The prep kit is normally included with the AED and can assist in the removal of these items.

✓ Some individuals may have implanted internal devices, such as pacemakers and defibrillators. These devices create a small prominence under the skin. If such devices are detected, the individual using the AED should make sure that the pads are not placed directly over these devices, because they may block the flow of energy.

❑ *Guidelines for Locating AEDs in a Health/Fitness Club Facility:*

• A critical step in the standard of care for use of an AED is the need to locate the AED where it can easily and rapidly be accessed in the event of a cardiac event. According to the AHA, this factor refers to the fact that an AED must be reachable within 1.5 minutes by a responder and must be applied in under four minutes from the onset time of a cardiac event. Accordingly, the club must consider these two time-related factors, when determining how many AEDs are needed and where they should be located in the facility.

> **A critical step in the standard of care for use of an AED is the need to locate the AED where it can easily and rapidly be accessed in the event of a cardiac event.**

• Clubs should determine which locations in the facility could be most easily accessed within a 1.5-minute walk. The average person who is walking at four mph can cover a distance of approximately 350 feet a minute, which translates to a distance of approximately 525 feet (175 yards) in 1.5 minutes.

• For clubs that have tennis facilities, the most suitable location in the tennis area for an AED would be the reception or reservation desk. If the desk cannot be reached in 1.5 minutes from some courts, then a second AED may be required and located at a second site. In most instances, a club with fewer than 20 courts will probably need only one AED, whereas a club with more than 20 courts might consider at least two AEDs. The highest risk areas in a health/fitness facility are normally the racquet courts, the steam, sauna and whirlpool areas, and the locker rooms.

• For clubs that offer fitness facilities, the most suitable location to locate an AED would be at the front desk. If any portion of the fitness facility cannot be accessed from the desk in 1.5 minutes, then at least one additional AED may be required and located at another appropriate site. Clubs that have two floors should consider positioning an AED on each floor. Other than the front desk, an AED might also be located in the exercise area, pool, or locker rooms. As a rule, the highest risk areas in an athletic facility are the locker rooms (where the steam, sauna, and whirlpool areas are located), the fitness center, group-exercise studios, and racquet courts.

The key point that must be emphasized when deciding where to position AEDs in a facility is to ensure that every AED can be easily accessed. In other words, the AED should be positioned in an open location that has limited traffic congestion, rather than locked or placed in a closet or other area that cannot be easily accessed.

20

Front-of-the-House Operations

Chapter Objectives

Health/fitness clubs are successful because of many factors, including their operating practices. Operating practices are those administrative policies, practices, procedures, and systems that enable a club to deliver its products and services in such as manner as to create memorable member experiences and drive financial profitability. This chapter examines the "best" industry practices involving front-of-the-house operations. These practices are particularly relevant to those departments within a club that involve direct interaction between the facility's employees and members, including the front-desk department, child-care department, fitness department, aquatics department, and racquet/tennis department. Not intended to be all-inclusive, the chapter reviews the most critical practices (i.e., the "best" practices) that club operators should address in their operations.

Defining an Operating Practice

Operating practices can be most easily defined as administrative policies, practices, procedures, and systems that enable and empower employees to deliver the club's products and services to its members as consistently as possible. Operating practices range from the policies governing scheduling appointments to the practice of conducting new member orientations. The more formalized these operating practices are, the easier it is for the club to consistently deliver its products and services. The health/fitness club industry has numerous well-thought-out and proven operating practices. As a result, no one best method for operating a club exists. Instead, there are benchmarks or best practices that can help clearly define what health/fitness club operators should do in order to run their business successfully. The most successful club operators divide operations into two important components: standards and systems. The operating standards are the minimum expectations that a club has for the delivery of a practice. These expectations provide a basic action framework for the staff. The systems are the tools that the staff can employ to meet the established standards or expectations.

No one best method for operating a club exists. Instead, there are benchmarks or best practices that can help clearly define what health/fitness club operators should do in order to run their business successfully.

Front-Desk (Reception) Department

The front-desk department at the majority of health/fitness clubs in the industry has four primary responsibilities: welcoming members and guests, scheduling appointments, answering phones, and disseminating club information. The degree to which the club is successful at each of these responsibilities is dependent to a great extent on the operating practices it has implemented.

> The practice of greeting members is especially important in the club business because it sets the tone for each member's or guest's overall experience in the club.

❑ *Welcoming Members and Guests.* The practice of greeting members is especially important in the club business because it sets the tone for each member's or guest's overall experience in the club. Successfully greeting members and guests depends on several factors, such as being able to make contact with each member/guest and calling them by name. It also requires being aware of their arrival and monitoring their access to the club. As a result, most club operators establish baseline policies and practices that are designed to drive the greeting process. Examples of some of the most effective operating practices or systems include:

• *Membership identification system.* The majority of clubs require members to show their membership card upon entry to the club. Not only does requiring members to present their card enable the staff to ensure that each visitor to the club is a member, more importantly, it provides a means for personally identifying and greeting each guest by name. Some clubs ask their members to show their card to front-desk staff, while others require members to swipe their card through a card reader. In Germany, instead of swiping the card, members place either their card or other object containing a computer chip against a device that can register the information present on the chip. In Brazil, many clubs take fingerprint scans; while in Turkey, a few clubs use either an eye/retina scan or other biometric scanning device to monitor member entry. These various systems usually drives a screen on the front-desk computer that displays basic information on the member, including the individual's name, the last time the person visited the club, the individual's activity interests, etc. A recent trend is to use fingerprint or eye scan technology to indentify members. If the visitor is an invited guest, clubs require the presentation of an authorized guest pass that identifies the name of the guest, the dates the guest pass is valid for, and the name of the club member or staff person who authorized the guest pass.

  The most important policy for clubs with regard to greeting members is to have standards concerning their expectations on how members should be greeted. At ClubCorp, for example, one basic standard was to greet each member by name within 10 seconds of their arrival. Another standard was to stand and smile when greeting a member or guest. On one hand, ClubCorp's standards set the framework for its employees, while, on the other hand, the actual systems for performing standard-related tasks, such as collecting cards, swiping cards, etc., were the practices that allowed the standard to be met at ClubCorp.

• *System for monitoring member and guest access.* Monitoring the access of members and guests is different than greeting them. Monitoring refers not only to being able to identify who is using the club, but also making sure that whoever is using the club is not exposing the club to any undue liability. The most critical step in monitoring access to the club is identifying if the visitor is a member or guest and whether that person is authorized to have access privileges. The majority of clubs utilize special technology to accomplish this step. Numerous software applications (e.g., Check Free/Aphelion, CSI, Motion Soft, Twin Oaks, and iGo Figure are examples of the many vendors that provide such software) enable staff to verify a member or guest's status, using existing databases that are stored on the software.

The monitoring process is important for several reasons. For example, it helps make sure that the club's facilities are made available to only those individuals who have paid for the privilege. It also provides a means to know who is in the club at any given time (an important factor from a risk-management perspective). In addition, it enables the club to determine overall club usage, information that can later be used to make other operating decisions. Knowing who is in the club can become extremely valuable in the event of an emergency or if someone needs to contact that individual. For those clubs that do not use software, the next best practice is to employ a sign-in log. A sign-in log involves having each visitor, member, or guest sign their name and list the time of their entry to the club.

Another operating practice involved in monitoring is to ensure that each non-member/guest has completed a pre-activity screening instrument and has signed a waiver (if appropriate) within the past 12 months. According to *ACSM's Health/Fitness Facility Standards and Guidelines, 4th Edition*, all club users must undergo pre-activity screening. Completing this requirement at the time of a person's entry to the club makes the most sense. At ClubCorp, the standard is to require each visitor, member, or guest to sign-in when they enter the facility and to have guests complete a pre-activity screening instrument at the same time and sign a waiver (if necessary).

❑ *Scheduling Appointments.* In most health/fitness clubs, the front-desk staff has the responsibility of making all reservations and appointments, including court reservations, appointments for personal training or massage sessions, class registrations, and event sign-ups. In some of the larger clubs, these functions are often handled by a separate reservation desk (e.g., East Bank Club, Chicago; Western Athletic Clubs, California; Lifetime Fitness, Eden Prairie, Minnesota and Telos Fitness, Dallas, Texas). Regardless of which personnel in the club are assigned responsibility for handling reservations and making appointments, standards and practices for performing those duties should be established.

• *Scheduling standards.* To ensure that the scheduling of appointments and reservations is handled properly, basic standards need to be established concerning what constitutes an appropriate reservation. In that regard, some of the key standards might include:

✓ *Having a set restriction concerning how far in advance appointments can be scheduled.* In most clubs, this standard can range from one

> The most critical step in monitoring access to the club is identifying if the visitor is a member or guest and whether that person is authorized to have access privileges.

day to as far as a month in advance. Within the industry, for example, some tennis clubs limit their reservations to seven days in advance, while others allow reservations to be made only one day in advance. The key is for the club to identify the appropriate time limit during which its membership can schedule appointments in advance.

✓ *Having a cancellation/no-show policy.* The most successful club operators establish clear cancellation and no-show policies concerning reservations and appointments. Such policies help establish clear value for the club's services and also help provide flexibility to accommodate other members and guests. A common practice in the industry is to have a 12-hour cancellation policy. In other words, those appointments that are cancelled more than 12 hours in advance result in no charge, while those that are terminated with less than 12 hours notice involve some form of penalty charge. A no-show policy involves establishing some type of consequence if an appointment does not show. For example, the club might charge a $10 fee for no-shows.

✓ *Specifying the information to be collected.* It is critical that clubs establish a standard concerning what information should be obtained when scheduling an appointment or reservation. For example, at ClubCorp, when an appointment is made for a tennis court, the staff must get the member's name, the member's membership number, the time and date of the appointment, the court the reservation is for, and the staff person who made the appointment. In addition, the ClubCorp staff person who made the reservation/appointment must initial the reservation.

> **It is critical that clubs establish a standard concerning what information should be obtained when scheduling an appointment or reservation.**

✓ *Having a procedure that confirms appointments and reservations.* Another essential standard is to develop and adhere to a firm practice of confirming all appointments. Some club operators require their staff to send a confirmation e-mail 24 hours in advance of the appointment, while others have one of their employees reconfirm the appoint by calling the individual who made the appointment.

✓ *Scheduling systems and practices.* Most clubs employ a paper reservation and scheduling system. These systems utilize pre-designed appointment books or reservation sheets that enable the necessary appointment information to be documented for each reservation and appointment. In recent years, many clubs have moved to software and Internet-based scheduling systems. Such systems provide incredible flexibility, since they allow members to schedule appointments and reservations through their own computer or smart phone, but also allow the club's staff to book reservations through the club's computers Not only do these web-based software systems allow appointments to be made more quickly, they also have the capability of printing out daily appointment and reservation sheets for the staff, as well as sending reminder emails and text messages directly to the member. Supplier companies, such as those mentioned previously for club check-in, have all developed good web-based, scheduling software. While no documented studies have been published regarding the frequency of using the web-based programs, empirical evidence exists that indicates between 10 and 50 percent of members schedule appointments through web-based programs.

❏ *Answering Phones.* For most independent club operators, the front desk is the location where all phones are answered and information from those calls is processed. Many larger clubs have a separate department (some larger companies have call centers) that is dedicated to answering the phone. The most recent trend in the club industry has been to automate the phone answering system so that callers never speak to a staff person; instead, calls are handled through a voicemail system. Those clubs that still view answering the phone as a primary responsibility of the front desk should establish standard practices for answering the phone. Examples of the more critical standards in this area include:

- *Specifying the number of rings before answering the phone.* At ClubCorp, for example, all phones must be answered within five rings. The key is for each club operator to establish a standard for this issue that is appropriate to the club.

- *Specifying the greeting.* Clubs should identify a standard way in which the phone should be answered by every staff person, for example, "Hello, this is the Racquet Club, Mary speaking, how may I assist you?" Customer research indicates that it is very important for a business to answer the phone in an appropriate manner. Accordingly, clubs must establish clear standards concerning how the phone will be answered.

- *Specifying how callers should be put on hold or forwarded and, if necessary, messages should be taken.* Every club should have a standard practice concerning how calls should be forwarded and how callers should be put on hold. For example, at ClubCorp, callers are never left on hold for more than 30 seconds, before being given the opportunity to speak with a staff person. In this instance, the primary goal is to make sure that callers know that their needs are being taken care of in a prompt manner. With regard to forwarding calls, clubs should also have a set policy concerning this practice. As such, the club standard might involve requiring the staff person who answered the phone to contact the requested staff person to notify that individual of the phone call before forwarding the call. If the staff person is not in, the outside caller should be informed and asked if that person wants to leave a message. Each club can establish its own policies concerning how to handle phone calls. However, if the club wants to provide great service, it should establish clear standards in this regard. Similar to forwarding calls and putting the caller on hold, when it comes to taking messages, clubs should ensure that they have a standard format for taking messages. At ClubCorp, the front-desk staff is expected to get the name of the caller, the time and date of the call, the name of the person the call is for, and to initial the message.

> **Clubs should identify a standard way in which the phone should be answered by every staff person.**

Clubs should establish standards and practices for handling the dissemination of information at the front desk.

❑ *Disseminating Club Information.* Another key responsibility of the front-desk staff is to disseminate information about the club. Front-desk staff are often expected to share important information about the club, either over the phone or in person. Accordingly, clubs should establish standards and practices for handling the dissemination of information at the front desk. Examples of basic standards and practices in this regard include:

- *Establishing what information can be disseminated.* Most clubs like to have their front-desk staff provide information about club programs and events. On the other hand, front-desk staff should never be required to give out membership information or employee/member information. Accordingly, club operators should develop a clear set of standards and/ or practices that clarify the information that can be provided through the front desk.

- *Making the information accessible.* Once the club has established what information may be distributed through the front desk, it then becomes the club's responsibility to make that information easily accessible. For example, at some clubs, the front-desk staff are provided with binders that include information on:
  - ✓ Quarterly events and program calendar
  - ✓ Monthly newsletters
  - ✓ Group-exercise class schedules
  - ✓ Basic club information (e.g., the location, operating hours, and general description of the club's facilities, programs, and services)
  - ✓ Daily information (e.g., what is scheduled to occur that day at the club)
  - ✓ Club phone numbers
  - ✓ Names of department heads
  - ✓ Emergency procedures and information
  - ✓ Club policies and rules

In the last few years, clubs have begun to push information through their websites, Facebook pages, Twitter pages, in-club kiosks, and customized smart-phone applications. As a result, front desk staff are not expected in those facilities to serve as the primary information distributors. Instead, they are expected to guide members and guests to the appropriate information resource.

Child-Care Department

In most health/fitness clubs, the child-care department provides what could reasonably be considered as short-term "babysitting" for parents who are participating in activities at the club. These "babysitting" activities differ from both licensed day care, which requires state licensure, and youth programming, which involves the delivery of organized and structured activity programs for children. Several policies and practices are very critical to the safe and successful operation of a child-care department, including:

❏ *Hours of Operation.* Clubs should inform their members when the child-care services will be available. Within the industry, these schedules can vary from club to club. For example, in some urban clubs, the hours that child-care services are available are scheduled around specific programs or times of the day, while in many of the suburban clubs that target the family market, these services are provided during the entire day.

❏ *Age Groups.* Clubs should make it crystal clear what age groups can be handled by the child-care department. Most clubs don't normally permit children below the age of six months or above the age of eight years to participate in their child-care programs. Many family-oriented clubs offer separate child-care areas for different age groups, such as a room for children who range in age from six months to 18 months, another for those from 19 months to three years, yet another for kids from three years to five years, and one for those from six years to eight years old. Every club should establish clear policies in this area. Many clubs also develop activity areas within the facility that are designed specifically for those children who are over the age of eight, but who are not yet teenagers (individuals who are often referred to as "tweeners").

❏ *Drop-Off and Time-Limit Policies.* Definitive guidelines concerning drop-off and time-limit stipulations are among the most important child-care policies and practices that a club can establish. Since most states have strict restrictions governing the amount of time and extent of child-care services, clubs must be aware of the relevant regulations involving those matters so that they don't find themselves delivering a service that requires state licensure. For example, most states place restrictions on a club's drop-off policies if the facility offers "babysitting" services. Examples of key, specific issues that should be addressed in this regard include:

> **Definitive guidelines concerning drop-off and time-limit stipulations are among the most important child-care policies and practices that a club can establish.**

- *Time limit.* In most states, the maximum time a child can be left in an environment, such as a child-care area in a health/fitness club, is four hours, before licensing is required. To be on the safe side, many clubs limit the hours that they will "watch" a child to two or three hours.

- *Parent's presence.* Because of state requirements, clubs must require that parents be on the premises at all times when their children are in the child-care area. As a result, clubs should communicate this fact to their members. Furthermore, clubs should make sure that the members indicate their presence when they sign their children in.

- *Sign in and sign out.* A standard practice in most clubs is to require the parents or guardians to sign their children in and out of the child-care area. This practice usually involves having the parent/guardian sign their name, identifying their child's name, note (in writing) the time of the drop-off, and indicate which part of the club they will be in. If the parent chooses to have someone other than themselves pick the child up, when they sign in, they must provide that person's name and a means of identification for that person. At the time of signing out, the parent must present themselves, sign a sheet indicating the time they picked the child up, and note their relationship to the child.

It is critical that every club spell out in detail what services are provided in the child-care area and how the children will be handled.

❑ *Services Provided.* It is critical that every club spell out in detail what services are provided in the child-care area and how the children will be handled. In that regard, the following should be addressed:

• *Food.* Clubs should establish a policy concerning the provision of food for children in the child-care area. Some club operators require that parents/guardians furnish all of the food and beverages that their children consume while in the child-care area, whereas others adopt policies that indicate that they will provide water, crackers, etc. for the children. All factors considered, the prudent approach for a club is to have a policy that requires the food to be provided by the parents or guardians.

• *Restroom practices.* Restroom policies are a very sensitive issue for clubs and parents. With some children still in diapers, clubs must have a policy regarding the changing of diapers. The safest approach is to state that the club will not change diapers and will notify parents in the event that a diaper has to be changed. Clubs also should have a policy that clearly states what the policy will be when an older child needs to use the restroom. In these circumstances, some clubs require that the parent/guardian handle the situation. Other clubs have a policy that mandates that an adult of the same gender must accompany the child to the restroom entry and stand outside the restroom while the child is using the facility. This latter approach involves a higher level of risk from a liability perspective. Another option involves the fact that many child-care areas currently have a separate children's restroom that cannot be locked from the inside. In these facilities, a child can use the restroom, while the child-care staff maintains supervision of the child without direct contact or interference. Some clubs conduct criminal background checks on all staff members who work in the child-care area (a prudent recommendation for any club operator) and share the fact that these individuals have satisfactorily cleared their background checks with the parents who bring their children to the club. Another very important part of any policy concerning the child-care area is to have a sheet that the parent or guardian must sign, indicating how they want the club to deal with this issue while their child is in the club's care.

• *Activities.* Clubs should include in their policies what activities are provided for children while they are in the care of the club, for example, arts and crafts, computers, video games, nap time, etc. These activities should be spelled out very clearly for parents/guardians.

❑ *Registration and Enrollment.* Every club should have a policy regarding what information should be obtained the first time that a child is left with the child-care department. In most instances, this step would involve:

• *Obtaining medical/health information.* Clubs should obtain a basic medical background on each child, including any allergies, medical-health issues, special-handling instructions, name of the child's physician, etc.

• *Getting family-background information.* Each parent/guardian should provide certain background information, such as their names, contact information (phone, e-mail, etc.), whom to contact in an emergency, etc.

- *Waiver or release.* Each parent/guardian should sign a waiver or release indicating that they are aware of the club's policies and practices and concur with them. The waiver/release sheet should include specific space that can be used to document any special requests of the parent concerning the child. It should be noted that in many parts of the U.S., courts do not recognize waivers that parents have signed on behalf of their children.
- *Special instructions.* Each club should have a form that allows the parent/guardian to identify any special requirements or practices they want addressed with their child.

❏ *Staff-to-Child Ratio.* If the club offers licensed day care, it is legally required to abide by certain child-to-staff ratios. These ratios vary, depending on the age of the children. Even though most clubs do not offer licensed day care, it is still important that all clubs have policies that address the ratio of staff-to-children in their child-care areas. While clubs should determine what is best for them concerning this factor, the following guidelines illustrate some of the practices that exist in the industry:

- Children under age two: no more than three children per adult.
- Children two to five: no more than five children per adult.
- Children five to eight: no more than six to seven children per adult.

❏ *Medical Situations.* It is extremely important that the club has a policy for handling any medical situations involving children in the child-care area. The two most important issues in this regard are handling children who are sick and their parents want to leave them in the child-care area and responding to a medical situation that arises while a child is under the care of the child-care department. In the case of a child being ill, clubs should have a firm policy concerning whether children who are ill can be left in the child-care area. Most clubs do not allow children who are ill to be left in the child-care area. This particular policy, while strict, helps prevent other children from catching an illness from the sick child. All factors considered, it is a well-advised policy to have in place. In the event of medical emergencies, the club should have a clear policy concerning what to do that is communicated to all staff and members. A critical part of that policy or practice should be to contact the parent or guardian immediately in the event of any emergency. Another key element of such a policy should be to have a signed form that indicates how the parent wants any emergency to be handled, if they cannot be reached immediately and the emergency requires prompt action.

> It is extremely important that the club has a policy for handling any medical situations involving children in the child-care area.

Fitness Department (Fitness and Group Exercise)

The fitness department is primarily responsible for making sure that each member and guest of the club is able to engage in a physical-activity program in a safe and effective manner. Although much of what this department does revolves around programming and risk management, a few operating practices are critical to the achievement of its goals, including pre-activity screening, fitness assessment, orienting new members/guests to the fitness facilities, exercise prescription and training, on-the-floor supervision, and equipment care and maintenance.

❑ *Pre-Activity Screening.* The purpose of pre-activity screening is to identify the physical and behavioral factors that will influence the member's/user's ability to participate safely in a physical-activity program. Clubs should establish policies and practices that ensure that each member/user receives such a pre-activity screening prior to participating in a physical-activity program. The two most common pre-activity screening tools are the Par-Q (physical-activity readiness questionnaire) and the medical history questionnaire (MHQ).

- *Par-Q.* The Par-Q is a simple, self-administered, one-page written instrument that screens for coronary-risk factors and identifies individuals who are at an increased risk of having a cardiovascular incident with the onset of moderate-to-vigorous physical activity due to their present coronary health status. The Par-Q was developed over 30 years ago as a basic, straightforward tool for identifying coronary heath risks. If the member completes this form, that individual can easily be identified as a person who has any risks that would require further assessment from a healthcare professional. If the club administers the Par-Q, then the staff can easily identify those individuals who will require further assessment from a healthcare professional or more careful guidance with their physical-activity program. This tool is designed to be used by both lay people and fitness professionals.

- *Medical history questionnaire (MHQ).* The MHQ is a more complete screening tool than the Par-Q and is expected to be administered by a qualified fitness professional. A MHQ allows a club not only to identify coronary health risks, but also to uncover other health-related issues that might compromise the member's/user's ability to exercise safely. The MHQ can come in a variety of formats, ranging from a short form that seeks information on the most basic health-related issues to a form that elicits information concerning past exercise patterns and related lifestyle behaviors. The results of a MHQ should be interpreted by a qualified fitness professional.

Clubs should determine which of the screening tools will work best for them. Once a tool is identified, the club should then establish a process by which each new member of the club completes the pre-activity screening assessments.

> Fitness assessments should be used with those club members for whom additional information is needed to properly design their exercise program or for those members/users who want to establish benchmarks for monitoring their body's responses to physical activity.

❑ *Fitness Assessment.* Assessing the members' level of fitness is a practice that clubs should consider undertaking. All factors considered, such a fitness assessment may not be appropriate for every member. Primarily, fitness assessments should be used with those club members for whom additional information is needed to properly design their exercise program or for those members/users who want to establish benchmarks for monitoring their body's responses to physical activity. Clubs should have a system in place that provides a clear path concerning which members/users should be channeled into the fitness-assessment process. Fitness-assessment systems tend to vary considerably and can include any or all of the following elements:

- *Cardiovascular assessments.* Cardiovascular assessments can be as simple as a three-minute step test or as complex as a physician-supervised, graded exercise test. Most clubs typically employ either a step test or a sub-maximal exercise test using a bicycle ergometer to evaluate a member's level of cardiovascular fitness.

- *Muscular strength and endurance assessments.* The industry benchmarks for assessing muscular strength and endurance are component-specific tests, such as a grip-strength test, one-minute sit-up test, 1RM or 10RM test with specific exercises, or timed push-up test. On the other hand, a few clubs utilize sport-specific tests to evaluate the muscular strength and endurance levels of their members.
- *Flexibility assessments.* The most common flexibility assessment is the sit-and-reach test. A number of clubs use a goniometer to measure joint-specific ranges of flexibility for the trunk and limbs.
- *Body-fat assessment.* Body-fat assessment may be the fitness measurement that is most desired and used by members. The assessment tools for this factor range from simple circumference measurements to skin-fold measurements with calipers to underwater weighing for more exact determination of body fat. In recent years, some clubs have opted to use bioelectric-impedance devices and technologically advanced apparatuses, such as the Body Pod, to assess body-fat levels.
- *Metabolism.* With the recent focus on the nation's obesity epidemic, many clubs have started to employ more health-oriented assessments, such as those that measure an individual's overall resting metabolism and caloric expenditure. Devices, such as the Body Gem, which is an indirect calorimeter, allow clubs to obtain relatively accurate measurements of a member's resting caloric expenditure. Such information can be used to provide better guidance with regard to weight-management efforts.

A club can offer other assessments to its members, depending on the level of sophistication the club wants to achieve. More detailed information on both pre-activity screening and fitness assessment is available in the most recent editions of both *ACSM's Guidelines for Exercise Testing and Prescription* and the *ACE Personal Trainer Manual*.

❑ *Fitness and Physical-Activity Orientation.* It is essential that every club has a system in place to orient each new member to its fitness and exercise facilities. The primary goal of this orientation process is to ensure that all members/users have the information and guidance that they need to safely use the club's facilities to pursue a program of physical activity. Some club operators design their orientation process to provide members/users with a brief introduction to their facilities and equipment, while other club operators view the orientation process as an opportunity to fully engage every new member into the club. Within the industry, clubs take several approaches to the orientation process, including the following:

- *Group orientations.* Many clubs schedule group orientations, which involve having new members attend a 30- to 60-minute session that is facilitated by a fitness professional. These sessions typically provide an overview of the club's equipment, a sample exercise program for working out with the equipment, and a brief explanation of how to use the

It is essential that every club has a system in place to orient each new member to its fitness and exercise facilities.

equipment. Not only are these sessions designed to get new member started, they are also intended to introduce them to other services the club offers. In the higher-end clubs, these group orientations may also include an overview of other departments and an introduction to other services offered by the facility.

- *Individual orientations.* An individual orientation is a more personalized approach that is employed by some clubs. An individual orientation allows a new member to spend time, one-on-one, with a fitness professional who provides a more personalized introduction to the club's fitness facilities and services. In some instances, these gatherings feature a single 30- to 60-minute session, while in other clubs, they are offered as a series of 30- to 60-minute sessions. The extent of these individual sessions might range from a tour of the fitness facilities and overview of the equipment to a complete exercise prescription and multiple personal-training sessions. The trend among many of the larger club operations (e.g., 24 Hour Fitness, Town Sports International, Equinox, etc.) is to offer new members a three-session, personal-training package at an introductory rate as a means of orienting them to the club's fitness facilities.

- *Self-directed orientations.* Over the past few years, several health/fitness operators, such as McFit based in Germany and The Gym Group in England, have moved toward self-directed orientations that utilize web-based software applications. In these clubs, members are directed to a website or internal kiosk, where they can view an orientation program and receive an initial exercise program to follow in the club. As such, in the next 5 to 10 years, this approach may become the orientation process of choice for many operators.

❑ *Exercise Prescription and Personal Training.* The process of providing members with an exercise prescription and personal-training session may be the most effective approach for integrating new members into the club. Over the last decade, clubs have moved away from the tendency to provide each new member with an exercise prescription. Instead, they have focused on promoting personal training. This trend, while a positive step for those individuals who can afford to utilize personal training (5 to 20 percent of the membership), creates a situation in which other members/users might be left without the guidance that they need to be successful with their physical-activity program. All factors considered, wise club operators should provide both of these systems for their members, given the fact that they build on and enhance each other's effectiveness and can help increase the overall level of member/user participation in the club's fitness offerings.

> The process of providing members with an exercise prescription and personal-training session may be the most effective approach for integrating new members into the club.

- *Exercise prescription.* An exercise prescription is a personalized-exercise plan that is based on the needs of the individual. An exercise prescription takes into account several factors, including the member's/user's health status, the person's level of inactivity/activity, and the individual's related lifestyle behaviors. Properly designed, it should serve as the foundation for a sound exercise and lifestyle program. Ideally, all members/users should receive a personalized exercise prescription that is documented for them on either an exercise card or a software program. The exercise prescription should then be used to provide personalized fitness instruction from a qualified professional. The process of providing new members with an exercise prescription often involves having someone from the fitness staff initially take the member through the exercise program at least once. After the initial session(s), the fitness staff should monitor the member's progress and, if needed, develop a revised program for the member. One of a club's primary goals should be to establish an exercise roadmap for members to follow and then to check their progress on a regular basis. Recently, many clubs have chosen to use web-based applications that make it easier to construct and monitor a member's exercise prescription.

- *Personal training.* All factors considered, personal training is more of a program than an actual operating practice. Nonetheless, personal training is an important system that clubs should incorporate into their operations. In recent years, personal training has developed into one of the leading sources of incremental revenue for the health/fitness club business. The original focus of personal training was to provide members/users with the opportunity to work closely with a fitness professional who could provide them with a personalized exercise prescription and ongoing motivation. Currently, many club operators (e.g., Equinox, 24 Hour Fitness, Western Athletic Clubs, Virgin Active, etc.) have sophisticated systems for introducing new members to personal training.

❑ *Fitness-Floor Supervision.* The process of supervising the fitness floor is an operational practice that can lead to improved membership retention, enhanced level of revenue, and a safer club environment. Fitness-floor supervision refers to the process of having the club's fitness staff regularly walk the fitness floor to assist members with their exercise programs and to answer any questions members may have about their fitness programs. According to the most recent edition of *ACSM's Health/Fitness Facility Standards and Guidelines*, clubs should have at least one fitness professional on duty at all times who is dedicated to supervising the fitness floor. Accordingly, clubs should have a floor-supervision system that ensures that a fitness professional is always available to assist members on the fitness floor. The activities involved in fitness-floor supervision may include one or more of the following:

> The process of supervising the fitness floor is an operational practice that can lead to improved membership retention, enhanced level of revenue, and a safer club environment.

- Answering questions for members who are having problems
- Correcting members with their exercise technique, when appropriate
- Teaching new exercises to members, if appropriate, to replace ones that they are currently performing
- Checking the status of the equipment to make sure it is working correctly
- Greeting new members
- Promoting other services and programs of the club
- Checking exercise cards and redesigning exercise programs
- Providing towels or water to the members
- Reinforcing the fact to members that they are exercising in a safe environment

Over the past few years, clubs have focused on offering personal training and have deemphasized the practice of maintaining a strong floor-supervision presence. One of the difficulties with this approach is that personal training typically reaches only 5 to 20 percent of the membership, while supervising the fitness floor can touch the needs of far more members. It is interesting to note that one of the primary complaints of members on the fitness floor, based on industry-based, member-retention research, is the lack of attention they receive and the difficulty of obtaining assistance without having to pay for it. The key point that must be emphasized is that clubs that focus on establishing a process for providing supervision of the fitness floor can reap substantial rewards, in terms of both member satisfaction and membership retention.

❏ *Equipment Care and Maintenance.* Another critical operating practice that the fitness department must have is an established system for monitoring and caring for the equipment on the fitness floor. By monitoring the condition of the equipment, the fitness department can help provide a safer and more convenient exercise environment. The process of monitoring and caring for the equipment should be a standard element of every fitness department's operating practices. In that regard, clubs should establish daily, weekly, monthly, and annual checklists for monitoring and caring for the equipment on the fitness floor. These checklists can serve as a means for the club to audit its equipment and ensure that all equipment is ready for use by the members. Almost without exception, all equipment manufacturers provide care and maintenance guidelines for their equipment. Figures 20-1 and 20-2 detail some of the important monitoring and care activities for fitness equipment.

Equipment	Daily Care	Weekly Care	Monthly Care	As Needed
Variable-Resistance Equipment	• Clean frames with mild soap and water. • Clean upholstery with mild soap and water.	• Check all cables and bolts and tighten as needed. • Check moving parts and adjust as needed.	• Lubricate the guide rods with lightweight oil.	• Repair and/or replace pads. • Replace cables if needed.
Free-Weight Benches and Accessories	• Clean frames with mild soap and water. • Clean upholstery with mild soap and water.	• Check all cables and bolts and tighten as needed. • Check moving parts and adjust as needed.		• Repair and/or replace pads. • Replace cables if needed.
Dumbbells and Bars	• Clean off bars with a dry cloth.	• Check all screws and bolts and tighten as needed.	• Use lightweight oil on a cloth to remove any rust.	• Repair and/or replace broken bars and dumbbells.

Figure 20-1. Care and maintenance guidelines for resistance equipment

Equipment	Daily Care	Weekly Care	Monthly Care	As Needed
Bicycles and Recumbent Bicycles	• Clean off control panel with a damp cloth. • Clean off seats with mild soap and water. • Clean housing with mild soap and water.	• Check equipment diagnostics on the control panel for any warnings or indications of problems. • Check all screws and bolts and tighten as needed. • If positioned on a carpet, vacuum underneath.	• Remove housing covering the bike and clean out any dust or lint.	• Refer to manufacturer's guidelines.
Elliptical Trainers and Stairclimbers	• Clean off control panel with a damp cloth. • Clean housing and pedals with mild soap and water.	• Check equipment diagnostics on the control panel for any warnings or indications of problems. • Check all screws and bolts and tighten as needed. • If positioned on a carpet, vacuum underneath.	• Remove housing covering the elliptical or stairclimber and clean out any dust or lint.	• Refer to manufacturer's guidelines.
Treadmills	• Clean off control panel with a damp cloth. • Clean housing with mild soap and water.	• Check equipment diagnostics on the control panel for any warnings or indications of problems. • Check all screws and bolts and tighten as needed. • If positioned on a carpet, vacuum underneath.	• Clean belts using a damp cloth. • Check belt/deck surface and lubricate as needed. • Check rollers and adjust if they're out of alignment.	• Replace belts if warranted. • Replace deck surfaces if diagnostics indicate. • Refer to manufacturer's guidelines.

Figure 20-2. Care and maintenance guidelines for cardiovascular equipment

Aquatics Department

The aquatics department requires strict attention to operating standards and systems. Much of this requirement stems from the fact that local health departments regulate many of the practices that are employed to operate commercial and public pools. Although not intended to cover every operating practice that is required to operate a pool environment, this section reviews the key operating practices and practices that are essential for the safe operation of an aquatics department, including:

❑ *Monitoring and Controlling Pool Chemistry and Temperature.* Maintaining the proper chemical balance in the pool is a crucial factor in member/ user safety, not to mention a strict requirement of most state and local departments of public health. Some health departments mandate that pool operators monitor and record pool chemistry and temperature at least three times a day, while others only require such monitoring once daily. In addition to monitoring the chemistry and temperature levels in the pool, most health departments have established guidelines for what constitutes appropriate chemical levels. The four primary chemical levels that should be monitored and maintained are:

> Most public/ commercial pools use either chlorine or bromine as the chemical agent to prevent harmful organisms from reaching unsatisfactory levels in the pool.

- *Chlorine or bromine level.* Most public/commercial pools use either chlorine or bromine as the chemical agent to prevent harmful organisms from reaching unsatisfactory levels in the pool. Chlorine, the most frequently used chemical, is added to the pool in one of two ways— either in tablet form (calcium or lithium) or in liquid form. In either instance, the chlorine level is controlled through automated systems that maintain the free chlorine level between one part per million (1 ppm) and three parts per million. According to the National Spa and Pool Institute (NSPI), the minimum level of free chlorine should be above 1 ppm. With regard to user safety and comfort, the level of chlorine should not exceed 3 ppm. Because chlorine is a highly dangerous chemical, the club's staff should take considerable care whenever they handle it.

  While bromine is used less frequently than chlorine, many individuals consider it to be a more effective and user-friendly chemical than chlorine. Bromine is colorless and odorless and, as a result, is not as irritating to the member/user. NSPI standards indicate that bromine levels should normally be maintained between 2 ppm and 4 ppm, with the most appropriate levels being between 2 ppm and 3 ppm. Most modern pool systems monitor the chemical levels and adjust them automatically, based on the requirements established by the operator. A highly recommended practice involves having pool operators hand-monitor the chlorine and bromine levels in the pools themselves, as a back-up to the automatic monitoring systems. A third system for introducing chlorine into pools has recently found favor with club operators. This option involves using a "salt water" system that breaks down salt into free chlorine that enters the pool.

- *Total alkalinity.* The alkalinity level is another important factor that should be monitored at least once daily. The NSPI standard for the total alkalinity level is between 80 and 100 ppm when a chlorine system is employed and between 100 and 120 ppm when bromine is used.

- *Calcium hardness*. The NSPI standard for calcium hardness is that the level should be between 200 and 400 ppm, with a minimum level of 150 ppm and a maximum level of 1,000 ppm.
- *PH (percent hydrogen)*. The recommended standard for pool pH is 7.4, with a range of 7.2 to 7.6 being ideal. If the pH falls below 7.2, then the pool water is becoming too acidic, and if it rises above 7.6, it is becoming too basic. Changes in a pool's pH level can be an indication that a chemical imbalance exists.

In addition to monitoring and maintaining the aforementioned chemical levels, pool operators should also monitor and control the temperature of the pool. According to industry practices, the temperature of the pool should be maintained within plus or minus two degrees of the temperature that is appropriate for the circumstances in the pool during the course of the day. The proper temperature for a pool depends on the activities that are being performed in the pool. While no universal standard exists, Figure 20-3 details temperature guidelines that are consistent with policies and practices in the industry.

❏ *Cleaning the Pool and Filters*. Next to monitoring and maintaining the pool chemistry, cleaning the pool is the second most important day-to-day operating practice that clubs should systemize. Clubs should establish a cleaning checklist that is audited on a daily, weekly, and monthly basis to ensure that all basic cleaning functions are undertaken as scheduled. Figure 20-4 provides a general overview of the most critical cleaning practices for commercial pools, each of which should be an integral part of a club's pool-operating practices.

❏ *Emergency and Safety Preparation*. The pool facilities are among the most likely areas of a club to experience incidents that place members and guests in harm's way. As a result, clubs should implement operating systems that allow for the safest possible environment for members and users. The previous chapter presented an overview of basic emergency preparedness factors, measures that are especially important in the pool area. Beyond these basic emergency-preparedness steps, clubs should also consider standardizing and executing the following pool-specific emergency and safety practices:
- *Posting all appropriate signage, per local and state codes*. This signage should address several key elements, including showering before entering

Activity	Temperature Range
Fitness and lap swimming	78 to 82 degrees Fahrenheit
Recreational swimming	82 to 86 degrees Fahrenheit
Aquatic exercise	82 to 88 degrees Fahrenheit
Children (under three years of age)	90 to 96 degrees Fahrenheit

Figure 20-3. Recommended pool temperatures, based on the activities that are being conducted in the pool

Cleaning Activity	Comments
Vacuuming the pool	Pools should be vacuumed daily, using either built-in vacuums or automatic vacuum systems. The best time to perform vacuuming is at closing to allow for the appropriate interlude (at least five hours) to pass before allowing members to use the pool.
Cleaning skimmers	This practice is only required in pool systems that use skimmers. Most modern pools use gutter systems. In busy pools, this task should be done on a daily basis.
Cleaning the walls and tile	If the pool surface is paint, vinyl, or fiberglass, then the cleaning should be done with a nylon brush. This process needs to be done at least monthly and more often in pools with heavy usage. In addition, the scum line should be cleaned on a regular basis, using a soft brush or cloth.
Backwashing the filter	Backwashing needs to occur on a regular basis. In very busy pools, this step can be as often as once a day, but more likely will need to be done weekly. The frequency of backwashing normally is based on the guidelines of the filter manufacturer and type of filter employed (sand, diatomaceous earth, or cartridge). A pressure rise of 5 psi is often an indicator that a filter needs to be backwashed.

Figure 20-4. Key pool-operating practices

the pool, not running on the pool deck, no diving, notices on pool depth, communications on pool supervision or lack thereof, the location of emergency/safety equipment, and information on contacting assistance.

- *Making sure that the proper safety equipment is positioned at poolside, and communicating its location to staff and members/users.* Most local and state governments have specific requirements concerning safety equipment in the pool area. Far too often, these requirements are insufficient. The proper safety equipment for a pool includes:
  - ✓ First aid kit
  - ✓ Automatic electronic defibrillator (AED)
  - ✓ Spinal board
  - ✓ A 25-foot rope attached to a ring buoy
  - ✓ Shepherd's crook
  - ✓ Extension poles (at least one)
  - ✓ Eyewash station
  - ✓ Blankets or similar wrap

- *Providing the necessary supervision and oversight of the pool area.* In many states, a lifeguard is not required for pools that are less than four and a half feet in depth. While the best operating practice is to provide a lifeguard during all hours that a pool is in operation, in those regions where one is not required, clubs should establish a monitoring system that ensures reasonable oversight of the pool area. Examples of such a system could include the following steps:
  - ✓ Using video equipment and monitors
  - ✓ Having staff do a walk-through of the pool every hour that the pool is open to members and guests
  - ✓ Using volunteer lifeguards during peak hours

- *Conducting weekly safety audits.* Clubs should develop an audit checklist that addresses such factors as safety equipment, pool chemistry, pool cleaning, and supervision, and is used to perform an audit on a weekly basis to make sure that the appropriate safety procedures are being taken, for example:

  ✓ *All pool chemicals are stored in a safe and secured area.* The chemicals used in pool care should be stored in a dry area, off the floor. Many of the chemicals used in pool care are highly volatile if they come in direct contact with moisture or other chemicals. The storage area should be secured, as well as only be accessible to authorized staff (e.g., staff trained in the handling of pool chemicals such as a certified pool operator).

  ✓ *All members/users sign in.* A highly recommended operating practice is to have every member/user sign in and out when using the pool. Limiting access to the pool area to authorized individuals can be a life-saving measure.

Tennis Department

The tennis department, like the other aforementioned departments, can also benefit from having structured operating systems that can help ensure the consistent delivery of a safe and enjoyable experience. Administering the tennis department often involves many of the same operating practices that other front-of-the-house departments employ. Several operating practices exist that are somewhat specific to the circumstances attendant to the tennis department, including:

❑ *Cleaning and Maintenance Practices.* In order for members to have a relatively safe and enjoyable experience with the club's tennis facilities, certain cleaning and maintenance practices are necessary. Above and beyond the normal cleaning practices that a club conducts, these steps include:

- *Checking light levels and adjusting them as needed.* The light levels at net height should be at least 40-foot candles, preferably closer to 75-foot candles (professional competitive level play often requires illumination levels as high as 125-foot candles). If the club has indoor courts, it should establish a practice of regularly monitoring light levels and replacing bulbs whenever the light levels fall below the minimum recommendation. As a rule, every few years, the light ballasts will need to be replaced.

- *Cleaning the courts surfaces of debris.* Cleaning the court surfaces of indoor hard courts typically involves vacuuming the courts at least once a day to remove ball fuzz. For outdoor hard courts, this task entails vacuuming or blowing off the courts on a regular basis, while for clay courts, it involves sweeping and watering the courts. Regardless of the type of court-playing surface or the method used to clean that surface, the key goal is to remove any loose impediment that could interfere with play or present a potential danger to the members/users.

Regardless of the type of court-playing surface or the method used to clean that surface, the key goal is to remove any loose impediment that could interfere with play or present a potential danger to the members/users.

- *Checking and adjusting the nets.* On a daily basis, the club staff should check the nets for damage and tension levels. Nets with holes should be repaired or replaced, and nets at the improper height should be adjusted.
- *Inspecting and repairing court surfaces.* Because hard courts often crack, they can present a danger to the member/user. Clay courts can have low spots or areas of hardening that can also present a danger. Accordingly, clubs should regularly inspect the court surfaces and make any appropriate repairs.

❑ *Scheduling Court Reservations.* Every club should establish operating policies and practices regarding the scheduling of tennis-court time. These policies and practices should be understood by the staff and clearly communicated to the club's members. Examples of reservation and scheduling practices and policies include:

- *Establishing limits for court time.* Most indoor courts normally schedule time in one-hour blocks, while outdoor courts employ 90-minute blocks.
- *Establishing advance reservation limits.* Clubs should set limits concerning how far in advance members/users can reserve a court. Most clubs in the industry permit reservations to be made up to one week in advance.
- *Establishing matchmaking services.* Many clubs develop practices that allow the club to arrange matches for members in those instances when the facilities are provided with sufficient notice.
- *Establishing a requirement for the basic information needed to reserve a court.* As a rule, this requirement involves obtaining several pieces of information, including name, member number, number of players, etc. This practice is very similar to front-desk operations.
- *Establishing permanent court-time policies.* Some clubs provide their members with a permanent court time, which refers to the practice of giving members the same reservation time slots each week. This practice requires careful consideration to ensure that too many members of the club are not precluded from playing because of other members are assigned the most desirable time slots.

❑ *Programming Functions.* Sound programming is the essence of a successful tennis program. The most successful tennis operators establish specific operating practices that govern their facility's approach to programming. In turn, these practices enable members to actively participate in those tennis programs that most interest them. Examples of operating practices often employed in the industry involving tennis programming include:

- Establishing and distributing an annual program calendar and booklet
- Having a matchmaking policy and detailed steps that should be taken for matchmaking to occur
- Having registration forms for each tennis program available in areas that members/users can easily access

The most successful tennis operators establish specific operating practices that govern their facility's approach to programming.

- Posting the guidelines and rules pertaining to each program. This step can involve employing a variety of tools, such as websites, Facebook page, newsletters, or printed program handbooks for members.

Key Points to Consider

It is important to note that a club's practices for front-of-the-house operations are not exclusive of other club practices, involving such diverse elements as programming, service delivery, and marketing. In many instances, what might be considered service delivery might actually be an operating practice, or what is considered programming could also be viewed as operations. Accordingly, the operating practices reviewed in this chapter involve those policies, practices, and systems that were not previously detailed in other chapters.

It is important to note that a club's practices for front-of-the-house operations are not exclusive of other club practices.

21

Heart-of-the-House Operations

Chapter Objectives

The previous chapter presented an overview of the basic operating practices and systems that are important to front-of-the-house departments (e.g., front desk, child-care, fitness, pool, and racquet/tennis). This chapter examines the "best" practices for "heart-of-the-house" operations. Heart-of-the-house operations encompass supporting areas of the club that may directly serve the members and users, or possibly may support the activities of staff serving in front-of-the-house roles. "Heart-of-the-house" operations in health/fitness clubs involve several departments, including locker rooms, laundry, housecleaning, and accounting. This chapter provides a detailed review of the key operating practices and systems for each of those departments.

Locker Rooms

The health/fitness club industry has a diverse array of locker-room offerings and operations. For example, some clubs have locker rooms that only offer changing areas and day-use lockers, while other facilities feature full-scale locker rooms that include such conveniences, as rental lockers, laundry services, and a full array of amenities. As a result of this diversity of offerings, the operating practices involving locker rooms tend to vary from club to club. This section on locker rooms initially presents an overview of basic locker-room operating models and then examines the key practices that clubs should adopt to facilitate operations in their locker rooms.

❏ *Types of Locker Rooms.** There are four basic types of locker rooms. The first type of operating set-up for locker rooms is the basic model that involves a changing area with day-use lockers (users bring their own locks), shower areas, and restrooms. Locker rooms in this category offer no towel service (although some clubs provide towels for a fee) or any type of amenity, such as soap or shampoo. In recent years, some of the "budget" club operators, such as McFit in Germany and the Gym Group in England, have started charging a

> The operating practices involving locker rooms tend to vary from club to club.

*It should be noted that some of the information in this section is also addressed in Chapter 17.

fee for the use of their showers. In most instances, this type of locker room is typically found in clubs that have a lower dues structure (e.g., normally under $40 a month), such as U.S chains LA Fitness and Planet Fitness.

The second type of locker room (this structure is the most common in the industry), consists of locker rooms that have changing areas with day-use lockers (the lockers have day-use access with cards, keys, digital locks, computer chips, or personal locks), showers, restrooms, sauna, steam and/or whirlpool (usually a combination of these), and several basic service amenities, such as towels, soap, and shampoo. This type of locker room arrangement typically exists in clubs that have monthly dues structures that range from $40 to $100 a month, such as U.S. chains 24 Hour Fitness, Lifetime Fitness, and Town Sports International, as well as global operators, such as Fitness First, England and Virgin Active, England.

The third type of operating structure for locker rooms, which appear mostly in premium and luxury clubs, such as U.S. operators Sports Club/ LA, Western Athletic Clubs, Wellbridge, and Tennis Corporation of America, entails locker rooms that include changing areas with both day-use lockers and rentable lockers (a combination of card access, chip card access, and keyed locks), showers, restrooms, sauna, steam and/or whirlpool (usually all three are provided), a full line of amenities, such as towels, soap, and shampoo, and services, such as laundry and shoe shines.

The fourth type of locker room operating structure is available in some of the top luxury clubs and club companies in the industry, such as the Houstonian, Houston, Texas; ClubCorp, U.S.; Sports Club/LA; and Pacific Athletic Club (operated by Western Athletic Clubs). This "executive" premier locker-room space includes premium lockers (i.e., full-height, rentable lockers), private showers, separate sauna, steam room and whirlpool, uniform and laundry service, shoe shines, lounges, coffee services, and more.

Each of the aforementioned operating structures has its advantages and disadvantages. On one end of the continuum is the simple locker-room structure that requires minimal staffing and work to maintain and brings in no incremental revenue (unless the limited funds generated by towel and shower fees are counted). On the other end of the continuum is the full-service locker room that involves considerable staffing and work to maintain, but concurrently produces significant revenue streams (for example, a few of the aforementioned luxury club operators generate as much as $500,000 annually from their locker rooms).

Members see cleanliness as one of the critical factors in choosing a club.

❑ Operating Practices for the Locker Room
  • *Cleaning and care of locker rooms.* According to research conducted by Roper Starch for IHRSA, members see cleanliness as one of the critical factors in choosing a club. This attribute becomes even more crucial when it comes to women, since they tend to see cleanliness as far more important than men when choosing to join or remain a club member. Since locker rooms typically have the most traffic of any area in the club (statistics indicate that members spend between 33 and 50 percent of

their time in the locker room), the value of maintaining the locker room in tip-top condition is heightened. Accordingly, club operators should establish a system that ensures that their facility's locker rooms are well maintained and clean at all times. Figure 21-1 illustrates the most important areas of cleaning in the locker room.

- *Maintaining the sauna, steam room, and whirlpool.* It is important that clubs that offer one or more of these amenities should care and monitor these areas on a regular basis. Accordingly, clubs should establish a system of standardized practices to help maintain these areas. Examples of standardized practices for the sauna, steam room, and whirlpool include the following:

✓ *Sauna*:

⇨ Monitor the temperature in the sauna every couple of hours and maintain it between 160 and 170 degrees Fahrenheit.

⇨ Make sure that a working clock and thermometer are present at all times in the sauna area.

⇨ Clean the surfaces daily.

⇨ Check the room every couple of hours to make sure no member is in harm's way.

⇨ Pick up all loose papers in the room.

⇨ Post appropriate signage regarding the precautions that members should take before entering and using the sauna (refer to the chapter on risk management for additional information).

⇨ Have a mechanism in place to shut down the sauna if the room's temperature rises too high.

Daily Activities	Bi-monthly	Monthly/Quarterly/Annually
• Remove trash and replace liners • Refill paper dispensers • Refill all soap and related dispensers • Dust all surfaces with a lint-free cloth • Spot clean all mirrors and glass surfaces • Spot clean locker surfaces, doors, and all exposed hardware • Clean and disinfect sinks, commodes, and urinals • Clean and disinfect sauna, steam room, and whirlpool • Vacuum carpets • Dust-mop or sweep wood surfaces • Wet mop and disinfect hard-floor	• Completely clean mirrors and glass surfaces • Clean all hard surfaces by scrubbing with a machine or similar brush • Clean and disinfect showers, steam room, sauna, and whirlpool completely • Clean and dust all HVAC grills and vents • Clean light fixtures • Empty and clean out all dispensers • Empty and clean out all waste repositories • Clean and polish all wood surfaces	• Refill air fresheners and dispensers (monthly) • Clean grout lines in showers (monthly) • Clean carpets with bonnet-style cleaner (quarterly) • Extraction clean carpets (annually) • Wash down all walls (annually)

Figure 21-1. Locker room cleaning and care chart

✓ *Steam room*:

⇨ Monitor the temperature in the steam room every couple of hours and maintain it between 100 and 110 degrees Fahrenheit.

⇨ Make sure that a working clock and thermometer are present at all times in the steam room.

⇨ Clean and scrub the steam room's surfaces, floors, and walls daily.

⇨ Make sure that a source of cold water is available in the steam room.

⇨ Check the steam room every couple of hours to make sure that no member is in harm's way.

⇨ Pick up all loose papers in the room.

⇨ Post appropriate signage regarding the precautions that members should take before entering the steam room (refer to the chapter on risk management for additional information).

⇨ Have a mechanism in place to shut down the steam room if the room's temperature rises too high.

✓ *Whirlpool*:

⇨ Monitor the temperature in the whirlpool every couple of hours and maintain it between 102 and 105 degrees Fahrenheit.

⇨ Monitor the pool chemistry (pH and chlorine levels) at least twice a day and maintain the proper balance (ph 7.2 to 7.4 and chlorine 1 ppm to 3 ppm)

⇨ Make sure that a working clock and thermometer are present in the area of the whirlpool at all times.

⇨ Empty and clean the whirlpool daily, including cleaning the scum line along the top edge of the whirlpool.

⇨ Check the whirlpool every couple of hours to make sure that no member is in harm's way.

⇨ Remove any unwanted containers that might be adjacent to the whirlpool.

⇨ Post appropriate signage regarding the precautions that members should take before entering the whirlpool (refer to the chapter on risk management for additional information).

⇨ Have a mechanism in place to shut down the whirlpool if the temperature in the whirlpool rises too high.

• *Locker assignments and usage.* As discussed previously, lockers are handled in one of three ways in most clubs. The first method allows members/users to bring their own locks to use with available lockers. The second option permits members to use available lockers, but requires the utilization of either an access card (usually the individual's membership card), token, or key. The third approach involves renting the lockers and providing the member/user with a combination for the locker or a card containing a chip that opens the locker. Among the more important practices that apply to each of these systems are the following:

> Monitor the temperature in the steam room every couple of hours and maintain it between 100 and 110 degrees Fahrenheit.

✓ *Available lockers, with the user's padlocks*:

⇨ Provide signage at the front-desk area, inside the locker room, and inside the lockers that indicate that the club is not responsible for items that the member leaves in the lockers.

⇨ Have a daily system in which the staff removes padlocks that remain on lockers at closing each evening.

⇨ Have a system in place where the staff removes any items remaining in the lockers at closing each evening.

✓ *Available lockers, accessed with a card, key, digital lock, chip card, or token*:

⇨ Provide signage at the front-desk area, inside the locker room, and inside the lockers that indicate that the club is not responsible for items that the member leaves in the lockers.

⇨ If members have to obtain the access card, key, or token from the club, have a system for requiring the user to leave personal identification or other item as collateral for the access item. The club employs this collateral to help motivate individuals to return the access tool before leaving the club.

⇨ Have a system in place where the staff checks the lockers at closing each evening and removes any remaining items.

⇨ Have a system in place that enables the staff to open the lockers if members lose their key or access card/token.

✓ *Rented lockers, accessed with a combination*:

⇨ Provide signage at the front-desk area, inside the locker room, and inside the lockers that indicates that the club is not responsible for items that the member leaves in the lockers.

⇨ Provide a system that ensures that each member registers for a locker. This step requires a process of obtaining specific information from the member, assigning a locker and combination, and initiating charges for the locker.

⇨ Provide a system to audit/monitor the rented and un-rented lockers each month to verify occupancy and charged fees.

⇨ Provide a system that allows members to forego their commitment to rent a locker. As part of this system, the club must have a method for ensuring that those lockers are not in use and have a process to make sure that the combination on all resigned lockers is changed before a locker is rented to another member.

⇨ Have a system in place where the staff checks the lockers after a resignation and removes any items that remain in the locker.

⇨ Have a system in place that enables the staff to open the lockers if members forget their combination.

• *Dispersing and handling amenities*. As discussed previously, many locker room operational set-ups offer various amenities to club members. In this instance, the most commonly provided amenities are towel service, basic personal-care items, shoe shines, and uniform services. Clubs

> Many locker room operational set-ups offer various amenities to club members. In this instance, the most commonly provided amenities are towel service, basic personal-care items, shoe shines, and uniform services.

should establish standardized systems for each of these practices to ensure that they are handled in a consistent, appropriate manner. These operational practices can address the following key factors:

✓ *Personal-care items.* Two of the items most frequently provided by clubs are soap and shampoo. Other personal-care items that some clubs offer include conditioner, body lotion, hair spray, shaving cream, and razors. With regard to personal-care items, the following operational practices can help ensure an orderly dispensing system:

⇨ Establish a practice of having the staff check all dispensers before each high-activity period and make sure that all dispensers are filled.

⇨ Establish a par-stock inventory practice. This requires the club to have the staff sign out and identify the quantity of items they remove from the inventory and place in the locker rooms. This process helps ensure that clubs do not fall low on their inventory and helps control potential inventory theft.

⇨ Establish consistency in the types of personal-care items that the facility provides. Many members perceive changes in personal-care items among the most disturbing actions that clubs can take.

✓ *Towels.* Towels are among the most worthwhile amenities that a club can offer its members. At the same time, if a club does not handle the disbursement of towels properly, it can present one of the greatest operating challenges that the staff might experience. The type of towels offered will depend on the dues structure and market position of the club. Clubs serving less affluent demographics and with lower price points normally offer import towels that weigh between six and eight pounds to the dozen, while clubs serving a more affluent demographic normally provide domestic towels that range in weight from 10 to 14 pounds to the dozen.

> **If a club does not handle the disbursement of towels properly, it can present one of the greatest operating challenges that the staff might experience.**

⇨ Establish a system for distributing towels. Some clubs, for example, distribute towels at the front desk and require users to pay for them, while other clubs leave the towels out in the locker rooms and allow members to use as many as they desire. The tendency for clubs that leave the towels out in the locker rooms is to charge higher dues.

⇨ Establish a system to monitor towel usage. If the club distributes towels at the front desk, this practice can also serve as a system for monitoring or controlling towel usage. Clubs that leave towels out in the locker room, however, should perform regular weekly inventory counts to maintain better control of their towels. These clubs should consider placing an abundance of towel bins in the locker-room areas to encourage members to leave the towels that they use in the club.

⇨ Establish a system where the staff monitors the locker rooms every few hours to pick up towels and replenish the supply of towels.

✓ *Shoe shines*. In many of the higher-end clubs (e.g., ClubCorp, Tennis Corporation of America, Western Athletic Clubs, and Sports Club/LA), shoe shines are an important locker-room amenity. Some of these clubs provide shoe shines purely as a value-added service, while others see it as a source of added incremental revenue. From an operating perspective, several key practices should be developed with regard to offering a shoe-shine service, including:

⇨ Establish a process for members/users leaving their shoes. Some clubs require that members take their shoes to a designated shoe-shine area, while others have members leave their shoes in front of their lockers, where the staff picks them up and returns them.

⇨ Establish a fee system for the members, where the members either charge the shoe-shine service to their membership or pay the locker room staff directly. In a few facilities, the service is provided on a complimentary basis.

✓ *Uniform service*. Providing uniforms (workout shorts, shirts, socks, and supporters—if needed) in the locker room has become an increasingly popular amenity, especially in urban clubs and clubs that serve a corporate market. Two distinct approaches exist with regard to offering uniform service. In one scenario, some clubs provide and wash the uniforms of members and employees (e.g., ClubCorp and Sports Club/LA). The other option involves clubs allowing their members (and in some cases, employees) to use their own workout apparel, which the club washes and cares for them. Both of these approaches require that clubs should establish practices that help ensure that this amenity is provided (delivered) in an appropriate manner. In that regard, the following steps can facilitate the process:

⇨ Establish a detailed delivery process if the club supplies the uniforms. Some clubs, for example leave the uniform items on shelves for members to select. In this situation, members wear the uniform and afterwards drop the used uniform in a bin to be washed. Other clubs issue each member a uniform and uniform bag. This practice involves having the member wear the uniform and afterwards place it in a bag that is left in a bin for washing. The bag is subsequently returned to the member's locker.

⇨ If the club washes the member's/user's personal workout apparel, establish rules and processes governing this practice. In this regard, clubs should specify what workout apparel the club will wash and whether the club will assume responsibility for any lost apparel (except for very unique circumstances, clubs should not be responsible for lost apparel). The club should also develop a system for handling personal workout apparel (e.g., the club provides laundry bags for members to use).

⇨ Establish a policy that limits the club's responsibility for replacing lost or damaged uniforms (e.g., one uniform per member per year if the club provides the uniform).

> Providing uniforms (workout shorts, shirts, socks, and supporters—if needed) in the locker room has become an increasingly popular amenity, especially in urban clubs and clubs that serve a corporate market.

Laundry

Laundry operations exist in approximately 50 percent of health/fitness clubs in the industry. As a rule, they are a standard service in those clubs that serve a more affluent member demographic. The laundry department's sole responsibility is to handle the laundry needs of the club, ranging from washing towels only to cleaning an array of items, such as towels, uniforms, sheets, table covers, etc. Although a few clubs employ outside laundry services for their towels and related items, the cost of these services and the quality of the towels normally provided by them does not always serve the best interests of either the club or the members/users. While laundry operations are not very complicated, if the right systems are not in place, clubs will likely discover that the laundry can cause far more difficulties than expected, particularly with regard to member satisfaction. Accordingly, clubs should standardize the most basic laundry practices to ensure that difficulties do not arise. Among the key practices involving the laundry are the following:

❑ *Have the Right Equipment.* If the club is going to have a laundry, it is essential that the facility has the equipment that the staff needs to handle the laundry demands of the club, for example, commercial-grade washer extractors and dryers. Most clubs will find that they need a minimum of one 50 to 60 pound washer extractor for every 1,500 memberships and twice that (100 to 120 pounds) in dryer capacity for every 1,500 memberships if they do towels only. If the club provides laundry service for uniforms, then the aforementioned equipment requirements will apply for every 1,000 memberships. In addition to an appropriate number of washers/extractors and dryers, clubs should have automated dispensing systems (machines that mix the cleaning agents and dispense them at the right time and in the right combination in the washers). Several companies, such as Ecolab, manufacture these systems.

❑ *Establish Task-Oriented Checklists.* Many clubs assign the responsibility of handling the laundry to the housecleaning department or earmark the duties involved to all staff members. Other clubs, such as the East Bank in Chicago or the Houstonian in Houston, have dedicated laundry staff. Figure 21-2 presents a list of those operational practices that should be established (and monitored through task-oriented checklists) to effectively manage the laundry.

Housecleaning

The cleaning and care of the overall facility is often one of the most overlooked elements of club operations. According to consumer research, the cleanliness of a facility is one of the most important factors that influence a person's decision to either join or remain a club member. Despite its importance to the consumer, the need to keep the facility clean and well-maintained is frequently neglected by club operators. In fact, cleaning the facility should not occur either by accident or as an afterthought. Rather, it should be a by-product of an established system of formalized practices that the club adheres to on a routine basis. Figures 21-3 to 21-5 provide an overview of the cleaning requirements

Laundry operations exist in approximately 50 percent of health/fitness clubs in the industry. As a rule, they are a standard service in those clubs that serve a more affluent member demographic.

Activity or Task	Frequency
Clean out dryer filter	After each drying cycle
Check cleaning-fluid levels for the washer	Before each load is put in
Adhere to recommended guidelines concerning specific number of items that can be placed in either the washer or dryer	Count before each load and the machine is started
Clean out behind washers and dryers	Daily
Follow cleaning and drying instructions, per manufacturer guidelines	Adhered to with each load
Fold towels and uniforms (clubs should outline their expectations)	After each load
Inventory towels	Daily, weekly, and monthly

Figure 21-2. Recommended operational practices involving the laundry

Facility Area	Cleaning Activity	Frequency
Fitness Floor	Remove trash	Daily
	Dust all horizontal surfaces	Daily
	Clean and disinfect vinyl pads on equipment	Daily
	Clean and disinfect equipment frames	Daily
	Vacuum carpets and clean stains	Daily
	Spot-clean mirrors	Daily
	Wash and disinfect hard-floor surfaces, including all rubber-floor surfaces	Daily
	Clean HVAC vents	Bi-monthly
	Clean light fixtures	Bi-monthly
	Vacuum and clean under all equipment	Bi-monthly
	Fully clean mirrors and glass surfaces	Bi-monthly
	Clean carpets	Quarterly or annually
	Clean wall surfaces thoroughly	Annually
Group-Exercise Studios	Remove any trash	Daily
	Dry mop wood floors	Daily
	Dust all horizontal surfaces	Daily
	Spot clean mirrors and glass surfaces	Daily
	Clean mirrors thoroughly	Daily
	Wet mop wood floors	Weekly
	Wash and disinfect rubber floor surfaces	Daily
	Clean HVAC ducts	Bi-monthly
	Clean light fixtures	Bi-monthly
	Clean the audio equipment	Bi-monthly
	Wash the solid-surface walls	Quarterly to annually
	Refinish wood-floor surfaces	Annually

Figure 21-3. Cleaning guidelines for fitness and group-exercise facilities

Facility Area	Cleaning Activity	Frequency
Gymnasium	Remove trash	Daily
	Dry mop and dust floors	Daily
	Dust all horizontal surfaces	Daily
	Spot clean all glass surfaces	Daily
	Clean all glass surfaces thoroughly	Weekly
	Tack/wet mop the wood floors	Weekly
	Clean HVAC filters	Bi-monthly
	Clean light fixtures	Bi-monthly
	Refinish wood floors	Every two years
Racquet Courts	Remove trash	Daily
	Dry mop and dust floors	Daily
	Dust horizontal surfaces	Daily
	Spot clean walls and glass surfaces	Daily
	Remove ball marks	Daily
	Tack or damp mop the floors	Weekly
	Thoroughly clean glass surfaces	Bi-monthly
	Clean HVAC vents	Bi-monthly
	Clean light fixtures	Bi-monthly
	Refinish floors (squash should be left unfinished, but sanded)	Annually
Tennis Courts	Remove trash	Daily
	Sweep/vacuum indoor hard courts	Daily
	Blow outdoor courts to remove debris	Daily
	Roll dry outdoor hard courts after rain	Daily
	Sweep courts and brush lines for clay courts	Daily
	Water clay courts	Daily
	Scrape dead material on clay courts	Weekly
	Patch low spots on clay courts	Weekly
	Jet broom and sweep hard courts	Weekly
	Pressure wash hard courts	Bi-annually
	Recondition clay courts (add surface material)	Semi-annually to annually
	Replace tape on clay courts	Every two to three years
	Resurface hard courts	Every three to four years
	Resurface clay courts	Every three to four years

Figure 21-4. Cleaning guidelines for gymnasiums, racquet courts, and tennis courts

Facility Area	Cleaning Activity	Frequency
Lobby and Circulation Areas	Remove trash	Daily
	Vacuum carpets	Daily
	Clean off walk and mats in lobby areas	Daily
	Wet mop hard-surface floors (granite, tile, etc.)	Daily
	Buff hard surfaces	Daily
	Dust horizontal surfaces	Daily
	Clean and polish furniture	Daily
	Clean and polish mirrors, sconces, etc.	Bi-monthly
	Clean light fixtures	Bi-monthly
	Clean HVAC vents	Bi-monthly
	Clean carpets	Quarterly to annually
	Strip and refinish wood floors	Annually
Massage Rooms	Remove trash	Daily
	Vacuum carpeted floors	Daily
	Dust horizontal surfaces	Daily
	Remove all soiled linen	Daily
	Clean and disinfect beds, tables, etc.	After each client
	Clean and polish furniture	Daily
	Wet mop the floors if wood or tile	Daily
	Clean light fixtures	Bi-monthly
	Clean HVAC vents	Bi-monthly
	Clean carpets	Annually
Offices	Remove trash	Daily
	Vacuum carpeted areas	Daily
	Dust horizontal surfaces	Daily
	Clean and polish furniture	Daily
	Wet mop the floors if wood or tile	Daily
	Clean light fixtures	Bi-monthly
	Clean HVAC vents	Bi-monthly
	Clean carpets	Annually

Figure 21-5. Cleaning guidelines for the lobby, massage rooms, and offices

for several of the key areas in a health/fitness club, including the fitness center, the group-exercise studio, gymnasium, racquet courts, tennis courts, offices, lobby and circulation areas, and massage rooms. (Note: cleaning guidelines for locker rooms and pools are not covered in these figures because they have been addressed in previous chapters.)

Accounting

Accounting operations are a sub-set of the financial management practices that were reviewed earlier in the book. As was noted, financial management encompasses a club's financial structuring and the types and kinds of reports the facility uses to monitor its overall financial performance. Accounting operations, on the other hand, are the processes, policies, and practices that the club employs to ensure that the money is handled in an appropriate manner, both on the revenue and the expense side. These processes, policies, and practices can normally be grouped into four distinct categories: accounts payable, accounts receivable, payroll functions, and financial reporting. Club operators have several resources available that can help them set up their accounting practices, including GAAP (generally accepted accounting practices) principles in the U.S. and IFRS (international financial reporting standards) in global markets, each of which are an accepted set of accounting principles, standards, and procedures that most (if not all) companies employ to compile their financial statements. In the United States, GAAP is administered by the Financial Standards Board that is headquartered in Norwich, Connecticut.

❏ *Accounts Payable.* Accounts payable refers to the policies and practices that govern how the club/facility pays its vendors and employees for services. Because accounts-payable practices focus on managing and making payments to the club's outside vendors, they are an integral element of controlling expenses. Figure 21-6 lists several of the most relevant accounts-payable practices that clubs can adopt to assist them in managing their finances.

Accounts Payable Practice	Description/Purpose
Expense reports	The expense-report process requires employees to complete an expense report with accompanying receipts for all business-related expenses. The reports should be approved by a supervisor before payment.
Check requests	The check-request process requires department heads to complete a form requesting any check for payment of a service provided by a vendor. This form is usually approved by the manager before a check can be issued.
Purchase orders	A purchase-order system requires that before any items are ordered, the items desired be priced beforehand and put on a purchase order for approval. Once approved, the items can be purchased. The purchase order then serves as a check-and-balance mechanism against the packing slip and invoice from a supplier.
Par-stock inventory system	Every supply the club uses and every item/product sold should have a par-stock that is inventoried regularly. A point-of-sale software system typically does this for retail operations, but clubs need their own system for supplies.
Check and invoice approval and payment	To provide better control, each club should have a process that requires at least two signatures on a check request or invoice before a check is cut. Furthermore, every check should be reviewed against the invoices and signatures by someone other than the accountant or bookkeeper before it is released.

Figure 21-6. Accounts payable practices

❏ *Accounts Receivable.* The accounts-receivable accounting operation involves the policies and practices that pertain to the billing and collection of funds from anyone (e.g., members) who uses the club's services. The primary focus of accounts-receivable accounting function is to ensure that the club receives all monies that are due for the services and benefits provided to anyone by the facility. Figure 21-7 illustrates several of the most relevant accounts receivable practices that clubs utilize to assist them in managing their finances.

❏ *Payroll Functions.* Payroll functions refer to the policies and practices governing a club's handling of all compensation and benefits involving both employees and independent contractors. The main focus of payroll activities is to ensure that employees and contractors receive the proper compensation for the services they have rendered. Figure 21-8 details several of the most relevant payroll-related practices that clubs employ to assist them in managing their finances.

Accounts Receivable Practice	Description/Purpose
Monthly member billing	Creating the monthly member statements if the club bills its members directly.
Daily charging activities	Applying all member charges to their member accounts in the event the club allows members to charge services on their membership account.
Monthly EFT and charge handling	Most clubs use electronic funds transfer to bill and collect member payments. Accounting needs to correctly set-up each member's account for proper billing and collection.
Bank reconciliation	This practice falls into both a payable and a receivable function, because it involves the daily undertaking of reconciling the books to make sure all deposits and debits are accounted for and that the bank account is liquid.
Accounts receivable collection	Accounting has the responsibility of monitoring the club's accounts that are outstanding and making sure all past-due funds are collected. This involves 30-, 60-, and 90-day policies and practices that are focused on prompt collection of all past-due funds.

Figure 21-7. Accounts receivable practices

Payroll Practice	Description/Purpose
Time sheets/time cards/time clock	Every club should have a system in place to set employee schedules, have the employees check-in, monitor the hours that employees work, provide reports on time worked, overtime hours, etc.
Preparing payroll and contractor checks	Involves preparing the payroll and contractor checks, and using the time-card and time-sheet information.
Monitoring overtime, vacation, and personal time	Most accounting departments are involved in monitoring overtime hours, vacation pay, and personal pay. In addition to monitoring, accounting handles all distributions of compensation related to those factors.
Employee benefits administration	Most accounting departments are responsible for the appropriate enrollment of employees in the club's benefit programs and handling the activities related to those benefits.

Figure 21-8. Payroll practices

❑ *Financial Reporting.* Financial reporting refers to the policies and practices that are involved in monitoring the club's overall financial performance. Financial reporting may also include activities that relate to the preparation of a club's budget and monitoring the facility's actual adherence to the budget (financial-wise). Figure 21-9 presents an overview of several of the most relevant financial-reporting practices that clubs can use to assist them in managing their finances.

Financial Reporting Practice	Description/Purpose
Daily sales sheets	Daily sales sheets allow clubs to monitor the total sales each day. A daily sales sheet encompasses a tally of each sale that occurs that day. The daily sales sheet should reflect each sale, what it was for, the amount of the sale, the category of sale, whether it was cash or charge, etc.
Daily, weekly, and monthly financial reports	Clubs should have specific reports that can help them better understand their finances, including daily sales report, daily payroll report, weekly/ monthly profit-and-loss statement, weekly/monthly balance-sheet report, weekly/monthly accounts-payable report, weekly/monthly accounts-receivable report, and monthly fixed-asset report.
Budget and forecast tools	Every club should have an annual budget for each department, as well as quarterly forecast reports for each department that reflect the expected revenue and expense outcomes of operations. Accounting is normally responsible for preparing and printing these reports, in conjunction with management.

Figure 21-9. Financial reporting practices

22

Club Spas

Chapter Objectives

Day spas have not always been such an important component of the club industry. As early as the mid-1990s, most club operators would have questioned the wisdom of devoting financial resources to build and operate a day spa. On the other hand, at the present time, most club operators are aware of the value of a day spa in serving the needs of the marketplace and helping to grow the club's overall operating revenues. In this chapter we will present an overview of the day-spa business as it applies to the successful operation of a health/fitness club. This overview addresses several factors attendant to the spa business and club spas in particular, including:

- Defining the types of spas that exist, particularly those in the health/fitness club industry
- Describing the individuals who like to engage in the spa experience and how understanding these populations can assist in operating a spa for a particular type of club
- Detailing the basic facility and equipment needs of a successful club spa
- Identifying the basic program and service elements needed for a successful club spa
- Discussing the most effective approaches to marketing a club spa
- Reviewing several of the key issues involving spa staff

General Spa-Industry Data

Most club operators are aware of the value of a day spa in serving the needs of the marketplace and helping to grow the club's overall operating revenues.

In 2009, the International Spa Association (ISPA) reported that at the end of 2009, approximately 20,600 spas existed in the United States, representing nearly a 70 percent increase over the previous five years. According to ISPA's research, the spa industry generated a total of $12.3 billion in revenue in 2009. While that statistic entailed a 9 percent increase over the previous five years, it was a 4.3 percent decrease from 2008 to 2009. Overall, spas experienced 143 million visits in 2008, an increase of seven million visits when compared to just five years earlier. On the other hand, when measured against 2008, it was a decline of nearly 17 million visits. According to the *ISPA 2008 Global Consumer Study*, among active U.S. spa goers, 82 percent utilize day spas. Besides the U.S., only England, Japan, and Singapore have as many as 65 percent of spa goers frequent day spas. It is interesting to note that U.S. spa goers rank third in terms of average annual spending on spas of $537, trailing Singapore residents who spend $937, and the approximately $850 annually spent by Italians who use spas.

According to the publication, the *IHRSA 2010 Profiles of Success*, 10.4 percent of health/fitness clubs in the U.S. and Canada offer spa treatments (42 percent have just massage services), while approximately 8 percent of facilities have a dedicated spa. From a financial perspective, the IHRSA report indicates that on average, club spa services contribute close to 9 percent of a club's total revenues.

Types of Spas

To many individuals, a spa is a retreat from the world; a place where they can escape from their normal daily regimen and pursue activities that they believe will help to enrich their lives. According to the International Spa Association (ISPA), spas have been in existence for a very, very long time. The original concept of a spa was derived from retreats that had hot springs and provided treatments that involved the use of these soothing hot-mineral springs. The original concept for spas emanated from baths filled with hot mineral waters that were believed to be beneficial for the body. Over the years, however, spas have evolved substantially, resulting in spas moving well beyond the original notion of hot-mineral baths.

> Spas provide several services, including massages, facials, body wraps, manicures, pedicures, salon services, yoga, meditation, nutrition counseling, and exercise classes.

Spas provide several services, including massages, facials, body wraps, manicures, pedicures, salon services, yoga, meditation, nutrition counseling, and exercise classes. The introduction of these multiple services into the spa environment has spawned numerous spa concepts. According to ISPA and as reflected in Figure 22-1, several primary types of spas exist, including:

❏ *Medical Spas*. Medical spas are spa facilities that provide services that are medically focused. These services encompass therapeutic and rehabilitative treatments (e.g., therapeutic massage, exfoliation, detoxification, botox treatments, microdermabrasion, etc.) that are integrated with more conventional medical services. According to the *ISPA 2010 U.S. Spa Industry Study*, medical spas represented approximately 8.7 percent of the total spa market, putting them third behind day spas and resort/hotel spas.

❏ *Resort/Hotel Spas*. Resort/hotel spas are spa facilities that are located in either a hotel or resort setting. The primary focus of these spas is to provide basic spa services (e.g., sauna, steam, whirlpool, massage) for hotel and resort guests. Resort spas, as compared to hotel-based spas, offer an incredible array of spas services, including body treatments, facials, manicures/pedicures, massage, and various wet-therapy modalities. According to the *ISPA 2010 U.S. Spa Industry Study*, resort/hotel spas are the second largest segment of the industry, representing 8.8 percent of the total spa market.

Figure 22-1. Types of spa facilities

❏ *Destination Spas.* Destination spas are spa facilities that are located on resort properties that offer a complete destination experience. These spas fully engage the visitor in a spa experience that includes such endeavors as dining, exercise, and spa treatments (e.g., massage, body wraps, facials, pedicures, hot mineral baths, etc.), among others. These spas usually bundle their services into packages that involve designated time periods. According to ISPA's research, destination spas represent less than one-half of one percent of the total spa market in the United States.

❏ *Mineral-Springs Spas.* Mineral-springs spas are spa facilities that offer spa services that incorporate the use of onsite sources, such as natural minerals, and naturally heated water and seawater, which are employed in hydrotherapy treatments. According to ISPA's 2010 survey, less than one-half of one percent of the total number of spas that exist in the United States marketplace are mineral-spring spas. Mineral spring spas are far more prevalent in Europe, especially in Germany.

❏ *Day Spas.* Day spas are spa facilities that focus on delivering easily completed spa services (e.g., hair, manicures, pedicures, facials, massage, etc.) that can be experienced in periods of 30 minutes to one day in length. Most day spas are located in affluent urban and suburban markets that serve individuals who want to have a spa experience without having to leave their community. Approximately 79 percent of the spas in the United States are classified as day spas.

❏ *Club Spas.* Club spas are day-spa facilities that are located within health/ fitness clubs that focus on providing basic spa services, such as massage, facials, manicures, sauna, steam, etc., to club members and guests. According to ISPA's research, club spas represent 2.8 percent of the entire spa industry.

As the aforementioned review of the various types of spas indicates, the spa industry affords individuals multiple opportunities to engage in the pleasant environment afforded by spa treatments. One of the underlying themes among all of these spa offerings is the fundamental focus on providing an experience that can help enrich the individual's life.

Spa Consumer Profile

In 2004 and 2006, ISPA sponsored research that was designed to identify the characteristics of the individuals who use spas. This research identified three primary profiles for spa consumers: periphery spa consumers, mid-level spa consumers, and core spa consumers.

❑ *Periphery Spa Consumers.* Periphery spa consumers are individuals who tend to be impressed by well-operated spas and whose primary expectations concerning the spa involve indulging in cosmetic services that make them feel special and look beautiful. These consumers are price-sensitive and tend to prefer the more superficial spa services (e.g., cosmetic or physical body). As a rule, they want to experience pleasurable and light spa services. These consumers are not into the wellness and spiritual aspects of spa services; rather they prefer massages, facials, and manicures. This consumer group is the predominant segment for which club-based spas should develop and target their facilities and services.

❑ *Mid-level Spa Consumers.* Mid-level spa consumers are people who tend to view going to spas as more of a wellness experience. These individuals want to achieve an emotional encounter, as well as experience the cosmetic and physical-body services that the periphery spa consumer typically pursues. These individuals prefer the isolation of a treatment room, seeking services such as massage, skin treatments, and body treatments. These consumers tend to be price-sensitive when the more esoteric services are involved. They are not as sensitive about price when it comes to less arcane services, such as massage, manicures, and facials. These consumers are interested in the therapist's credentials. In most instances, this group is a secondary market for club spas. Individuals who comprise this group also want to be able to customize their experience.

❑ *Core Spa Consumers.* Core spa consumers are individuals who have "adopted" the spa lifestyle. They tend to view the spa experience as being an essential part of their overall wellness routine. These consumers place a high level of importance on the entire spa experience, not just the actual treatment. They measure the spa experience, starting with their arrival, and continuing through the treatment that they receive and concluding when they depart. All factors considered, these individuals are the most demanding of the consumers who utilize the services of club spas. As a rule, they prefer not to interact with periphery and mid-level consumers. While individuals in this group will use a club spa, they also tend to expect to receive services and achieve experiences that are counter to the largest audience for the services offered by club spas. These customers want to customize their experience.

With regard to spas, the club industry has the greatest opportunity to be successful when they provide spa experiences that appeal primarily to periphery spa consumers and to mid-level consumers to a lesser degree. As such, the group of core spa users is relatively small. In reality, if that group is targeted, it will often drive away the other two consumer audiences.

Research has identified three primary profiles for spa consumers: periphery spa consumers, mid-level spa consumers, and core spa consumers.

According to the *ISPA 2010 U.S. Spa Industry Study*, approximately 80 percent of all spa goers are women. In their *2008 Global Consumer Study*, ISPA indicated that the two largest age-driven demographic segments for spa goers were those individuals over the age of 55 and those people between the ages of 18 and 34. Over 50 percent of spa consumers are married, while 57 percent are employed full-time or part-time. The average household income of a spa consumer, based on ISPA data from 2006, was $72,000 annually (it should be noted that this is almost identical to the average household income of the average health/fitness club member). In essence, the demographic profile of a spa consumer closely parallels the demographics of health/fitness club members, with one notable exception—women are more likely to be spa consumers than club members.

A Profile of Why Consumers Use Spas

Industry research shows that spa consumers at all levels indicate that they have three primary rationales for using a spa: indulgence, escape, and work.

> **Industry research shows that spa consumers at all levels indicate that they have three primary rationales for using a spa: indulgence, escape, and work.**

❏ *Indulgence.* The most self-centered of the reasons for using a spa, indulgence is the primary driver for periphery consumers and a secondary driver for mid-level consumers. Accordingly, it is the factor that clubs should focus on when they design their spas. When consumers refer to indulgence, they often inject such talk by mentioning such factors as fun, playfulness, decadent, pampering, heavenly, joy, enjoyment, and personal time. As a rule, women, more than men, are willing to indulge themselves. Indulgence is highly dependent on household cash flow. In that regard, when the expendable income level of peripheral and mid-level consumers declines, they are less likely to engage in indulgent activities. The most common spa services that are categorized as indulgent are massages, facials, aromatherapy, body scrubs, and thermal treatments.

❏ *Escape.* Escape is the primary driver to use a spa for those consumers who are not engaging in spa services merely as a means to an end. In this instance, escape refers to achieving an experience that allows consumers to remove themselves from the everyday occurrences of life. This process entails a blend of mind and body factors. Escapist experiences involve spa treatments that create an environment that is characterized by a sense of calmness, respite, tranquility, seclusion, etc. This driver is likely to be one of the major reasons why mid-level or core consumers utilize a spa. The most common escapist spa experiences include body scrubs, body wraps, aromatherapy, and hydrotherapy.

❏ *Work.* Work is a driver for using a spa that is grounded in the desire of individuals to make improvements in themselves, whether it is to look better, feel better, or balance their life. Mid-level consumers and core consumers are more likely to be driven to utilize spas by work than either indulgence or escape, because they tend to see spas as being a more integral element in their overall lifestyle.

Spa Visit Motivators

In the *ISPA 2008 Global Consumer Study*, researchers looked at the various "motivators" that generate traffic for a spa. In the U.S., the three primary reasons consumers visit a spa are first, to relax and relieve stress, second, to be pampered, and finally, to enhance overall health and well-being. When it comes to actually having an enjoyable and uplifting spa experience, consumers indicate that the leading factors are: a stress-free environment, the expertise of staff, and the overall atmosphere of the spa.

It should be emphasized that the aforementioned factors for influencing consumer spa behavior fluctuate based on the nation of origin, but, in general, the leading influencers remain similar. As to what actually drives spa consumers to the door of a spa, in the U.S., the top three drivers were referral from a friend (45 percent), an offer of complimentary products or bonus services (38 percent), and the recommendation of a healthcare professional (30 percent). These three motivators vary considerably from nation to nation. For example, in France, the opportunity to receive a complimentary product or bonus service is the leading motivator (45 percent), while in Australia, a gift certificate (60 percent) is the most likely factor to drive spa traffic.

Club Spa Facilities and Features

According to the *ISPA 2010 U.S. Spa Industry Report*, the average day spa occupies 2,655 square feet and has 6.6 treatment rooms. The typical club spa can encompass one or more types of treatment spaces, including massage rooms, facial rooms, multipurpose-treatment rooms, wet-treatment rooms, manicure and pedicure spaces, relaxation space, and reception area/retail space. It should also be noted that one of the most recent trends in spa facilities is the inclusion of rooms where couples can receive massages, facials, and wet treatments (approximately 38 percent of spas offer couple treatment rooms). Each of the various types of treatment spaces in spa facilities has its own unique features.

> One of the most recent trends in spa facilities is the inclusion of rooms where couples can receive massages, facials, and wet treatments.

❑ *Multipurpose-Treatment Rooms.* Multipurpose-treatment rooms are available in 62 percent of spas, while 67 percent of spas offer massage rooms. Body treatments and massage services are the predominate treatment offered by day spas, with 94 percent offering body treatment services and 88 percent massage services. From a consumer perspective, 81 percent of U.S consumers take massage, while facial services are the third most popular treatment, with 42 percent of consumers receiving a facial. As a result, multipurpose rooms need to be designed to accommodate the delivery of a variety of spa-related activities, including massage services, body treatments, and facials. These rooms typically range in size from 100 to 120 square feet. Couples rooms are usually larger—150 to 200 square feet. As a rule, multi-purpose treatment rooms include:

- Indirect lighting that is controlled through dimmer switches
- Floor surfaces that are easily washable and provide cushioning for the therapists. The best surfaces are soft vinyl floors or treated wood floors.

Some surfaces, such as tile, are relatively easy to clean, but are not good for the therapists. On the other hand, carpeting can be difficult to keep clean. Recently, the use of cork as a flooring surface has grown in popularity.

- Built-in sound systems that can be controlled by the therapists
- Built-in millwork that includes a hard counter surface, sink, storage spaces, and retail-display cabinetry
- Wall surfaces that can easily be cleaned, as well as being able to help provide a soothing environment
- Individual room thermostats that can help maintain the proper air temperature
- Added sound attenuation construction to reduce transmission of sound

All factors considered, multipurpose treatment rooms are the most important spaces in the club spa, because they are in areas in which peripheral spa consumers are most likely to engage in spa services. The typical treatment room accounts for 52 percent of spa revenues.

❑ *Wet-Treatment Rooms.* In the spa industry, the average wet-treatment area consists of one to two rooms (18 percent of spas have rooms for Vichy showers and 16 percent for hydrotherapy). Wet-treatment rooms are utilized primarily for spa treatments that involve the use of water. Among the treatments that are performed in these rooms are body wraps, body scrubs, and hydrotherapy treatments (16 percent of spas have hydrotherapy space), which involve such implements as hydrotherapy tubs, Vichy showers (18 percent of spas have space for Vichy showers), Scottish hose (less than 2 percent of spas have space allocated for the Scottish hose), etc. In the U.S., approximately 22 percent of spa services are wet treatments (body scrubs, wraps, hydrotherapy, etc.). These rooms typically range in size from 120 to 150 square feet, while rooms for couples are closer to 200 square feet. As a rule, these rooms include:

- Indirect and direct lighting, both on dimmer switches
- Floor and wall surface that is water resistant and easy to clean. The most suitable surface for the floors and walls is tile (e.g., ceramic or porcelain). At the least, the walls in these areas need to have a four-foot wainscot of tile. Custom vinyl surfaces can also be used, in lieu of tile.
- Built-in shower and additional water faucet fixtures. The additional fixtures can be used for hydrotherapy tubs or Vichy showers.
- Floor drains
- Built-in sound systems that can be controlled by the therapists
- Built-in millwork that includes a hard counter surface, sink, storage spaces, and retail-display cabinetry
- Added sound attenuation construction to reduce the transmission of sound

Because wet-treatment rooms mostly appeal to mid-level and core consumers, they are not essential to the successful operation of a club spa.

> All factors considered, multipurpose treatment rooms are the most important spaces in the club spa, because they are in areas in which peripheral spa consumers are most likely to engage in spa services.

❏ *Manicure and Pedicure Spaces.* The manicure and pedicure spaces require a more social and open atmosphere than do the multipurpose and wet-treatment rooms, which need to be private. These spaces not only are designed to provide manicures and pedicures, but also to facilitate social interaction between the therapists and customers. These spaces typically include the following features:

- *Pedicure space* (in the spa industry, the average pedicure space has three stations):
  - ✓ Approximately 50 to 60 square feet per pedicure station (chair, foot bath, and therapist chair)
  - ✓ Floor and wall surfaces that are water resistant and easy to clean. The most suitable surface for the floors and walls is tile (e.g., ceramic or porcelain). At the least, the walls in this area should have a four-foot wainscot of tile. Custom vinyl surfaces can also be used in lieu of tile.
  - ✓ Floor drains
  - ✓ Soft, yet bright, lighting
  - ✓ Built-in sound systems that can be controlled by the therapists
  - ✓ Dedicated negative exhaust system to help pull fumes out of the space
- *Manicure space* (in the spa industry, the average manicure space has four stations):
  - ✓ Approximately 40 to 60 square feet per manicure station (table and two chairs)
  - ✓ Floor surfaces that are either carpet or a solid material (e.g., vinyl, wood, or tile)
  - ✓ Lighting that is soft, yet bright

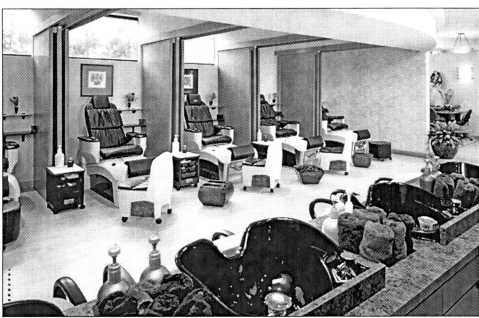

Spa pedicure space, The Atlantic Club, NJ

Ohlson Lavoie Collaborative, Denver, CO

✓ Built-in sound systems that can be controlled by the therapists

✓ Dedicated negative exhaust system to help pull fumes out of the space

Individuals consider manicure and pedicure services as both an indulgence and work. Accordingly, the services offered in these spaces tend to appeal equally to core spa consumers and peripheral spa consumers. In the U.S., manicures and pedicures are the second most frequently used spa services, with 45 percent of spa goers receiving one or both of these treatments. Club-based spas should view these spaces as being somewhat less essential than multipurpose treatment rooms.

❏ *Relaxation Space.* A relaxation space is most commonly found in club spas that have more than six treatment rooms. The relaxation room serves as a transition space between the treatment rooms and the rest of the club, an area in which the client is allowed to relax prior to entering a treatment room, or wind down after a treatment, before returning to the locker room or leaving the spa. Some of the larger club spas have both a men's and a women's relaxation area. As a rule, these rooms typically range in size from 100 to 400 square feet and include the following features:

> **The relaxation room serves as a transition space between the treatment rooms and the rest of the club, an area in which the client is allowed to relax prior to entering a treatment room, or wind down after a treatment, before returning to the locker room or leaving the spa.**

• Soft floor surfaces (e.g., carpet or wood with throw carpets)

• Indirect soft lighting

• Sound attenuation construction that facilitates a quiet environment

• Millwork with display cabinets, hard-surface countertops, and built-in refrigerators

• Built-in sound system

Relaxation rooms appeal mostly to core spa consumers and, as a result, are not an essential element when developing club spas. On the other hand, if the club wants to appeal to core consumers, then relaxation rooms are a must.

❏ *Reception Area/Retail Space.* A reception area/retail space is not normally incorporated into the design of most club-based spas. These spaces, which provide a separate entry and retail space specifically for the spa, are normally not required, unless the club spa is designed to drive a large non-member level of business. This space normally consists of a reception desk, retail displays (e.g., wall-mounted cabinets, floor displays, etc.), and a soft-seating area. This space typically features:

• Wood, granite, or similar hard surface flooring

• Extensive millwork with retail displays

• Indirect soft lighting

• Custom wall treatments and furniture

• Sound system

In addition, if the club spa has more than four treatment rooms, then a separate storage and employee room should be provided. Such an area can be used for several purposes, including storing the various treatment supplies, preparing the treatment materials, and serving as a location for therapists to relax.

Club Spa Space Requirements

A club spa can be simply as small as a single multipurpose treatment room or as large as a 20-room, full-service facility. The typical fitness club has between one and four treatment rooms, with two treatment rooms being the norm (compared to an average of 6.6 treatment spaces in a day spa). A few club companies, such as Lifetime Fitness, Sports Club/LA, DMB Sports, and Western Athletic Clubs, offer club spas that encompass from 6 to 12 treatment rooms, while other club operations have spas that consist of over 20 rooms (e.g., Houstonian in Houston, Texas and Exhale). When developing a club spa, facilities should evaluate several factors, including the following:

- *Internal Market Demand.* How many current club members would be interested in using spa services? Typically, a club that serves either a family market or a predominately female market will have greater demand for spa services. Anecdotal data from the club industry indicates that between 5 percent and 10 percent of a facility's members will use spa services on a regular basis, with some luxury club operators reporting usage levels of 15 percent to 25 percent. For example, if a club has 3,000 members, it could expect that approximately 300 of those members will become active spa goers.
- *External Market Demand.* How large is the non-member market, and what type of traffic can be generated? Many club operators report that in mature club spas (spas open a few years), approximately 50 percent of their business comes from non-members, while in the beginning, club members may encompass 70 percent to 80 percent of the client base.
- *Target Audience.* Which spa consumer group will be the club's desired audience?
- *Available Space in the Facility.* What space is available for renovation or conversion to spa-related services?
- *Costs of Development.* What will it cost to develop a spa, and what will be the expected return on the investment?

While no actual club-industry averages exist for how many rooms should be incorporated into a club spa, a list of the general guidelines on how to proceed in this regard includes the following:

- Provide a minimum of one treatment room/station per 1,000 memberships and a maximum of two treatment rooms/stations per 1,000 memberships. For example, if the club has 3,000 memberships, it should have a minimum of three treatment rooms and a maximum of six treatment rooms.
- For club spas that have no more than four treatment rooms, all of them should be designed as multipurpose treatment areas. If a facility has more than four treatment rooms, it should consider providing one wet-treatment room (only if its intent is to appeal to mid-level and core consumers). In most instances, a club spa will never need more than one wet-treatment room.
- The club spa should include relaxation space if the facility has at least six treatment rooms and the decision has been made that the spa is

The typical fitness club has between one and four treatment rooms, with two treatment rooms being the norm.

going to target core spa consumers. If the spa facility wants to attract a relatively large number of women, the club should consider having both a women's and a men's relaxation room.

- As a rule, manicure and pedicure areas normally never have to exceed two stations each, unless the club is offering a full-service spa that attempts to appeal to all levels of spa consumers. In the event that the club has a full-service spa, the number of spaces for pedicures and manicures depends upon the assumed traffic level.
- Depending on the number of specialized rooms (e.g., treatment areas, manicure/pedicure spaces, and relaxation rooms) that are included in the club spa, the typical club spa facility ranges in size from 600 to 2,000 square feet. It should also be noted that the median free-standing day spa in the United States is 2,655 square feet, according to statistics provided by ISPA.

Club Spa Equipment

The variety and quantity of equipment in a club spa is dependent upon the services provided by the spa and the facility spaces that exist. Figure 22-2 presents a list of the basic equipment requirements in the various types of club-spa areas.

Multipurpose Treatment Room	Wet Treatment Room	Manicure/Pedicure Space	Relaxation Room
• Massage/facial table (adjustable) • Therapists stool • Bolster pads • Stone heater and stones • Warmers for oils and lotions • Hydro collator • Paraffin heater/ bath • Facial system (rotary brush, vapo-steamer, vacuum/spray, high-frequency galvanic stimulator, and magnifying lamp) • Towel-heater cabinet • Sterilizer/autoclave • Mixing bowls • Blankets and sheets	• Wet/dry table • Vichy shower unit • Hydrotherapy tub (optional) • Heat lamp • Hydro collator • Mixing bowls • Paraffin heater/bath • Shower • Step stool • Therapist stool	• Manicure table • Task chairs • Pedicure chair with footbath • Nail-drying station • Foot spa • Pedicure stool • Paraffin heater/bath • Storage cart	• Soft seating (sofas and chairs) • Coffee table • Magazine racks • Refrigerator • Cabinets for retail displays and storage • Dispenser system for drinks

Figure 22-2. Equipment options for a club spa

Club Spa Service Offerings

The three leading service offerings in the U.S.-based spa industry are massages (81 percent), manicures/pedicures (45 percent), and facials (42 percent). From a revenue perspective, massage/bodywork treatments drive approximately 32 percent of spa revenue, and skin treatments, including facials, account for approximately 25 percent of revenue, followed by retail sales, which generate 12 percent of revenue and manicures/pedicures, which contribute 8 percent of revenue (refer to Figure 22-3).

The services that a club spa provides depend upon several factors, including the market it intends to serve (periphery, mid-level, or core), the space it has available, and its overall revenue and profitability goals. Industry research indicates that club spas should focus most on those consumers who are seeking indulgences (first) and escapes (second). As a result, providing massage, manicure/pedicure, and facial services should be a top priority for clubs with a spa. Since 10 percent to 20 percent (12 percent on average) of spa revenues typically come from retail sales, clubs should also consider allocating space to this function.

❑ *Massage Services.* Massage encompasses a vast array of treatments, ranging from soothing massage modalities to therapeutic modalities. The most frequently offered massage services include:
  • *Swedish massage.* A gentle relaxing massage modality that focuses on enhancing circulation and relaxing the musculature.
  • *Sports massage.* A more therapeutic massage modality that centers on addressing specific sport/activity-related issues. This type of massage

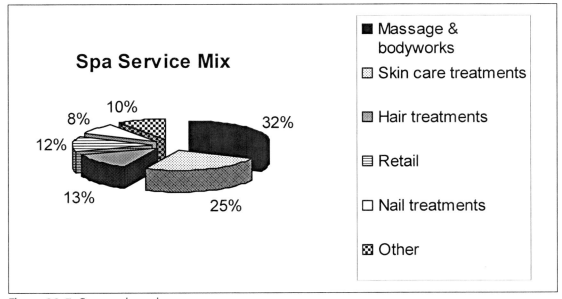

Figure 22-3. Spa service mix

tends to involve deeper massage, designed to release deep tension and break up scar tissue.

- *Trigger-point massage.* A modality based on Asian massage techniques that focus on applying pressure to specific trigger points to release tension. While this type of massage can be painful at first, it is excellent as a therapeutic modality.
- *Hot-stone massage.* A modality that employs pre-heated stones, placed along the musculature, to help release tension. The stones are moved periodically to other areas of the body's surface.
- *Aromatherapy massage.* A modality that involves the use of aromatic oils, in combination with Swedish massage techniques. Some individuals consider this type of massage to be both relaxing and therapeutic.

In addition to the aforementioned massage techniques, a host of more esoteric techniques exist that vary in popularity, depending upon the facility's geographic location. These activities include such techniques as Thai massage, reflexology, bamboo massage, and shiatsu. Most massage treatments involve time periods ranging from 25 to 90 minutes.

> The most common type of club-spa facials encompass the use of special lotions to exfoliate the skin, followed by gentle massage, and finally, the application of lotions to hydrate the skin.

❏ *Facial Services.* Facials involve a combination of treatment applications, including exfoliation, detoxification, hydrating, and massage. The most common type of club-spa facials encompass the use of special lotions to exfoliate the skin, followed by gentle massage, and finally, the application of lotions to hydrate the skin. Recently, day and club spas have begun to utilize microderm abrasion to provide a more thorough exfoliation of the skin surface. It is common for spas to provide special names for their various facial treatments, based on the lotions and techniques used, for example, executive facials, spa facials, European facials, eye-contour treatments, acne treatments, back facials, facial peels, fruit-based facials, facial masks, make-up applications, etc.

❏ *Body Treatments and Wet Treatments.* Body treatments and wet treatments are services that the majority of club spas provide in their wet treatment rooms. The body treatments normally involve some use of water, while wet treatments (as the term implies) directly incorporate the use of water. The most frequently offered body and wet treatments include the following:

- *Body scrubs.* Body scrubs are treatments that involve the use of brushes, sponges, and/or lotions to exfoliate the targeted skin surface. Some of the most common types of body-scrub treatments are deep-sea salt scrubs, body polish, essential oil scrubs, Turkish body scrubs, and fruit-based body scrubs.
- *Body wraps.* Body wraps are treatments that involve wrapping the entire body or a segment of the body with special products, such as seaweed or mud. These treatments focus on both detoxification and exfoliation. Examples include herbal wrap, mud wrap, essential oil wrap, spirulina wrap, silk wraps, etc.
- *Hydrotherapy tub treatments.* These are treatments that are conducted in a hydrotherapy tub and involve the use of water jets to stimulate and massage the body.

- *Vichy shower and Scottish hose treatments.* The Vichy shower involves the use of multiple water jets to massage the body. In most cases, the client is prone on a wet table while the Vichy treatment is conducted. A Scottish hose is a more intense water treatment that involves the use of a powerful water jet that is sprayed on the body to create intense stimulation of the skin and underlying body tissues.

❑ *Other Services That Club Spas Can Offer.* In addition to certain basic services, such as massage, facials, and body treatments, club spas should also consider providing the following services, based on the audience to which they are attempting to appeal:
- Manicures
- Pedicures
- Waxing (a fast-growing service-treatment segment)
- Paraffin treatments for the hands and feet
- Cosmetic application (assisting clients in the proper use and application of cosmetics)
- Spray-on tanning

One of the newest service trends in the spa industry is to offer shorter treatment sessions. Because the time demands of consumers have intensified, spa operators have developed new treatment approaches that involve durations of 30 minutes or less. Not only do these shorter treatment sessions accommodate consumer time restraints, they also provide consumers with an opportunity to spend less on their treatments.

Club Spa Financial Parameters

The price that club spas place on their services depends upon many factors, including the geographic region in which the spa is located, the club's initial investment in the spa facility, the target audience, the surrounding demographics, and the role the spa plays in the club's overall business strategy. Clubs should always conduct the proper market research before establishing the services that they will offer and the prices that they will charge for those services. Club-based spas, on average, offer their services at a lower price point than day spas, resort/hotel spas, and destination spas. If the club is trying to grow the business and appeal to periphery spa consumers, the price points for its services must be carefully considered, since this group of consumers is extremely price sensitive. According to the *ISPA 2010 Spa Industry Study*, the average price of a spa treatment was $83, with a massage going at $85, a facial at $91, body treatments at $95, and nail service (manicure/pedicure) at $42. Figure 22-4 illustrates the general ranges for several of the most common club-spa service price points.

According to 2010 ISPA research, the average freestanding day spa generated $490,000 in 2009 with average revenue per square foot of $185 and average revenue per employee of nearly $35,000. Based on these metrics, a day spa could expect to generate close to $75,000 per treatment room annually. As such, the average club spa can expect to generate between

Clubs should always conduct the proper market research before establishing the services that they will offer and the prices that they will charge for those services.

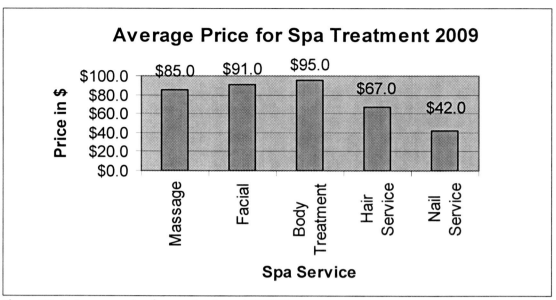

Figure 22-4. Average price for spa treatment (2009)

$3,000 and $6,000 a month per treatment room and, $1,000 to $3,000 a month per manicure/pedicure station.

In 2009, the profit margins of spas varied significantly. Approximately 20 percent of spas reported a profit margin exceeding 20 percent, while 23 percent reported profit margins of between 10 percent and 20 percent. Unfortunately, 27 percent of day spas actually lost money in 2009. A club spa should operate with a higher profit margin than a free-standing spa, since it does not have the same expenses associated with its operation. The primary expense for a club spa would be employee compensation, which, according to ISPA, represents on average 47 percent of revenues and in 38 percent of spas, represents over 55 percent of total revenues. Accordingly, a well-operated club spa should experience profit margins ranging from 20 percent to 30 percent of revenues.

Marketing the Club Spa

The marketing efforts of a club spa depend, in large part, on the audience that the club is attempting to attract. Ideally, a mature club spa should pull 50 percent of its clients from the club's existing membership base and 50 percent from non-members who either reside or work within the locale of the club's primary market. This duality of markets requires a club to pursue two distinct approaches to marketing. First, it must establish a marketing approach that effectively draws members from its target market. Second, it must develop a marketing strategy that attracts non-members to the spa without impacting any sense of overall exclusivity of the club that the facility might be attempting to establish. Club operators who view the spa as a prospecting source for membership often incorporate efforts to promote the spa to non-members as part of their overall membership marketing campaign. Several successful strategies can be employed to help market club-spa services, including:

❑ Strategies Used to Market the Spa to Members:

- *New-member coupons.* When individuals first become a member, many clubs provide them with a coupon for either a complimentary spa service or a spa service at a discounted rate. Clubs that offer a discount rate should quote the discount in absolute dollars, rather than percentages. According to 2010 ISPA data, 63 percent of spas offered first-time users a discount.

- *Club displays.* Some of the best efforts to market the spa involve internal spa displays that touch the various senses, by incorporating visual, auditory, touch, and smell elements.

- *Spa demonstrations.* Clubs can program monthly or even weekly demonstrations that offer members the opportunity to experience the club's spa services on a complimentary basis. For example, the club's complimentary spa offerings could include five-minute chair massages, one nail manicure, aromatherapy, etc. According to research conducted by ISPA, receiving complimentary products and services, or add-ons to existing services is one of the top three drivers of day-spa usage.

- *Special classes.* Many clubs have found that offering special classes, such as massage classes for couples or classes in skin care, can help introduce members to the club's spa services.

- *Posters/flyers.* The use of custom-designed posters and flyers that are displayed in appropriate areas of the club can also help bring attention to the club's spa services.

- *Member spa-appreciation programs.* Generating additional business from existing clients is often as important as bringing in new clients. One means of generating repeat spa business is to leverage the loyalty of existing clients by offering member appreciation and loyalty programs. In 2010, 60 percent of spas offered special incentive programs to generate additional traffic from existing clients.

- *Member referral programs.* According to the *ISPA 2008 Global Consumer Study,* the leading global driver of spa visits was referral from a friend (45 percent of spa goers). As a result, implementing some form of a program around member/client referral would seem critical to a spa's success. According to 2010 industry data, 64 percent of spas in 2010 offered incentive programs for members and clients who referred others.

- *Special-event invitations.* Special days and holidays, such as Valentine's Day, Mother's Day, birthdays, etc., represent great opportunities for attracting members to the club's spa services. Clubs can send special invitations and gift certificates to their members during these time periods to help attract them to the spa.

- *Spa brochures.* Producing an attractive spa brochure that can be displayed in the club, as well as distributed to the membership, can be another excellent marketing tool.

- *Spa website.* Developing a website for the spa that is directly linked to the club's spa website can be helpful by providing a source of updated information on the spa's services (e.g., spa menu) and by possibly allowing on-line scheduling of appointments for the spa.

Special days and holidays, such as Valentine's Day, Mother's Day, birthdays, etc., represent great opportunities for attracting members to the club's spa services.

- *Social media sites.* With the recent advent of social media sites as marketing venues, club spas should consider creating special Facebook and YouTube pages to promote their spas services. Social media sites offer a unique and highly effective means of sharing client and member testimonials about a club's services, as well as providing a means to provide greater education about the facility's spa services.

❑ *Strategies Used to Market the Spa to Non-Members:*
- *Spa brochures.* Producing an attractive spa brochure that can be distributed to the market via direct mail and retail displays can be an excellent marketing tool.
- *Direct-mail invitations/certificates.* Targeted direct-mail invitations and gift certificates can be employed to attract non-members to the club spa.
- *Spa fairs.* Special massage events, involving local businesses or local community groups, can be conducted that can provide targeted consumers with a sampling experience of the club's spa services.
- *Special-event invitations and coupons.* Special days and holidays, such as Valentine's Day, Mother's Day, Father's Day, Christmas, birthdays, etc., represent great opportunities for attracting non-members to the club's spa services. Clubs can send special invitations and gift certificates to targeted non-member audiences during these time periods that are designed to help draw them into the spa.
- *Member-sponsor program.* Clubs can develop a sponsorship program that rewards members for inviting non-members to the club to engage in spa services. For example, each time a member brings in a nonmember, the member could be given a special discount or a credit against the normal price for spa services. According to ISPA, approximately 64 percent of spas offered referral incentive programs in 2009.
- *Club website.* Clubs can create a spa website that is linked to the club's primary website. This spa site can provide updated information on services and allow online appointment scheduling of the spa's services for non-members. If feasible, the website could also be linked to search engines for spas.
- *Social media sites.* With the recent advent of social media sites as marketing venues, club spas should consider creating special Facebook and YouTube pages to promote their spas services to the public. Social media sites offer a unique and highly effective means of for sharing client testimonials about your services, as well as providing a means to provide greater public education about your spa services.

> **Clubs can develop a sponsorship program that rewards members for inviting non-members to the club to engage in spa services.**

In addition to the aforementioned strategies concerning the most effective approaches for promoting a facility's spa services, clubs can also employ less-targeted marketing approaches, such as newspaper ads, magazine ads, and radio spots, to make non-members in the marketplace aware of the spa-related offerings in their facilities.

Club Spa Staff

According to the most recent data released by ISPA, the average day spa has 14 employees, of which 5.7 are full-time employees, 5.7 are part-time, and 2.7 are contracted providers. On average, spas spend 47 percent of their revenues on employee related expenses, with 38 percent of spas allocating over 55 percent of their revenue to employee related costs, and 16 percent allocating over 65 percent of revenues to employee related costs. The typical spa director earns between $30,000 and $75,000 annually, with 38 percent earning between $30,000 and $50,000 and 22 percent earning between $50,000 and $75,000 annually. The average spa technician earns between $20,000 and $50,000 annually (64 percent), while less than 3 percent earn over $75,000 annually.

Club operators have two basic options concerning the most effective approach for staffing their spa. They can either hire employees (full-time or part-time) to operate the spa (approximately 80 percent of workers are either full-time or part-time employees according to ISPA) or recruit independent contractors to do the job (approximately 20 percent of workers). The benefits and limitations of these two options are reflected in Figure 22-5. Once the decision has been made to utilize either employees or independent contractors, the next decision that has to be made involves the make-up of the staff and the compensation that should be accorded to each of the designated positions. The most common job roles in a club spa, the accompanying compensation ranges, and the job skill requirements for those positions are shown in Figure 22-6.

Some of the larger club spas, in addition to having a spa director, spa therapists, and estheticians, also have receptionists. For most club spas, the receptionist's responsibilities can easily be filled by other staff members during times when they are not performing treatment sessions.

Employees		Independent Contractors	
Benefit	**Downside**	**Benefit**	**Downside**
• The club has control of schedules, hours, pricing, and services. • Employees will blend with the overall club culture. • Employees will likely take more ownership in connecting the spa with the rest of the club. • Performance-based compensation can be established that supports spa and club goals.	• Added costs related to benefits • Possibly not as recognized in the community	• No payroll or payroll costs involved • Ability to use well-known business operator from the community • Costs are more directly tied to revenues generated; no downtime costs. • Potentially lower operating costs	• Less likely to have an integration of the spa with the club • The club has limited control of services and pricing. • The club has potentially less opportunity to generate revenues.

Figure 22-5. Benefits and downsides of hiring employees vs. using independent contractors in a club spa

Position	Compensation	Competency	Role
Spa director (normally in club spas with greater than four treatment rooms)	Base salary range of $18,000 to $40,000, plus commission on retail sales (two to five percent) and commission on total spa gross revenues or net revenues. Therapists are paid a commission on any treatment sessions they perform.	College degree or spa experience; either licensed massage therapist or licensed esthetician preferred.	Supervises the spa and is responsible for all aspects of the spa's operation. In smaller spas, this individual also performs treatments.
Massage therapist	Commission for services ranges from 35% to 60% of revenue generated. Range of 40% to 50% is most common. Base wage of six to eight dollars an hour during administrative times.	Licensed registered or certified by the state in massage therapy (varies by state); previous work experience.	Performs all massage treatments and also can do other body treatments, such as body scrubs, body wraps, etc., if they have undergone the appropriate training.
Spa therapist	Commission for services ranges from 35% to 60% of revenue generated. Range of 40% to 50% is most common. Base wage of six to eight dollars an hour during administrative times.	Licensed as a massage therapist or esthetician preferred. No licensing is required in most states for those individuals who conduct body wraps, scrubs, etc., if they have undergone the appropriate training.	Performs the body treatments and wet treatments, except does not do any massage or facial work; appropriate training in modalities required.
Esthetician	Commission for services ranges from 35% to 60% of revenue generated. Range of 40% to 50% is most common. Base wage of six to eight dollars an hour during administrative times.	Licensed by the state as an esthetician; previous work experience.	Performs all manicures, pedicures, and facials; can also conduct body-treatment sessions if they have undergone the appropriate training.

Figure 22-6. Club spa staff positions, compensation, and credentials (based on research conducted by ISPA)

Key Points to Consider

Club spas have been one of the fastest growing amenities in the club business, with those club operators who have spas reporting that approximately 9 percent of the club's revenue is derived from spa services. As the population continues to age (e.g., baby boomers) and the demands on an individual's time increases, a club spa that provides a refuge for personal indulgences and escapes will remain as both a valuable revenue source and an effective tool to enhance membership retention for health/fitness clubs.

23

Sports Performance Centers

Chapter Objectives

In the last decade or so, sports-performance programming and sports performance centers have become new elements in the health/fitness facility experience offering. Since sports-performance centers are such a new arena of programming for health/fitness facilities and because relatively little has been written about them, this chapter provides an overview of this niche industry, which has increasingly become an important component of the overall club industry product mix.

Introduction to Sports Performance Programming

The sports-conditioning and sports-performance industry is a relatively young industry, having its roots in the early 1990s. The industry can trace its roots to the expansive growth in youth and adult sports participation that occurred in the late 1980s and early 1990s.

Within the context of health/fitness clubs, sports-conditioning and sports-performance training involves the modalities, protocols, and programs that focus on enhancing an individual's ability to perform in athletic-related activities at a peak level, while encountering the challenges and stresses inherent in either a competitive or a recreational sports environment. Such training is also designed to serve as a mechanism for reducing the risk of injury due to sports participation. As a rule, sports conditioning and performance training provides movement modalities, protocols, and programs that are designed to enhance sport-specific attributes, such as acceleration, agility, balance, core stability, power, recovery, speed, and strength. In addition, because documented evidence shows that corporate executives and homemakers sometimes experience stresses equal to or exceeding those of competitive athletes, the value of sports-conditioning and sports-performance centers for aiding those target groups has helped lead to a further expansion of this industry segment.

As a rule, sports conditioning and performance training provides movement modalities, protocols, and programs that are designed to enhance sport-specific attributes, such as acceleration, agility, balance, core stability, power, recovery, speed, and strength.

The franchising model being employed by many of the sports-performance center operators is very similar to the model used in the health/ fitness club industry.

All factors considered, the sports-performance industry is in its infancy. As such, the industry represents a crossover of two more established industries—the health/fitness club industry and the healthcare/physical therapy industry. The influence of the health/fitness club industry is reflected in programs such as agility training, core conditioning, speed training, and strength training, which are fitness-based modalities. In addition, the use of certified personal trainers, pay-as-you-go packages, and monthly fees can also be traced back to the health/fitness club industry. Finally, the franchising model being employed by many of the sports-performance center operators is very similar to the model used in the health/fitness club industry. The healthcare industry (in particular, the physical therapy industry) has also influenced the practices of those in the athletic and sports-performance business. Because many sports-performance centers feature programs and services that are dependent upon the expertise of certain healthcare professionals, physical therapists, physical-therapy assistants, athletic trainers, chiropractors, and nutritionists also play a role in this emerging industry.

The Primary Forces Driving the Sports-Conditioning and Sports-Performance Industry

Participation in organized sports has grown significantly since the mid-90s both for youth between the ages of six and 17 and for adults, ages 35 and older. According to data provided by both American Sports Data and the Sporting Goods Manufacturing Association, competitive and recreational sports are a huge business in this country, driving over 40 billion participation days of activity annually. According to statistics from 2003, 33 percent of adults ages 35 to 54 and 30 percent of adults over the age of 55 participate in frequent fitness, sports or outdoor activity. Concurrently, approximately 41 million young people participate in frequent fitness, sports, or outdoor activity. An estimated 30 to 40 million youth participate in organized sports. The fastest growing segment of participation, having grown in excess of 200 percent the past 10 years, is the baby-boomer population (those over the age of 46), representing over 78 million people. The second fastest growth segment, growing at almost 200 percent, are echo boomers (the millennial generation, encompassing individuals between the ages of 6 and 30), representing approximately 77 million people.

Youth Sports Participation

According to the most recently available data on sports participation, approximately 75 percent of boys and 69 percent of girls between the ages of six and 17 participate in organized and team sports. Approximately 54 percent or 26 million have been actively involved in at least one organized sport activity. Figure 23-1 shows some general statistics regarding the types of organized sports in which youth, ages six to 17, currently participate. In addition to the sports listed in Figure 23-1, over two million youth under the age of 17 participate in gymnastics, while another two million participate in some form of martial arts.

Overall		Boys		Girls	
Baseball/softball	11 million	Baseball	7.0 million	Soccer	4.2 million
Basketball	10 million	Basketball	6.2 million	Softball	4.1 million
Soccer	9.6 million	Soccer	5.4 million	Basketball	3.8 million
		Football	2.9 million	Volleyball	2.0 million
				Cheerleading	1.8 million

Figure 23-1. Youth sports participation practices

Sports participation among youth has been driven, in large part, by the parents of these young people. According to a recent survey conducted by sports-participation researchers, nearly 99 percent of parents surveyed indicated that they believed that sports participation promotes physical fitness. This belief may, in part, be fueled by the mounting evidence that shows that over one-third of today's American youth are obese, and, nearly 50 percent of today's youth are overweight. Furthermore, several recently conducted studies indicate that youth-sports participation may fulfill a number of important developmental needs for youth, including:

- Sports participation is fun and provides instant gratification for the child.
- Sports participation fulfills the "affiliative" need of youth, which involves such factors as friendship, sense of belonging, and social connection.
- Sports can provide physical exercise, which can promote improved health.
- Sports can help youth with the development of self-esteem, self-confidence, and positive social values.

According to the National Association for Sport and Physical Education (NASPE), participation in organized sports and fitness activities is particularly important for middle school-aged youth (e.g., ages 10 to 14). NASPE-sponsored research shows that recreational and organized sports participation improves motor skills, physical fitness, physical and social growth, and self-esteem for middle school-aged youth. While many experts in the field of child development differ on which of these four drivers of sports participation are actually critical factors, the resulting outcomes are evident. Youth are currently far more likely to be actively engaged in at least one organized sports activity. In fact, it is the Association's position that all middle school-aged youth should, at least, have the opportunity to participate in organized sports and physical activity.

A strong indicator of youth sports-activity participation can be traced to population demographics. According to research, 33 percent of parents who enroll their youth in organized sports activities have household incomes in excess of $75,000 annually. In addition, the parents of youth engaged in organized sports are far more likely to have a college education, be a white-collar professional, and have two family members in professional careers. If the data on youth-sports participation is closely examined, a hypothesis could be made that youth-sports participation is partially a result of an affluent, competitive, and results-driven adult population that seeks to provide its children with experiences that simulate the competitive and results-driven world of which they are a part. Another indication of the growth in sports participation is reflected in data recently released by the National Federation of State High School Associations that show enormous increases in the number of students actively engaged in high school sports. It is interesting to note that Texas has over 740,000 students involved in organized school sponsored sports, which is 70,000 more than California, the second most active state, and over twice as many as New York—the third most active state for high school sport participation.

The burgeoning youth sports-participation market is not the only driver in the growth of sports performance based training programs and centers. Parents also see sports-performance conditioning as a way to provide their children with a competitive edge, as well as a means of increasing the chances that their children will receive a college scholarship and even have professional sports careers.

Colleges and universities have also contributed to the growth of specialized athletic and sports conditioning. Most colleges and even some high schools currently employ certified sports conditioning specialists (e.g., individuals certified by the National Strength and Conditioning Association). As this practice has evolved at the college and university level, it has created an ever-increasing demand at the high school and junior high school level for similar programs. This push has subsequently manifested itself in individuals as young as six years of age. Many coaches and parents believe that specialized training that focuses on improving agility, balance, quickness, speed, and strength can help youth perform better, which in turn, will have a positive impact on age-group recognition, and the possibility of receiving a college scholarship and/or having a professional sports career. The desire to have youth excel at their given sport activity at earlier and earlier ages is a significant and important driver of the demand for sports-conditioning and performance programs.

Preventing Sports-Related Injuries in Youth

> Fifty-five percent of all school injuries are related to sports participation, of which 62 percent occur during practice.

Approximately 3.5 million children under the age of 18 receive medical treatment each year for sports-related injuries. Most of these injuries are attributed to collisions, falls, and overexertion. Overuse injuries account for nearly 50 percent of all sports injuries at the middle and high-school level (ages 11 to 18). Interestingly, 55 percent of all school injuries are related to sports participation, of which 62 percent occur during practice. The majority of these injuries are typically treated in sports-medicine clinics, rather than in hospitals.

Football generates the greatest number of sports injuries among youth. As can be seen in Figure 23-2, however, football is by no means the only sport that results in significant levels of injury to American youth. When the date is broken down further, youth between the ages of six and 14 account for 40 percent of all hospital-reported sports injuries. From the ages of six to nine, girls are the most frequently injured, while boys between the ages of 10 and 14 are most often injured and most seriously injured.

Sport	% of Participants Injured
Football	28%
Basketball	15%
Soccer	22%
Baseball	25%
Softball	12%

Figure 23-2. Youth sports with the highest incidence of sports injuries

The Role of Sports-Conditioning Programs for Youth

According to a policy sheet written by the American Academy of Pediatrics (AAP), youth-sports injuries can be reduced when several important steps are taken, including:
- Matching the skills of the child to the demands of the particular sport
- Providing proper physical conditioning for the child before they participate
- Grouping children by skill level
- Ensuring that youth receive a physical exam before participating

Sports-conditioning and performance centers can play a critical role with two of the AAP recommendations. First, these centers can be involved in matching the specific demand of a sport to the skills and maturation level of the child. Second, these centers can provide the proper conditioning programs for reducing the likelihood of injury due to inadequate physical preparation.

In addition to being able to play a role in injury prevention, sports-performance programs and centers can play an important role in helping a child recover from a sports injury and helping prepare them for a safe reintroduction to their sport. Finally, sports-performance programs and centers can play an important role in building the basic components of fitness that allow for enhanced sports performance. By employing scientifically based steps for safely developing such athletic-related attributes as agility, speed, strength, and core stability, these programs can assist young people in reaching new performance heights in a relatively risk-free and time-efficient manner.

It is important to note that according to data in the publication, the *IHRSA 2010 Profiles of Success*, approximately 10 percent of health/fitness club memberships are held by youth under the age of 18. Accordingly, sports-performance centers are fulfilling a market niche that other health/fitness programs have generally been unable to capitalize on to this point.

Adult Sports Participation

As discussed previously in this chapter, participation in fitness and sports activities has increased dramatically among two groups of adults in particular—those between the ages of 35 and 54 and those over the age of 55. The largest increase in participation has been in fitness-related activities, such as resistance training, walking, group-exercise classes, etc, followed by increased participation in recreational sports, such as tennis, basketball, dancing, trekking, bicycling, etc. Researchers believe that several significant factors have contributed to this growth in fitness and sports participation, including the desire for older adults to feel and look younger, the desire of individuals to prevent major illness as they age, the desire of people to enjoy activities that they enjoyed when they were young adults, and the desire of individuals to remain active throughout their life.

Unfortunately, as many of these adults begin participating in fitness and sports activities for the first time in years, they experience a higher incidence of discomfort and injury. According to the research, baby boomers generate a more significant number of sports injuries than any other segment of the population. From 1991 to 1998, sports injuries among baby boomers increased by over 33 percent. Even more alarmingly, for adults over the age of 65, the number of sports injuries during this time period increased by 54 percent. The majority of the sports injuries in these adult populations can be attributed to such factors as muscle imbalances, a lack of flexibility, problems with balance and agility, core strength weakness, and improper preparation for the targeted sport activity.

The Role of Sports-Conditioning Programs for Adults

Based on the data reviewed in the previous section, sports-conditioning programs can fulfill several important roles for the adult population, particularly for baby boomers.

- Because adults should have access to a trained professional who understands the physical limitations of aging and the demands placed on the musculoskeletal system, as people age, physical therapists and certified-fitness specialists in this arena may be the most qualified individuals to fulfill this responsibility.

- Programs that focus on agility, balance, and core strength are critical to allowing older adults to safely and enjoyably participate in fitness and sports. These are factors in which most sports-conditioning programs specialize.

- Reducing the risk of injury and providing services that assist in the road to recovery from injury are important to active older adults. These are roles that sports-conditioning programs can play.

- For the older adult whose desire it is to continue engaging in competitive sports and activities, the conditioning expertise provided by sports-conditioning programs can be critical.

Overview of the Sports Conditioning Industry

In existence since the early 1990s, the sports-conditioning industry is currently evolving from an entrepreneurial industry, led by independent single-business operators and single-franchise operators, to a maturing industry, led by franchise organizations. The two dominant players in this particular market are

Programs that focus on agility, balance, and core strength are critical to allowing older adults to safely and enjoyably participate in fitness and sports.

Velocity Sports, based in Georgia, and Athletic Republic (e.g., formerly Frappier Acceleration Training), based out of North Dakota. Velocity currently has over 50 franchised locations in the United States, while Athletic Republic has franchised its program to over 160 locations in the United States, making it the leading sports-performance center franchise in the world. In addition to these two market-leaders, several other franchise business models have arisen in the past five years, including Centers for Athletic Performance (CAP), High Impact Training (HIT), Competitive Athlete Training Zone (CATZ), and Parisi Speed School. The Parisi Speed School, which has emerged as a major player in the market by focusing its efforts on the health/fitness facility industry, currently has over 65 club-based programs in operation around the United States, making it the second largest sports-performance center franchise in the U.S.

A Profile of the Market for Sports-Conditioning Programs in Health/Fitness Club Facilities

The primary market for sports-conditioning programs in the health/fitness club industry can be described as follows:

- Middle-school age boys and girls (e.g., 10 to 14 years old). This group may comprise as much as 50 percent of the total audience in many markets.
- High school-age boys and girls (e.g., 15 to 18 years old). This group may comprise approximately 20 percent of the audience.
- Youth-age boys and girls (e.g., 6 to 10 years old). This group comprises approximately 10 percent to 15 percent of the audience in most markets.
- College and professional athletes (e.g., 18 and older individuals who participate in high-level amateur or professional competition). This group might comprise as much as 5 percent to 10 percent of the audience, depending on the specific market that exists in a particular area.
- Recreational adult athletes (e.g., individuals over the age of 18 who engage in athletic endeavors that are recreational in nature). Depending on the specific market, this audience might range from 5 percent to 15 percent of the total.

The top predictor of sports-performance center success is based on the estimated number of student athletes (e.g., athletes in middle-school and high-school sports) who reside within a 20-minute driving distance of the site location. Sports-participation statistics indicate that approximately 55 percent of high school students and an estimated 30 percent of all middle-school students participate in some form of sport activity. According to antidotal research from the leading franchise operators, one meaningful benchmark for success is based on having an eligible student-athlete population of at least 1,500, and preferably 4,000, within the desired market area. Based on this antidotal data, the ideal market should have a student population of 12,000. Some unpublished research indicates that sports-performance centers are found to attract between 3 percent and 5 percent of the eligible youth population between the ages of 10 and 18, who reside in households earning over $75,000 annually.

> The top predictor of sports-performance center success is based on the estimated number of student athletes (e.g., athletes in middle-school and high-school sports) who reside within a 20-minute driving distance of the site location.

A second important predictor of success in the sports-performance center segment of the industry is based on the average household income of the targeted demographic area, especially those served by the identified schools. Households with an average income in excess of $75,000 are the most attractive market, since one-in-three of these households will have youth involved in sports participation.

Sports-Performance Center Metrics

In general, the sports-performance industry does not publish benchmark metric data. The data that is available is based on a survey of a small sample of successful operators. As a result, the metrics presented in this section may not be statistically valid, but are reflective of what the top operators in the business produce.

> The majority of sports-performance centers offer training packages ranging in duration from 12 sessions to 26 sessions, with packages of 20 sessions being the most popular.

Sports-performance centers range in size from 1,500 square feet to over 20,000 square feet, with the majority ranging in size from 3,000 to 5,000 square feet. A typical center tends to have between 20 and 90 clients a month, with the months of May, June, July, and August being the busiest. Unpublished research indicates that between 50 percent and 60 percent of client traffic in these centers is attributed to these four months of the year. On an annual basis, the average center sees about 500 clients over the course of the year. Client traffic is generated through a blend of private- and small-group training (e.g., less than six clients) and larger-group sessions (e.g., 12 to 20 clients). The majority of sports-performance centers offer training packages ranging in duration from 12 sessions to 26 sessions, with packages of 20 sessions being the most popular. A typical training package of 20 sessions costs between $400 and $1,000 dollars, with an average package price of approximately $700. Furthermore, the average annual revenue per client is just over $600, and the average revenue per client visit is slightly over $25. As such, from a health/fitness club industry perspective, the revenue generation capability of sports-performance centers is in the neighborhood of $100 per square foot per year.

The Essential Components of a Sports-Performance Center

❑ *Facility.* As previously discussed in this chapter, the average free-standing sports-performance center ranges in size from 3,000 to 5,000 square feet. Centers located within an existing club environment might range from as small as 800 square feet to as large as 5,000 square feet. The typical free-standing facility could include one or more the following components:
  • Indoor running track (20 to 60 yards)
  • Sport court
  • Indoor sport-turf surface
  • Open space for functional equipment (e.g., ladders, cones, hurdles, medicine balls, running cords, etc.)
  • Treadmills (e.g., super treadmills that go as fast as 25 miles per hour)
  • Resistance equipment (both circuit and free-weight oriented)
  • Custom plyometric equipment

- Locker rooms
- Classroom for video tapin g and viewing

❑ *Equipment.* Most, if not all, of the existing sports-performance centers utilize the following equipment and accessories:
- Plyometric benches and boxes
- Hurdles
- Ladders
- Cones
- Bands, tubes, and cords
- Chutes and sleds
- Weighted vests
- Super treadmills
- Resistance equipment (e.g., free weights, functional plate-loaded, and selectorized)
- Medicine balls and exercise balls
- Foam rollers
- Kettlebells
- Customized floor surfaces (e.g., rubber track, indoor turf, etc.)

❑ *Conditioning Concept.* The majority of sports-performance programs focus on a blend of training modalities that concentrate on the development of acceleration, high-end speed, agility, core stability, power, movement mechanics, and neuromuscular coordination. Among the techniques featured in these efforts are active stretching, plyometric training, hyper-speed training, power training with resistance and body weight, balance training, and cord training.

❑ *Program Packages Built Around Either a Specific Sports Theme or a Particular Age Group-Oriented Need.* In this regard, age-group programs are normally offered for youth 6 to 11, 12 to 18, and adults. The most commonly themed programs are targeted at speed development, jumping development, or sports-specific attributed geared toward a particular activity, such as football, basketball, baseball, soccer, volleyball, hockey, etc. The most successful performance programs appear to be driven by a focus on acceleration, speed, and power production. Among sports, football tends to represent the largest audience, although the most involved athletic endeavor can vary by market.

The most successful performance programs appear to be driven by a focus on acceleration, speed, and power production.

❑ *Packages Bundled by the Number of Sessions Offered.* Typical package durations range from 12 sessions to 26 sessions. Many of the national sports-performance programs offer guaranteed performance-improvement results, if a certain number of sessions are attended.

❑ *Small-Group Personal Coaching Sessions.* A majority of the sports-performance programs feature scheduled sessions that involve groups, ranging from two to a dozen athletes. Although numerous programs offer customized personal-performance training, it is not the primary business driver. Most scheduled sessions last between 60 to 90 minutes.

❏ *Team Field Programs.* Many of the leading national programs offer structured conditioning programs for teams (e.g., youth teams, middle-school teams, high-school teams, etc.). These programs are made available in a variety of formats, ranging from one day to several weeks. As a rule, most of these programs are conducted at a team's location.

❏ *Sports-Performance Camps and Academies.* During certain times of the year, many sports-performance centers offer specialized camps (e.g., one day to two weeks) that are targeted at a specific sport or skill (e.g., basketball, soccer, jump, speed, etc.).

❏ *Certified Trainers.* The franchised programs require staff to go through both on-line, video, classroom, and hands-on training before delivering their programs. In most cases, the programs have a prerequisite that the trainer must have an undergraduate degree in exercise science, athletic training, or physical therapy. In addition, many programs employ staff who have a master degree. Among the numerous health/fitness industry certifying organizations, NSCA and NASM certifications appear to be the most frequently seen in the sports-conditioning arena.

❏ *Software-Based Monitoring.* It has become a standard operating practice for the programs to use software to design and monitor the programs for the athletes.

Marketing Sports-Performance Centers

Marketing, especially grass-roots marketing, is critical to the development and operation of a successful sports-conditioning and performance center. As previously discussed in this chapter, the primary audiences for such services are youth at the middle-school and high-school level. As a result, club operators must develop an effective marketing strategy that enables it to attract these young athletes. Among the strategies that have proven successful in reaching this particular target audience are the following:

- Advertisements in local papers and magazines
- Contacting the local schools and talking with the coaches
- Conducting in-service training clinics for coaches
- Conducting workshops and seminars for parent groups
- Conducting testing and one-day trial programs for the local middle-school and high-school coaches
- Contacting and working with the local youth-sport leagues. Getting involved with the coaches and parents groups associated with these programs.
- Getting involved with the local booster and sport-league associations
- Sponsoring sports teams in the community
- Aligning with local college or professional athletes/teams. Getting a local professional and/or college team/athlete to be a spokesperson for the center.
- Interactive websites and social media pages.

> Marketing, especially grass-roots marketing, is critical to the development and operation of a successful sports-conditioning and performance center.

- Contacting local physician groups and physical-therapy groups that see kids with sports-related injuries
- Direct mail or email blasts to local youth-sports team organizers, parent groups, and coaches. Most direct mail is followed by phone calls and visits.

An Overview of Six Leading Sports-Performance Operations

❑ *Athletic Republic.* Athletic Republic, formerly Frappier Acceleration, was founded in 1990 by John Frappier, an exercise physiologist and established expert in the area of training athletes. The Athletic Republic business model was developed around specialized exercises, exercise protocols, and equipment which have benefits that have been documented through research to have a positive impact on sports performance. Rather than creating a franchise business model, Frappier initially established a licensing model that allowed local entrepreneurs to purchase a license for his program and then incorporate it into a business model, which they could adapt to their local market. In 2006, the company went to a franchise model and, a year later, changed its name to Athletic Republic. Over the past 15 years, over 100,000 athletes at 165 Athletic Republic licensed facilities have completed at least one level of the program. The Athletic Republic model consists of the following elements:

- Eight trademarked pieces of training equipment (e.g., treadmill, plyometric leg press, etc.) to support the program modules
- Multiple-stage acceleration program modules that are designed to accommodate mechanics, neuromuscular coordination, anaerobic and aerobic conditioning, muscle physiology, and posture. Modules are available in individual and group formats.
- Facility spaces ranging from 2,500 square feet to 7,500 square feet
- Custom software program for athlete testing and monitoring
- Video-analysis system using custom software
- The primary target audience is middle school-age student athletes.
- Sessions are conducted in either a private or group format, with groups ranging from two to eight athletes.
- Single-session pricing varies from $25 to $40.
- Packaged programs vary in length from eight sessions to 25 sessions.
- Specialized training and certified staff who deliver the programs

❑ *Parisi Speed School.* The Parisi Speed School was initially developed in 1993 with a free-standing sports-performance and personal-training center (initially operated with a Frappier license). Parisi opened a second center in 1998. By 2005, Parisi had a total of four locations. In 2005, Parisi went forward with the development of a franchise model that allowed health/fitness facilities to franchise a Parisi Speed School. As of 2011, a total of 65 Parisi franchise locations were either open or committed to opening. Parisi is most noted for its work in preparing athletes for the annual NFL combine. The Parisi business model consists of the following elements:

Parisi is most noted for its work in preparing athletes for the annual NFL combine.

- Three custom-program levels that are designed for three distinct athlete groups (Fast, Fit, and Fun for 7 to 11 year olds, Total Performance for 12 to 18 year olds, and Reach Peak for elite athletes over the age of 18).
- Speed camps
- NFL combine program
- Team training newsletter and program
- Video store, with tapes for training various level athletes
- A space of at least 2,500 square feet
- Utilizes existing ground-based equipment and has affiliations with vendors for functional equipment and treadmills.

❑ *Velocity Sports Performance.* Velocity Sports was founded in 1999 by Loren Seagrave, an internationally recognized track and field coach who specialized in training student-athletes. After opening his first center in Atlanta, Seagrave saw the potential of bringing his new model of performance training to other markets and retained specialists in franchising to assist him. Over the last 12 years, Velocity has grown to approximately 50 franchises in 29 states. The Velocity business model consists of the following elements:

- 8,500 to 15,000 square feet of total pace (some facilities are as large as 30,000 square feet)
- 7,500 to 12,000 square feet dedicated to sports conditioning
- Indoor turf field, indoor basketball court/sport court, 60-meter track, weight room, and lockers
- Basic conditioning accessories (e.g., bands, cones, ladders, plyometric benches, etc.)
- Structured programs for different levels of athletes, both individual and group
- A primary target audience of 12 to 16 year old student athletes (e.g., encompassing approximately 60 percent of its market share)
- Packaged programs of 12, 18, and 24 sessions, with each session lasting 90 minutes
- Sessions conducted in a group format, with the number of athletes per class ranging from 2 to 10
- An average session cost of $25 to $35. The packaged programs range from $444 for a 12-week package to $1,275 for 75 sessions. Franchises may differ in their pricing.

❑ *High-Intensity Training Centers (HIT).* HIT was founded in 2003 by Terry Shepherd, Ph.D., after 20 years as an exercise physiologist and university professor. The first HIT center was opened in Huntington, West Virginia. In late 2003, Dr. Shepherd brought on business partners to create a franchise business model for HIT. The headquarters for HIT were then relocated to Dublin, Ohio. The HIT business platform is built around an integrated-performance model consisting of the following elements:

- Speed-up—a sports-enhancement program for athletes of all ages
- Lighten-up—a weight-loss program

The HIT business platform is built around an integrated-performance model.

- Hit Fit—a generalized fitness program for recreational athletes
- EYEMETRIX—a visual-training program

❑ *Competitive Athlete Training Zone (CATZ).* CATZ first opened in 1996, with its first training center located in Pasadena, California. The CATZ program was developed by certified conditioning specialists and physical therapists. It utilizes existing equipment to create specialized training protocols that are designed to help improve the agility, speed, and power of athletes. The CATZ program consists of distinct workout protocols built around specific sports and are targeted at youth from the ages of 8 to 18. The CATZ philosophy focuses on developing athleticism, training movement not muscle, training sports-specific movements, and creating movements that simulate the chaos of sports. The CATZ business model is similar to Velocity and HIT. CATZ currently has eight sites throughout the U.S.

❑ *Centers for Athletic Performance (CAP).* CAP is a relatively new entrant into the athletic- and sports-training industry. CAP has developed proprietary programs that focus on developing speed and agility through strength training and functional sports-performance training, based on the principles involved in explosive strength training. Its program offering consists of modules for strength, speed and power/explosiveness, and mobility. These program modules are available in either individual or group formats and are packaged for various interests and skill levels of sports enthusiasts and athletes.

OVERVIEW OF THE INTERNATIONAL HEALTH/FITNESS CLUB MARKET

Body Tech, Columbia

Part Eight

24

Overview of the International Health/ Fitness Club Market

Chapter Objectives

Understanding the dynamics of the international market can help facilitate a greater understanding of the competencies involved in managing and leading a successful health/fitness club business. As of 2010, the global health/fitness industry was a $70 billion industry, serving nearly 120 million members in over 128,000 different clubs. Compared to the turn of the 21st century when the U.S. market was the dominant force in the industry, currently, the U.S. represents less than 25 percent of clubs and 30 percent of industry revenue in the world. Looking at the world market for fitness, it can be said that the top five markets account for approximately 52 percent of the total number of health/ fitness facilities (U.S., Brazil, Italy, South Korea, and Canada) and 57 percent of the global industry revenue (U.S., United Kingdom, Spain, Italy, and Japan). This chapter presents a basic overview of the international health/fitness club market that includes not only a brief history of the international health/fitness club industry, but also a discussion of the current dynamics of the market. Chapters 25, 26, and 27 delve into the Asian, European, and Latin American markets in greater detail.

Historical Perspective

❏ *The Early Years*. Similar to the domestic U.S. market, private clubs (particularly athletic-oriented clubs) evolved in the international arena in the 1800s. One of the earliest health/fitness clubs to open in Europe was Turnverein, opened in 1811, which was operated by Frederick Jahn. In 1848, Hippolyte Triat inaugurated Gymnase Triat in Paris, France, which was a club dedicated to men in pursuit of physical culture. In addition to these two landmark clubs, the Lille Athletic Club, Lille, France, was started in 1885 by Edmond Desbonnet; the Vienna Athletic Club, Vienna, Austria, commenced operations in the 1880s; the Athletic and Cycling Club of Saint Petersburg, Russia was opened in the 1880s; the London YMCA, England, opened for

As of 2010, the global health/fitness industry was a $70 billion industry, serving nearly 120 million members in over 128,000 different clubs.

Bill Pearl Enterprises

The Lille Athletic Club in Lille, France, founded by Edmond Desbonnet in 1885

business in the 1880s; and Louis Durlacher, also known as Professor Atilla, started his famous gym in Belgium also in the 1880s. These early clubs were predominately oriented toward men and provided a physical-activity environment that was based on gymnastics, sport, and martial arts (e.g., boxing, wrestling, etc.). In addition, these clubs introduced the world to organized group exercise, along with the use of barbells and dumbbells.

The earliest United Kingdom clubs were organized around social relationships and athletic endeavors, such as court tennis, cricket, squash, snooker, and lawn tennis. One of the first facilities in this regard was the All-England Lawn Tennis and Croquet Club, which was founded in 1868 and began operations in 1877, just outside London. The Fitzwilliam Lawn Tennis Club in Dublin, Ireland, which was founded in 1877, lays claim to actually operating as a club before the aforementioned All-England Club. In the late 1880s, the London YMCA began operations. It was one of the first clubs in England to offer exercise classes and a fully-equipped gymnasium. These facilities were representative of the earliest form of recreational sports-driven clubs (e.g., multi-purpose sports clubs) that subsequently were developed in the United Kingdom. With a strong social component, these facilities provided men with the opportunity to engage in physical activity. The programming focus in these clubs tended to involve either physical-culture activities (e.g., physique improvement, combat sports, and acrobatics) or court sports (e.g., court tennis, squash, tennis, etc.). As such, these early European efforts led to the development of America's first social/athletic clubs, such as the Olympic Club in San Francisco, California and the New York Athletic Club in New York, New York. Subsequently, the concept of social/athletic was also exported to Asia by expatriates, thus creating this type of club in Hong Kong and other major Asian markets.

❑ *The Modern Era.* The birth of the modern era of the international health/ fitness club industry occurred in Europe about twenty years after Vic Tanny introduced America to the modern health club. (Note: The modern era is defined as the period during which health/fitness clubs became part of the culture and opened their doors to the general public to provide a means of improving physical health.) One important delineating factor of the modern era with regard to the global market was the formation of companies dedicated to operating multiple clubs to serve the fitness and sports needs of the marketplace. In 1967, Keiser Training became the first German company to emerge as a multiple-site operator. About this same time period, health/fitness clubs also began to take root in Japan and somewhat later in other Asian countries. In fact, several organized health/ fitness club operations were established throughout Asia during the 60s and 70s. Clark Hatch International opened its first club in Tokyo in 1965, and over the next few decades, would go on to operate over 100 clubs throughout Asia. Central Sports, which opened in 1969 and The People Company, which started in 1973, have since become two of the largest club companies in the world. However, it wasn't until the late 1970s and early 1980s that health/fitness clubs became a significant business venture in the international arena. It is interesting to note that this scenario coincided closely with the consequential changes that were occurring in the United States marketplace.

In the early 1980s, club groups, such as Archer Leisure, Vardon Leisure, David Lloyd Leisure in the United Kingdom, and DIC in Japan, entered the market, followed a few years later by health/fitness industry groups, such as G&P Gockel in Germany, Health and Racquet in South Africa, and Living Well in the United Kingdom. During the same period, the health/fitness club industry also began to take off in a number of other segments of the international market, including Spain, Sweden, Norway, Italy, and the Netherlands. The 1980s also ushered in the beginning of large-scale operators, which in turn drove the international industry.

The real renaissance of the health/ fitness club industry internationally occurred in the 1990s.

The real renaissance of the health/fitness club industry internationally occurred in the 1990s. The international health/fitness club market exploded during this decade, with England, Germany, France, South Africa, and Japan experiencing the most significant growth. Figure 24-1 illustrates the enormous growth that occurred in the various international markets over the past decade.

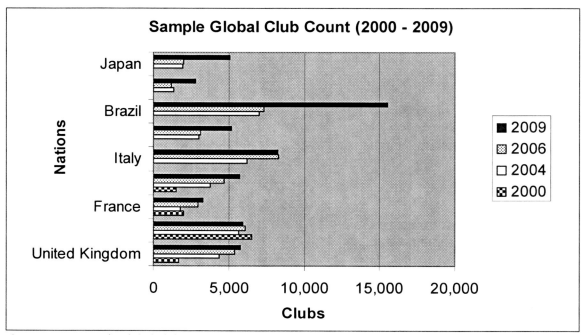

Figure 24-1. Sample global club count (2000-2009)

In the 1990s, the United Kingdom was the center of attention in the international health/fitness club market because of the explosion of quality facility operations in England, such as David Lloyd Leisure, Esporta, Holmes Place, Cannons, Dragons, and LA Fitness. These various operations featured business models that took British consumers by storm and created an incredible buzz in the financial markets. David Lloyd Leisure was sold to Whitbread for approximately $350 million dollars, which, at the time, involved a high multiple of earnings and became the benchmark that the financial markets in England employed to judge the other up-and-coming health/fitness club operations. Besides David Lloyd, companies, such as Cannons, Holmes Place, Esporta, and Fitness First, also went public in the late 1990s and were very well received by Britain's financial markets.

During the later half of the 1990,s several of these businesses traded at 30 to 40 times earnings, far in excess of the four to eight times earnings multiples that were the norm in the United States. One of the most unique factors about the British market, other than the incredible multiples on earnings, was the fact that they did not experience the price wars and discounting practices that had plagued the United States (in 2010, however this situation was not the case). During this period, the market in the United Kingdom focused on establishing quality benchmarks and avoiding the price markdowns and strong sales tactics that the U.S. industry experienced during its early years. In addition, British clubs were able to work closely with England's national health insurance group to create several important synergies for the market.

During this period, British clubs could be grouped into three basic categories, based on price and amenities. Clubs, such as Fitness First and LA Fitness, were what would be termed in the U.S. domestic market as affordable and convenient fitness-only facilities. Focused primarily on fitness-related activities, this group of facilities operated smaller, well-outfitted ventures that were both convenient and affordable to the masses, particularly to single individuals. In contrast, a number of British health/fitness operations, such as Esporta, were structured on a larger multipurpose-club model, one that targeted families, and provided slightly more amenities and services at a higher price. In the United States, such a facility would be called a mid-price level, family-fitness club. The third type of facility focused on the high end of the market. This group featured full-service, multipurpose clubs that offered both great programming and exceptional service. These high-end operations emphasized an appropriate blend of fitness, recreation, and social interaction (e.g., David Lloyd Leisure, Cannons, Holmes Place).

During the 1990s, the health/fitness club industry also began to thrive in other European countries, such as Germany, Italy, Belgium, France, Sweden, and South Africa. For example, a French company, Compagnie Gymnase, grew to 116 clubs by the mid-to-late 1990s. A significant portion of Compagnie Gymnase's clubs were subsequently sold to Club Med, which, in turn, branded them as Club Med Gyms. A chain in South Africa, Health and Racquet, reached over 60 clubs by the mid-to-late 1990s. Eventually, this chain expanded into both Europe and Australia (under the brand name Healthlands). However, because of legal and financial problems, it had to divest of its holdings. At the present time, the former Health and Racquet clubs in South Africa and Europe are operated by Virgin Active, which had created its own unique brand of health/fitness clubs during this same period.

In markets such as Germany, Italy, Spain, and Sweden, several smaller multiple-club companies opened their doors and brought a number of innovative (for their respective areas) programming emphases to their respective markets. For example, Keiser training opened small clubs in Germany that focused entirely on delivering a resistance-training environment. 24 Hour Fitness made its presence in the international market by purchasing several facilities in the Scandinavian region (e.g., Denmark, Norway, and Sweden). At one point, 24 Hour Fitness had approximately 70 clubs in the Scandinavian region. Subsequently, these clubs were sold to Nordic Capital and became a part of the SATS club group, a publicly held company of over 100 clubs.

During the late 1990s, Fitness First, based in London, seized a dominant position in the Australian market, by purchasing the clubs that were formerly operated by Health and Racquet of South Africa (e.g., Heathlands). Starting with approximately 15 clubs, Fitness First has grown its Australian club's holdings to over 70 strong, and currently represents one of its most profitable markets. Before Fitness First entered the Australian market, most of the health/fitness clubs down under were either small independent operators with less than 10 clubs or community swimming centers that were operated by the local government bodies. In an attempt to emulate Fitness First's success in Australia, a second major player in the industry, Fernwood, a women's-only chain, emerged in Australia. During the early part of the 21st century, a third major player emerged in the Australian market—Zest.

> During the 1990s, the health/fitness club industry also began to thrive in other European countries, such as Germany, Italy, Belgium, France, Sweden, and South Africa.

Since the 1990s, Japan has strengthened its dominant position as a commanding factor in the international health/fitness club industry. At the present time, three companies—DIC, Central Sports, and Konami (formerly, the clubs operated by the People Company)—operate close to 25 percent of the health/fitness facilities in the Japanese marketplace and generate close to 40 percent of the total revenue produced by clubs in the market. These Japanese operations feature facilities that provide exceptional fitness, group-exercise, and swimming programming. Swimming is an extremely popular activity in Japanese clubs, as is group exercise.

> During the 1990s, the Asian market (exclusive of Japan) was primarily driven by small fitness centers that were located in hotels and residential developments.

During the 1990s, the Asian market (exclusive of Japan) was primarily driven by small fitness centers that were located in hotels and residential developments. One of the first individuals to recognize the opportunities that existed in Asia was Clark Hatch, who has since opened over 100 clubs in markets such as Singapore, Hong Kong, Malaysia, Thailand, and the Philippines, most of which, if not all, are associated with hotel properties. During the later half of the 1990s, some U.S. entrepreneurs also decided to enter the larger Asian markets. For example, California Fitness, founded by Ray Wilson, became one of the first health/fitness club chains to enter Hong Kong. In fact, its first facility reached over 12,000 members in its first year of operation. Another organization that established a presence in Asia was 24 Hour Fitness, which created a subsidiary that operated those aforementioned California Fitness clubs. In addition to 24 Hour Fitness, Fitness First, based in London, and Gold's Gym and Bally's from the U.S. have made significant inroads into the emerging Asian market. Currently, the prevailing approach to the Asian market seems to be franchising, a philosophy espoused by Fitness First, which is making a strategic move into the Asian markets. In India, the largest operator is a locally based company.

Similar to Europe and Asia, South America also witnessed the emergence of the health/fitness club market in the 1980s, with the opening of Companhia Athletica and Runner/SA—both in Brazil. Currently, these are two of the leading operators in the Brazilian market. Since 2001, IHRSA has been involved as a cosponsor of Fitness Brazil, one of the largest global conferences for health/fitness club owners and operators—a true sign that the South American market has achieved noteworthy status.

By 2010, the international markets represent approximately 64 percent of the total membership base, 64 percent of the total membership base and approximately 77 percent of the gross revenues in the global health/fitness club industry. In other words, what was once considered primarily a North American industry, has developed into an international industry, one in which North America—particularly the United States—is just another player in a global marketplace. Figure 24-2 presents a quantitative overview of the international industry from a revenue perspective, showing the changes in revenue from 2006 to 2009.

❑ *The Future.* In 2006, IHRSA reported that, with regard to the global marketplace, one of the goals of the health/fitness industry was to reach 120 million club members by the year 2010, with 50 million in the United States and 70 million in the various international markets. As of 2010,

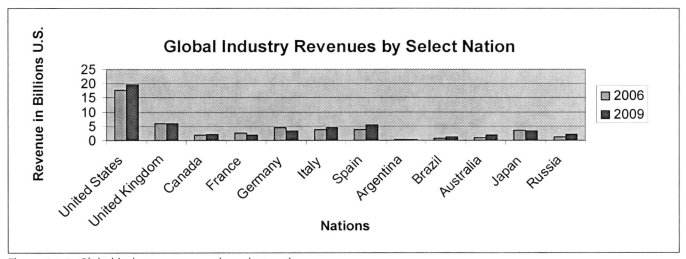

Figure 24-2. Global industry revenues by select nation

health/fitness clubs worldwide had an estimated 120 million members, with approximately 45 million in the United States and 75 million internationally. What once seemed a lofty goal for the global health/fitness club industry has now been achieved, and, in the case of the international market (i.e., non-U.S.), has been exceeded. In fact, the real number could easily reach 130 to 140 million by 2015.

The future of the international health/fitness club industry appears to be as promising as its past. In that regard, the following trends should have a substantial impact on the growth of the international marketplace over the next decade:

❑ *Club Consolidation and Strategic Acquisitions.* The health/fitness club industry in the United Kingdom and mainland Europe has stagnated over the past three to four years, with the total number of clubs in the U.K., Italy, Germany, Sweden, etc. remaining relatively flat. This situation is due in part to the global economic downturn of 2008 and 2009, as well as the consolidation that has occurred in many markets (e.g., England, Germany, Netherlands, etc.). The rapid expansion in the European industry that occurred in an earlier part of this century caused many clubs to reach a point where further growth in their home markets was a challenge, and expansion outside their local markets would lead to in further challenges to the profitability of the overall organization. As a result, several European based companies, such as Fitness First, retrenched in their core markets (U.K. and Germany) and sold off assets in less-profitable markets (e.g., Spain, France, Italy), while others actively pursued consolidation in strategic markets. Virgin Active in the U.K. has recently acquired both Holmes Place and Esporta in the U.K, resulting in it more than doubling its base of clubs. Health City, based in the Netherlands, recently acquired over 100 Fitness First clubs in several European markets (France, Italy, and Spain). Fitness First, while selling off assets in countries, such as France and Italy, has pursued further acquisitions and consolidation in Germany, where it is attempting to acquire some of Germany's top regional players. As of 2011, each of these companies has become firmly established as the "top dogs" in Europe, based on the number of clubs that it operates.

❑ *Development of New Business Models.* In the last five years, a new business model has taken Europe by storm, and currently seems to be taking hold in other nations across the globe. The key element of this new business model is the development of "budget" clubs. Budget clubs are differentiated from other club business models by the following attributes: low price that is typically half of the average market price, pure gym models (no pools, no group-exercise studios, no saunas, etc.), limited-to-no staffing, limited-to-no amenities (no towels, pay for showers, etc.), 24-hour access most, if not all, days of the week, and a heavy reliance on technology for servicing the customer (e.g., use of technology for everything from signing up people for membership to providing exercise prescriptions). Two of the leading players in this new business segment are McFit, based in Germany, and the Gym Group, based in the United Kingdom. McFit currently operates over 140 clubs in Germany, with plans in place to open clubs in Spain and other mainland European countries. The Gym Group, which manages over a half dozen clubs in England, has plans to rapidly expand throughout the U.K. The budget-club market has recently taken hold in Australia, and over the next few years, will become a prominent business model in all regions of the globe.

❑ *Emerging Franchise Models.* Franchising has become one of the newest trends in the global fitness market. Curves started the international love affair with franchise models, and over the past few years, several other firms have leaped on the opportunity. Anytime Fitness, a fitness-only club model based out of the U.S. with over 1,300 franchises globally, has made significant inroads into Asia, South America, and Europe. Viva Fit, a women's-only group, based out of Portugal, currently operates well over 100 franchises in Portugal and Spain, but has recently signed on to open franchises in both Asia and the Middle East. Fitness First, based out of the U.K., is an organization that typically owns and operates its clubs. On the other hand, it has developed franchise agreements for Asia (e.g., India, China, etc.) and the Middle East. Mrs. Sporty, a German-based women's-only chain, has over 300 franchise locations in Germany.

Franchising has become one of the newest trends in the global fitness market.

❑ *An Emerging Global Middle Class; Market Penetration Opportunities.* At the present time, the international market, as a whole, only penetrates approximately three percent of the eligible world population. While the level of penetration in Western Europe is higher, ranging from around 4 percent to approximately 19 percent, the overall European average (approximately 7.5 percent to 8 percent in the E.U.) is still well below the 16 percent level that exists in the United States. In Eastern Europe and Russia, the levels of market penetration range from less than 1 percent to a high of 3 percent. In the Asian and South Pacific markets, penetration rates range from less than 1 percent to over 12 percent, with large markets, such as China, India, and Indonesia, reaching between 1 percent and 3 percent of the eligible market. These statistics reflect the fact that a huge opportunity exists to provide a product that can tap into these relatively underserved and emerging middle-class markets. One of the challenges will be creating a workable model that fits within the cultural and financial conditions attendant to each specific country. For example, in the United States, the average annual club dues—as a percentage of per capital income—are 1.9 percent and .85 to 1 percent of household income for those individuals who are club members. In contrast, in Europe, the average annual dues are just over 2 percent of the per capita income. In Eastern Europe and Asia, dues represent an even larger percentage of the average citizen's household income.

In order to make fitness more accessible in the global marketplace, two factors have to happen. First, many of these markets have to see a continued growth of a middle class, with expendable income growing. At the present time, the middle class is defined by the World Bank as earning between $10 and $20 a day (under $5,500 annually), while Goldman Sachs, in a recent report, believes it should be defined as earning between $6,000 and $30,000 a year (it should be noted that in developed nations, middle class encompasses between $17,000 and $70,000 annually and in the U.S., between $20,000 and $100,000 a year). According to various sources the global middle class will add two billion people over the next 20 years. The question becomes, what incomes must be present for the emerging middle class to afford a club membership? Second, clubs will need to create new business models that can attract the emerging middle class and then will need to be prepared to change that offering as the per-capita income of people grows. The new budget clubs sprouting up in Europe and around the globe may be the answer to penetrating this emerging global middle class. What is known is that since the definition of middle class varies by market, the models that operators develop must also diverge in order to appeal to those respective markets.

The new budget clubs sprouting up in Europe and around the globe may be the answer to penetrating the emerging global middle class.

❏ *Tackling a Growing Health Problem*. With regard to obesity, the global marketplace is confronted with similar challenges. In the last decade, the level of obesity has increased in every country, in both genders, and across all age groups, races, and types of backgrounds, to a point where it is currently a worldwide epidemic. In fact, obesity represents one of the two most significant global opportunities for the health/fitness club industry to have a meaningful impact on the health of the planet. Leveraging this opportunity will require close cooperation between club operators and the various global political institutions.

❏ *Growing Older*. Statistics indicate that the population of the world is aging. In fact, the over-50 population is projected to be the largest segment of the world's population over the next 10 to 15 years, with countries such as the U.S., Japan, Italy, Germany, and England having a significant portion of their population over the age of 50. It is predicted that by the year 2050 there will be approximately two billion global citizens age 60 and older. The efforts that international clubs undertake to target this market will, in large part, determine their financial success in the coming decade.

❏ *Growing Up*. The under-30 population (i.e., the Millennial generation) may represent the biggest challenge for the health/fitness club industry. Possibly, the most globally influenced group of individuals in the history of mankind because of the world to which they have been subjected (e.g., mass media, Internet, smart phones, social media, etc.), this relatively young population has been raised on fast foods, video games, and sedentary living, as well as the addictive and celebrity fantasy realm of social media and ever-evolving technology. The challenge is to find a fitness model that appeals to this young audience and engages them in physical activity. It is a challenge that will benefit from the combined wisdom and innovation of the industry's international partners.

❑ *Moving Toward the Establishment of "Clans."* The global marketplace is fusing. Borders are being eliminated by the Internet and social media. News and information are becoming readily available 24/7, due to modern technology. This intent-driven fusion of global cultures has also seen an emergence of clans, niches, and cult brands. People, while becoming connected to a larger population of global citizens, are also seeking out relatively small groups that reflect their specific interests and desires. In the future, the global club industry's growth will depend on the ability of operators to morph from "karaoke" operators to businesses that are able to fulfill the needs of specific audiences (e.g., clans, micro-audiences, niches, etc.) and create what one modern business guru defines as "cult" brands.

(Note: Additional information on the global health/fitness club marketplace is readily available from IHRSA.)

In the future, the global club industry's growth will depend on the ability of operators to morph from "karaoke" operators to businesses that are able to fulfill the needs of specific audiences.

25

The Asian Health/ Fitness Club Market

Chapter Objectives

This chapter provides an overview of the Asian health/fitness club market and the implications this information holds for the health/fitness industry in Asia and throughout the world. Following the introduction, a closer look at the dynamics of the Asian health/fitness club industry is taken, including some of the differences that exist between Asia and other global club markets. The chapter features ideas, insights, and information on the opportunities and challenges that may arise for Asian health/fitness club operators over the next decade.

Overview of the Asian Market

The Asian continent is comprised of 48 separate countries that have an estimated combined population of 3,879,000,000 people, equivalent to 44 percent of the world's population. The 48 nations that make up the continent of Asia include countries, such as China, India, Japan, South Korea, Georgia, Cambodia, Azerbaijan, Afghanistan, Singapore, and Thailand, to name a few. In fact, three of these Asian nations are among the six largest in the world—China, Indonesia, and India—and have a combined population that exceeds 2.7 billion people. The enormity of Asia may be hard to visualize until it is compared to the total population of Europe, which is approximately 820 million, North America, which is just over 347 million, and Latin America, which has approximately 597 million people. The Asian market is nearly five times as large as the next biggest market, Europe, and over 10 times larger than the North American market.

According to the IHRSA 2010 Global Report, there are an estimated 16,840 clubs in the 12 Asian-Pacific countries surveyed in the study. These 16,840 clubs serve an estimated population of 12,974,000 members or approximately three tenths of a percent of the entire Asian population. Of course, the IHRSA data only applies to the 12 countries surveyed, rather than the 48 countries that make up Asia. Even when the population of these 12 countries is taken into consideration, the health/fitness club industry in Asia has still penetrated less than one percent of the entire Asian population. In contrast, Europe has

The Asian continent is comprised of 48 separate countries that have an estimated combined population of 3,879,000,000 people, equivalent to 44 percent of the world's population.

Asia is an extremely fertile territory for the development of the health/fitness club industry.

over 48,000 clubs that serve approximately 5.2 percent of the population, and North America has just over 38,000 clubs that service approximately 15 percent of the population. This cursory review suggests that Asia is an extremely fertile territory for the development of the health/fitness club industry. The most significant challenges for the health/fitness club industry in Asia are knocking down government-built barriers to a free-market economy and identifying ways to provide a health/fitness club experience to relatively large populations of people with limited economic resources.

Overview of the Health/Fitness Club Industry in Asia

❏ *Clubs, Members, and Penetration.* As indicated in the previous section, the Asian health/fitness club market is comprised of approximately 16,840 clubs (approximately 90 percent growth in the past five years) clubs that serve approximately 12,974,000 (approximately 20 percent growth in the past five years) members and generate total annual gross revenue of approximately 8.5 billion U.S. dollars. Figures 25-1 and 25-2 illustrate the number of clubs and revenue contributions of the various nations in the published report, the *IHRSA 2010 Global Report*, which included the Asian market. The data clearly shows that the Asian market is in its infancy, given that the total number of clubs and the total estimated revenues generated by facilities on this continent are significantly below those of Europe, Latin America, and North America. As a reflection of its relative state of infancy, the entire Asian market is not much larger than that of Brazil (e.g., based on club count).

While the Asian market, as a whole, may be considered in its infancy, nations, such as Japan and South Korea, represent an entirely different dynamic. These two nations more closely align with the health/fitness club markets in Europe and North America. Figure 25-3 provides a visual representation of the composition of the market, by club count, for Asia in 2006 and again in 2009. As of 2009, South Korea and Japan account for 68 percent of the clubs in the Asian market, with Korea accounting for 38 percent and Japan accounting for nearly 30 percent of all of the clubs in Asia. When revenue contributions are considered, Japan alone contributes 40 percent of the total revenue generated by clubs in Asia, with South Korea second at 27 percent. Over the past five years, South Korea has been the most actively growing market in Asia.

A final, somewhat telling, statistic about both the maturity of the health/ fitness club industry in Asia and its potential for future growth, is the data on market-penetration. As a whole, the Asian health/fitness club industry has penetrated less than 1 percent of the eligible population, which, when compared to Europe at 5 percent and North America at slightly over 15 percent, indicates a significant upside (refer to Figure 25-4 for the estimated penetration percentages for the various nations in Asia). The most successful market, in terms of market penetration, is South Korea, with an estimated 7.2 percent penetration, followed by Japan, with a 3.2 percent penetration of the market. Interestingly enough, Japan, which operates approximately 30 percent of the clubs in Asia and generates 40 percent of the market's total revenue, has only been able to reach 3.2 percent of its population.

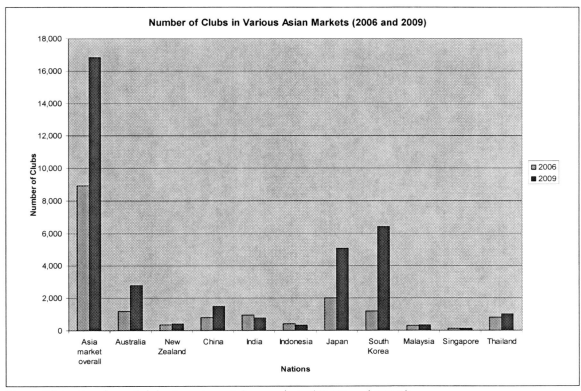

Figure 25-1. Number of clubs in various Asian markets (2006 and 2009)

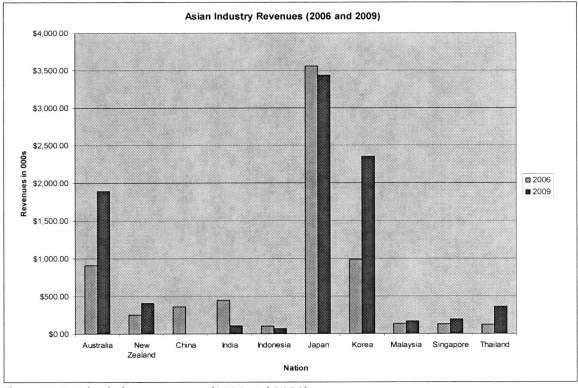

Figure 25-2. Asian industry revenues (2006 and 2009)

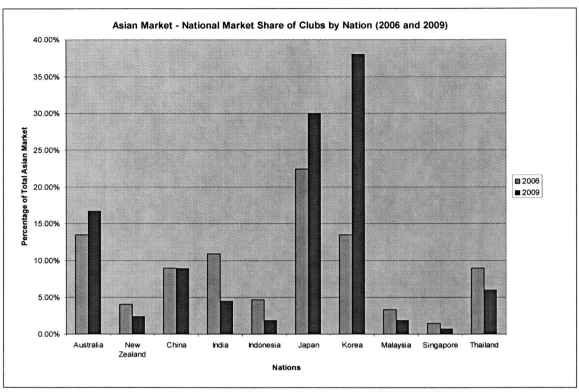

Figure 25-3. Asian market—national market share of clubs by nation (2006 and 2009)

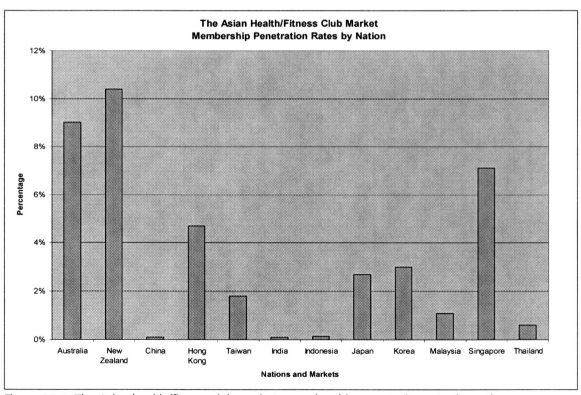

Figure 25-4. The Asian health/fitness club market—membership penetration rates by nation

In Asia, the average monthly dues for a health/fitness club ranges from a low of $24 a month in India to $79 a month in Vietnam (2008 data). Comparatively speaking, the average monthly dues in the majority of Asian markets are considerably lower than the averages for both Europe and the U.S. For example, in Asia, where the low end of the monthly-dues spectrum is $24, it is half as much as in Europe (e.g., $50). At the other end of the pricing spectrum, Vietnam has the highest average dues seen in Asia—$79. Russia has the highest monthly-dues average in Europe—$80 (U.S.).

Figure 25-5 provides an overview of the average dues pricing for the 12 nations included in the *2008 IHRSA Asia Pacific Market Report*. While the monthly dues prices for clubs across the various Asian nations is lower than those of both the European and North American markets, the actual cost of membership as a percentage of annual per-capita income is significantly higher in Asia than either Europe or North America. The percentage of per-capita income allocated to annual health/fitness club dues ranges from a low of approximately 2.2 percent in Japan to just slightly over 36 percent in Vietnam (refer to Figure 25-6 for the dues pricing to per-capita-income percentages in several Asian nations). These percentages are considerably higher than the average dues that exist in both Europe and North America. For example, in Europe, average annual dues run around 2 percent of per-capita income, with a high of approximately 8 percent to 10 percent in Russia. In contrast, the average in Asia is approximately 50 percent higher. In the case of Vietnam, it is 400 percent higher than the percentage that Russia has.

The reasons for these unique and wide-ranging variances in market penetration, membership pricing, and overall industry size for the various Asian nations can be traced back to several possible factors, including:

- *Disposable income of the populace.* Per capita earnings across Asia tend to be significantly lower than in either Europe or North America. Hong Kong, Japan, Singapore, South Korea, and Taiwan are the only nations where the per-capita income exceeds $20,000 annually (excluding Asia nations that are located in the Middle East). Only Japan, Singapore, and Taiwan have average per-capita income levels at or above $30,000 annually. In contrast, Europe and North America have average per-capita incomes of $30,000 and over. What may be even more telling is that China and India, the two most populous nations in the world, and two of the globe's fastest emerging economies (China is now the second largest economy, after the U.S.), have average per-capita incomes of under $6,500 and $3,000 respectively, on an annual basis. When the fact is considered that the middle class has been defined in some quarters as $10 to $20 a day, and by others as between $6,000 and $30,000 annually, the per capita incomes for China and India indicate that the average citizen is really not in a position to afford a fitness club. When the per-capita incomes are so low, it is easy to understand why the Asian operators have had less success penetrating the market than operators in Europe and the Americas. In those nations where the per-capita income approaches European and North American levels (e.g.,

Comparatively speaking, the average monthly dues in the majority of Asian markets are considerably lower than the averages for both Europe and the U.S.

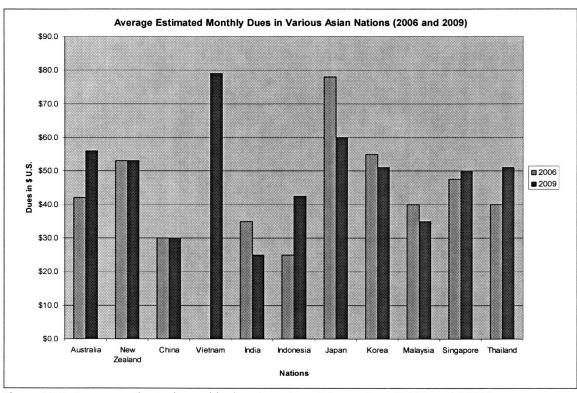

Figure 25-5. Average estimated monthly dues in various Asian nations (2006 and 2009)

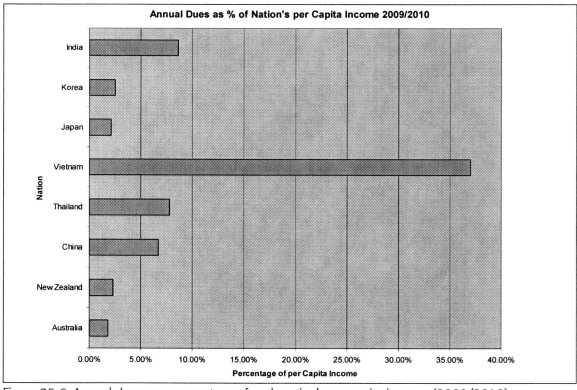

Figure 25-6. Annual dues as a percentage of each nation's per capita income (2009/2010)

Hong Kong, Japan, South Korea, Singapore, and Taiwan), club operators have experienced more success.

- *Cultural factors.* Cultural traditions definitely impact the ability to rapidly grow the Asian market. For example, in China, Hong Kong, and Taiwan, many older adults still practice martial arts in the parks and use this as their basic form of physical activity. As such, this segment of the older population does not perceive the same need for joining a health/fitness club as older adults in Europe and North America do. In many Asian cultures, physical work and activity are a natural part of their day, and, in many cases, these people expend more calories during the course of the day than do many active health/fitness club users in either Europe or North America. The health/fitness club market in many of the Asian nations (e.g., with the exception of Japan) is primarily the fitness environment of choice for the young and the affluent populace.

- *Industry longevity.* The Asian market is relatively new when compared to the markets in either Europe or North America, although the Japanese health/fitness club market has been in existence since the mid-1960s. In fact, the leading Japanese companies, such as Central Sports and Konami, opened for business in the late 1960s and early 1970s, which places them in the same approximate timeline category as the most mature operators in Europe and North America. Clark Hatch, a company that manages over 100 facilities throughout Asia, most of which are located in hotels, entered the Asian market in 1965, nearly 20 years later than Vic Tanny introduced the modern health club to the U.S. As a consequence, the health/fitness club industries in Japan and Taiwan had a significant edge over other Asia nations when it came to establishing a foothold for their businesses.

  On the other end of the spectrum, the health/fitness club industry is relatively new to countries such as China, India, and Malaysia. In these countries, the industry has been around for less than 20 years and, in many cases, less than 10 (e.g., it should be noted that in many Asian nations, member-owned athletic clubs that serve expatriate populations and the very affluent have been in existence for decades). From a historical viewpoint, compared to both the European and the U.S. club industries, the early development years for the Asian health/fitness club industry have been relatively slow. Once a strong foothold has been established in a given country, however, the industry has taken off.

- *Domestic operators.* One of the factors that has driven the growth and success of the health/fitness club industries in North America and Europe has been the passion and determination of domestic entrepreneurs. When the industry is grown organically (i.e., local business entrepreneurs take the lead in developing the club business), the industry is far more likely to achieve faster growth. In China, India, and Japan, local entrepreneurs launched the health/fitness club industry (e.g., Central Sports, Konami, Renaissance in Japan, and Talwalkar Fitness in India). As a result of these pioneering local operators, their businesses and the industry in their respective countries have been able to grow in a manner that is similar to health/fitness clubs in Europe and North America.

The health/fitness club market in many of the Asian nations (e.g., with the exception of Japan) is primarily the fitness environment of choice for the young and the affluent populace.

The perception of being foreign can be a particularly difficult hurdle to overcome in the international market, especially in Asia.

Besides the aforementioned examples, most of the Asian market has either been developed by either expatriate companies (i.e., companies whose headquarters are based outside of Asia) or been grown by local entrepreneurs using expatriate franchises (i.e., local business operators who purchase an international franchise). An examination of the various markets in Asia shows that many of the leading companies in that area of the world are expatriate-branded companies (e.g., Bally, World Gym, 24 Hour Fitness-California Fitness, Fitness First, and Gold's).

While each of the various business models provide an excellent brand for local owners to build on, the consumers in those markets still perceive these brands as foreign brands, and, in many instances, do not trust them. The perception of being foreign can be a particularly difficult hurdle to overcome in the international market, especially in Asia. All factors considered, as more local businessmen and women begin taking the lead in developing their own organic brands, at that point, the industry in the many undersized markets throughout Asia will begin to prosper.

Membership Characteristics

Data pertaining to the general membership characteristics of the Asian market are not as readily available as they are for North America and Europe. While the age, gender, and general-usage demographics of club members in Europe and the U.S. have been published by IHRSA in its various reports (e.g., the *2010 IHRSA European Market Report* and the *IHRSA 2010 Profiles of Success*), no such data concerning Asia has been released. Based on anecdotal evidence gleaned from personal observations by the author made during visits to Asia and information obtained from conversations with a few of the leading health/fitness club operators in the respective Asian markets, certain membership features of these markets can be formulated. In that regard, a list of key observations about the membership characteristics of the Asian market includes the following:

- In Japan, the gender profile of membership leans toward women. While an exact percentage is not available, it is estimated that the gender blend of the Japanese market closely parallels that of several European nations and the United States, with women comprising in the neighborhood of 50 percent to 55 percent (and possibly higher) of the market. From a usage perspective, group fitness and swimming are among the most popular activities in the clubs. Japanese club consumers are more accepting of technology as part of the club experience than their counterparts in the U.S.

- In China, the membership base swings heavily toward a younger age demographic, similar to several European countries, where the 18 to 34 age group is the largest segment. Prior to 1995, the Chinese market was essentially made up of a few hotel-based clubs and expatriate private clubs. Only in the last 10 to 15 years has the industry really taken off, in large part due to the introduction of foreign franchise models. As a result, health/fitness club membership in China, which formerly were the domain of the affluent, have only recently become attractive to the rapidly emerging young middle class. Group-exercise classes are extremely popular, and similar to both North America and Europe, women are the predominant participants in these programs.

The Leading Players in the Asian Health/Fitness Club Market

When the Asian market is viewed on a nation-by-nation basis, it is evident that in each of these national markets, a small number of health/fitness club companies hold a considerable share of the overall club market. For the nations profiled in the *IHRSA 2008 Asia Pacific Market Report,* the top five club companies in those nations control anywhere from 1 percent of the market to 33 percent of the market, with nine of those nations having over 10 percent of their market controlled by the top five companies, and four of those nations (Australia, Japan, Singapore, and Taiwan) having over 20 percent of the market controlled by the top five companies (refer to Figure 25-7). In fact, the top players in Singapore and Taiwan control more than 30 percent of the market.

In contrast, among the nations in the European Union, in only five nations, do the top five companies hold greater than 10 percent market share. In fact, two of the largest club companies, Fitness First and Virgin Active, have only 3 percent and 2 percent of the clubs in their markets. In the U.S., the top five players hold less than 4 percent of the total market. What these numbers clearly indicate is that in the various Asia nations, more so than in either the European nations or the U.S., the market has been, and possibly will continue to be, influenced and controlled by a small segment of relatively large and highly successful operators.

The Asian continent is quite different than either the European continent or the North American continent when it comes to the total market share being

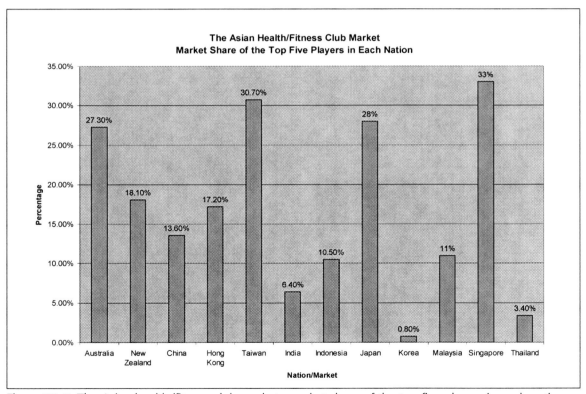

Figure 25-7. The Asian health/fitness club market—market share of the top five players in each nation

controlled by the major club companies. In Asia, approximately 7.4 percent of the club market is held by seven companies (refer to Figure 25-8 for a comparison of the largest companies by club count for 2006 and 2008), while the remaining 92.6 percent is held by smaller national companies and independent operators. In comparison, the top seven club companies in Europe control approximately 2 percent of the market, while in the United States, the top seven club companies control approximately 4 percent of the market. This data suggests that a small number of highly successful club companies can play a significant leadership role in shaping the trends and practices in both a single nation and across the entire Asian market.

The largest player in Asia, both with regard to the number of clubs it operates and the revenue it generates, is Konami, with 327 clubs and 2009 revenues of approximately $950 million (U.S.). The second largest player in Asia is Central Sports, with 154 clubs and 2009 revenues of approximately $465 million (U.S.). In comparison, the two largest players in Europe are Fitness First, with revenues of approximately $1 billion (U.S.) and Virgin Active, with revenues of approximately $800 million (U.S.), based on accounting for revenue from its recent acquisition of Esporta. In the U.S., the two largest players are 24 Hour Fitness, with revenues of approximately $1.3 billion (U.S.) and Lifetime Fitness with revenues of approximately $1 billion (U.S.). What this data indicates is that the top two players in the Asian market are on similar ground as the top two players in Europe and the U.S.

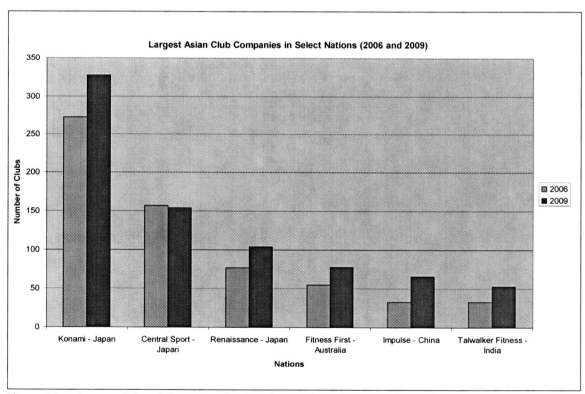

Figure 25-8. Largest Asian club companies in select nations (2006 and 2009)

The Asian market has not encountered the same level of merger and acquisition activity as its European counterparts or the large influx of private equity that club operators in both Europe and North America have experienced. The Asian environment for mergers or acquisitions does not seem as opportunistic as it is in Europe and North America. While private equity has helped foster development in Asia, most of the developmental funds for the Asian industry have been provided by European-based operators, such as Fitness First, with clubs in Australia, India, and Indonesia, and 24 Hour Fitness, with a strong presence in both Hong Kong and China (e.g., California Fitness). Some of the smaller nationally based operators (i.e., local ownership, not foreign) have utilized equity infusion from Asian-based firms and investors to help foster their organic growth. As of yet, private-equity firms have not been involved in the Asian market to the degree that they have been in the European and North American markets. While the private-equity side of the Asian market is significantly less active than the markets in Europe and North America, the presence of publicly listed Asian operators is quite similar. The three largest Japanese companies—Konami, Central Sports, and Renaissance—are all publicly listed. In the U.S., Lifetime Fitness and Town Sports International are publicly listed, while in Europe, SATS is publicly listed, while Fitness First is considering a listing in the near future.

> While the private-equity side of the Asian market is significantly less active than the markets in Europe and North America, the presence of publicly listed Asian operators is quite similar.

Opportunities and Challenges for the Asian Market

❑ *Opportunities*
  • *Market penetration.* As an industry in its infancy, with the exception of the Japanese and Taiwanese markets, the Asian club industry has an incredible future ahead of it. As the statistics show, with less than 1 percent of the Asian market served by health/fitness clubs, the opportunity for new business development is immense. In fact, in both China and India, whose combined population is over 2.7 billion, the opportunities are enormous. These two nations are among two of the four largest expanding markets in the global economy (e.g., part of the BRIC, along with Brazil and Russia). Imagine the opportunities for club operators if market penetration in these countries were even to approach 3 to 5 percent; then take these penetration percentages and expand them across the entire Asian continent.

  • *Attracting investment capital.* As the economies in Asia continue to develop and with the rapid expansion of the emerging middle class, its citizens will likely realize greater economic freedom, including more discretionary income. As the economic landscape improves, investors will want to capitalize on the opportunity to bring the health/fitness club experience to an audience that hereto has never had the ability or the inherent desire to join a health/fitness club.

❑ *Challenges*
  • *Economic clout.* The most significant hurdle for the Asian market involves the economic conditions and earning power of its citizens. In many Asian nations, there is a very small population of affluent citizens and

a very large group of poor citizens. Until a larger segment of the Asian population achieves the Western definition of middle-class status, the health/fitness club industry in that area of the world will have a difficult time achieving rapid growth. In nations, such as China and India, a rapidly emerging middle class exists, which, in part, is driving the current growth in those markets.

- *Cultural barriers.* In many Asian nations, membership in a health/fitness club is not part of the cultural tradition. Those citizens who parallel the baby boomer generation in the U.S. do not see the same value in club usage as the baby boomers in the U.S. and Europe. In addition, cultural traditions around family, gender, and physical-activity practices are all potential hurdles that the industry will need to overcome if it is to achieve the same popularity that it has experienced in Europe and the U.S.

- *Organic growth.* As occurred in Europe and the U.S., when local business leaders take the lead in developing the industry, the industry prospers far more significantly than it does when foreign companies take the lead. In that regard, the primary challenge for the Asian health/fitness club market is to follow the lead of companies such as Central Sports, Konami, and Renaissance in Japan. These companies were neither developed nor operated by foreign companies. As a result, they have been able to garner greater brand trust with the citizens of their respective nations. The challenge for the Asian market, which is also an opportunity in waiting, is to look toward organic growth fueled by investment from local investors versus allowing so much foreign franchising and management.

- *Talent availability.* Finding adequate personnel to staff and manage a health/fitness club is a global challenge, not just an issue facing Asia. Nonetheless, in order for the industry to achieve significant growth, the operators in Asia will have to identify and execute strategies to quickly develop fitness professionals who can step in and manage a club.

Concluding Thoughts

If the current trends continue for the next 10 to 20 years, little doubt exists that Asia will emerge as a global leader in the health/ fitness club industry.

Asia is the largest geographic populace in the world. This continent represents approximately 44 percent of the world population. Japan and China are already global economic powers, while India and Korea are becoming or may already be considered global economic powers. The combination of populace size and growing economic clout suggest a market that, in the next 20 years, may become the largest health/fitness club market in the world. The Asian club market is an emerging and dynamic business environment that is being shown the way to responsible growth by excellent operators, such as Central Sports, Konami, Renaissance, Talwalkar Fitness, and Fitness First, among others. In several countries, such as Japan, South Korea, Singapore, and Taiwan, the industry is well-established and serves as a template for entrepreneurs in other Asian markets who wish to build successful and profitable health/fitness club empires. If the current trends continue for the next 10 to 20 years, little doubt exists that Asia will emerge as a global leader in the health/fitness club industry.

26

The European Health/ Fitness Club Market

Chapter Objectives

This chapter provides an overview of the European market and the implications that this data holds for the health/fitness club industry in Europe and for the industry in the rest of the world. The chapter then examines the dynamics of the European health/fitness club industry, including review of the primary differences that exist between the European health/fitness club market and the North American club market, particularly the U.S. club market. The chapter offers ideas, insights, and information on the opportunities and challenges that may arise for European health/fitness club operators over the next decade.

Overview of the European Market

Europe is a continent of 52 nations, with an estimated population of 816,426,246 people, equivalent to 11.7 percent of the world's population. The 52 nations of Europe range from Gibraltar, with approximately 26,000 residents, to Russia, with a population of over 140,000,000. In comparison, North America, consisting of only two nations, has an estimated population of 347,354,870, equivalent to 5 percent of the world population. When viewed in this perspective, Europe represents a market that is over two times as large as that of North America. As these numbers indicate, Europe is an important and influential player in the current and future development of the global health/fitness club industry. In fact, the European market now generates slightly over 31 billion in revenue, which is more revenue than is generated by the industry in North America. In fact, Europe is the largest fitness market in the world. According to the latest global industry report from IHRSA, there are an estimated 48,000 clubs on the European continent. These facilities collectively have approximately 42.5 million members or 5 percent of the continent's population. Furthermore, for those countries that are part of the European union, the market penetration percentage approaches 8 percent. In contrast, North America has approximately 38,000 clubs, representing an estimated 53,200,000 members or 15 percent of the total population. From an absolute

Europe represents a market that is over two times as large as that of North America.

quantitative perspective, Europe has 26 percent more clubs than North America and nearly an equivalent number of members, and yet the market penetration in Europe is only a third of that in North America. This comparative statistic represents both a unique challenge and an incredible opportunity for European health/fitness club operators. The challenge for Europe is to achieve levels of membership penetration that are comparable to those in the North American market. It should be noted that several nations (e.g., nations, such as the Netherlands, Norway, and Spain) already have achieved penetration rates that either equal or exceed those seen in North America. The opportunity for Europe is that if it is able to achieve the same penetration rates as those that occur in North America, then the number of health/fitness club members in Europe could triple to approximately 120 million or equivalent to the global goals established by IHRSA for 2010. Furthermore, the revenues flowing to the health/fitness club industry in Europe would also triple, which would result in revenues growing from the current 2010 estimate of just over $31 billion (U.S.) to over $90 billion (U.S.).

Overview of the Health/Fitness Club Industry in Europe

❑ *Clubs, Members, and Membership Penetration.* As indicated in the previous section, the European health/fitness club market is comprised of over 48,000 clubs and 42 million members that generate gross revenues of approximately $31 billion (U.S.) annually. One of the more unique features of the European market is the level of maturity and sophistication that exists across the continent. Several nations, such as the United Kingdom, Spain, Sweden, Netherlands, and Norway, have already achieved market penetration levels equal to or exceeding those seen in the more mature U.S. market, while concurrently, emerging Eastern European nations, such as Estonia, Hungary, and Poland, have market penetration rates that are comparable to developing nations in Asia and Latin America. Figures 26-1 to 26-3 provide a visual perspective of these dynamics by showing the number of clubs, the number of club members, and the membership-penetration rates, respectfully, for select European markets. What these figures clearly indicate is that in many of the Western European nations (e.g., Netherlands, Spain, and United Kingdom), health/fitness club membership is as much a part of the daily routine for citizens as it is in the United States. In Eastern European nations, on the other hand, the health/fitness club industry is in its infancy.

> One of the more unique features of the European market is the level of maturity and sophistication that exists across the continent.

The European nation with the largest number of clubs is Italy (8,500), followed closely by Germany with slightly over 5,900 health/fitness facilities, and then the United Kingdom with just over 5,800 clubs. While Italy can lay claim to having the most health/fitness clubs, Spain takes top honors, with regard to the number of club members, at just over 7.5 million, with the U.K. and Germany a close second and third at 7.3million and 7 million, respectively. As industry insiders have come to understand in the United States, the most important measure of the health/fitness club industry's success is not the total number of members, but the percentage of residents within a market who have adopted the health/fitness club lifestyle. Based

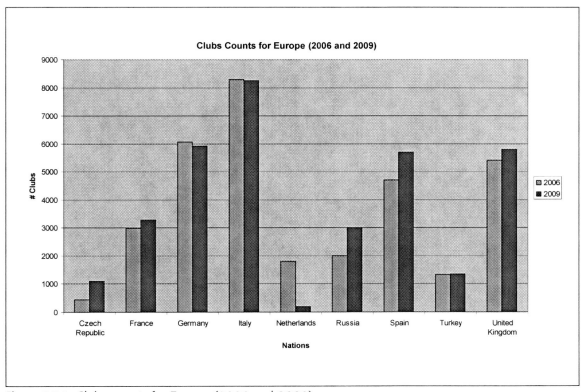

Figure 26-1. Clubs counts for Europe (2006 and 2009)

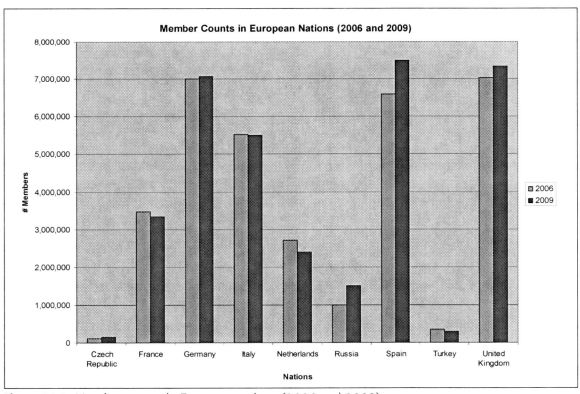

Figure 26-2. Member counts in European nations (2006 and 2009)

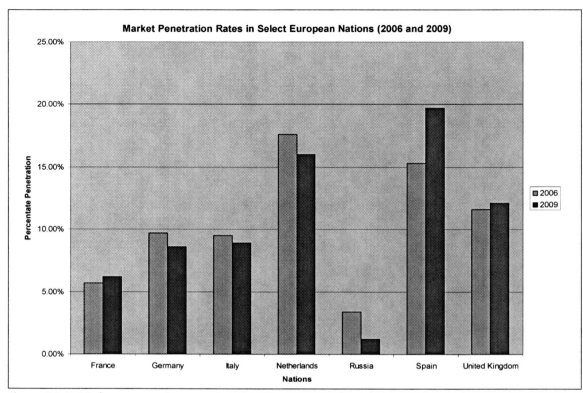

Figure 26-3. Market penetration rates in select European nations (2006 and 2009)

on this dynamic, Spain has the highest market-penetration level, having attracted approximately 19 percent of the market for memberships, followed closely by several Scandinavian nations and the Netherlands, each of which has been able to attract over 14 percent of its population as members.

A number of factors affect the dichotomy in club membership penetration across Europe, including the economic environment, the enormous difference in sports-culture, the level of professionalism of the club operators, and the organization of the industry. With regard to the latter dynamic, many countries do not yet have a well-organized, regionally based association of either health/fitness club professionals or facilities. With regard to the economic environment in Western Europe, a free market economy has existed for centuries. As a result, many citizens in these countries have sufficient expendable income to put toward club memberships. The average per-capita income, per the *IHRSA 2010 European Health Club Report*, ranges from 10,500 Euros (Russia) to 40,000 Euros (Norway), which if converted to $U.S., would be similar to the income ranges that exist across the various states in the U.S.

In the European Union (a consortium of countries that does not include all 52 European nations), the average per-capita income is approximately 23,758 Euro, equivalent to $33,784 U.S. This figure is approximately 17 percent less per-capita income than in the U.S. In Eastern Europe, a free-market economy is newer. In fact, in many cases, it is less than 20 years old. As a result, economic conditions are evolving, a situation which results in a polar economic climate (e.g., affluent and poor populations) and a slowly emerging middle class. As the middle class continues to grow in Eastern Europe, so will membership levels in health/fitness clubs.

In Europe, the average monthly health/fitness club dues vary by nation, from a low of around 40 Euros (approximately $57 U.S.) in Germany up to an average of 60 Euros (approximately $85 U.S.) in Russia and Spain (refer to Figure 26-4 for a comparison of average monthly dues by European countries). The average monthly dues prices shown in Figure 26-4 include the value added tax (VAT) that club members must pay on top of the quoted dues price (VAT is a form of taxation that is similar to the sales tax that some municipalities in the U.S. place on health/fitness club memberships and ranges from 12 percent to 23 percent across Europe).

Comparatively speaking, the average monthly dues paid by most Europeans for a health/fitness club membership represent a significantly higher percentage of their per-capita income than in the U.S. For example, in the U.S., according to the publication, the *IHRSA 2010 Profiles of Success*, the average annual dues for a health/fitness club in the U.S. are $720 annually. This figure represents approximately 1.7 percent of the average per-capita income for a U.S. citizen. In comparison, the average dues in Germany are equal to 2 percent of per-capita income, in Spain they are equal to 3 percent of per capita income, and in Russia are equal to slightly over 7 percent of per-capita income (refer to Figure 26-5 for national comparisons). This single measure indicates that in Europe, the average

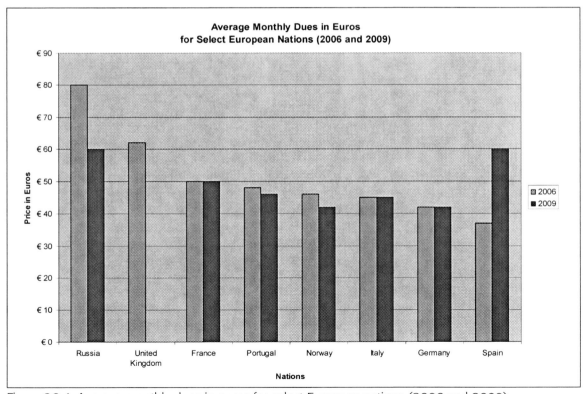

Figure 26-4. Average monthly dues in euros for select European nations (2006 and 2009)

It could be argued that one reason Europeans are willing to set aside a larger portion of their earnings for health/fitness club membership than U.S. citizens is because citizens in Europe are accustomed to paying higher prices for other products and services.

citizen is willing to put a larger portion of his earnings toward a health/fitness club membership. The rationale for this situation has not been set forth in any of the industry literature, and any conjecture as to why this discrepancy exists would be purely hypothetical. Nonetheless, it could be argued that one reason Europeans are willing to set aside a larger portion of their earnings for health/fitness club membership than U.S. citizens is because citizens in Europe are accustomed to paying higher prices for other products and services, in many cases as the result of VAT and import fees.

Two other factors impact the competitive atmosphere, and in particular club pricing, for the health/fitness club industry in Europe. One is the strong development of local-authority (i.e., city/village operated) fitness facilities in countries like the U.K. and Spain, where a large portion of the market is public and costs are kept low. The other is the birth and rapid growth of budget-clubs, which charge half the dues price of the average health/fitness club. Among the leading budget-club operators in Europe are McFit, Pure Fitness, and Jumpers in Germany, the Gym Group and Fitspace in England, and Health City in the Netherlands. The budget-club segment, while emerging in Germany in the late 90s, has only become as a significant club segment during the past five years.

❑ *Membership Characteristics.* In Europe, gender involvement in the health/fitness club experience varies widely. In many cases, it is significantly different than what exists in the U.S (refer to Figure 26-6 that is based on 2006 data). For example, in the U.S, according to the publication, the *IHRSA 2010 Profiles of Success*, approximately 48 percent of club membership is composed of women. In Europe, while the overall average for gender participation across all nations is comparatively close to that of the U.S., the mix by nation is considerably different. In France and Italy, for example, 66 percent and 58 percent of club members, respectfully, are women, while in Germany approximately 50 percent of members are female. In Spain and the United Kingdom, statistics indicate that approximately 53 percent and 54 percent of members. respectively, are female.

Such differences in gender participation could logically be expected to play a significant role in driving the design, marketing, and programming of European health/fitness clubs, given that club operators must offer an experience that is appealing to the largest user audience. Not surprisingly, some of the gender differences actually play a significant role in the club's product offering. For example, in France and Italy, where 6 out of 10 club members are women, group exercise is far and away the most popular activity (e.g., 69 percent and 65 percent of users participate).

In Germany, a completely different dynamic exists. For example, in Germany, club membership is almost evenly distributed between men and women, which is different than previously when men actually represented nearly 60 percent of the market. Despite having an equal number of women and past demographic in which men were the majority, strength training is the most popular form of club activity in Germany (e.g., 87 percent of activity). Similar to the U.S., Europeans exhibit activity tendencies based on

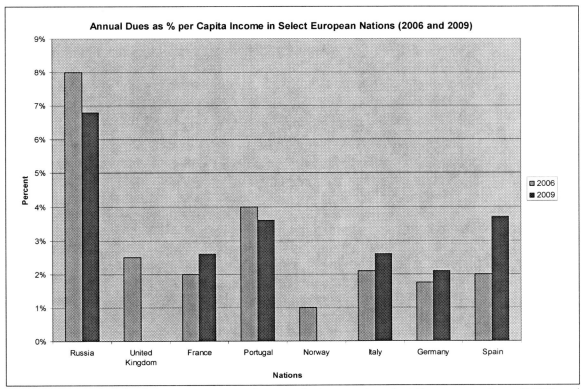

Figure 26-5. Annual dues as a percentage of per capita income in select European nations (2006 and 2009)

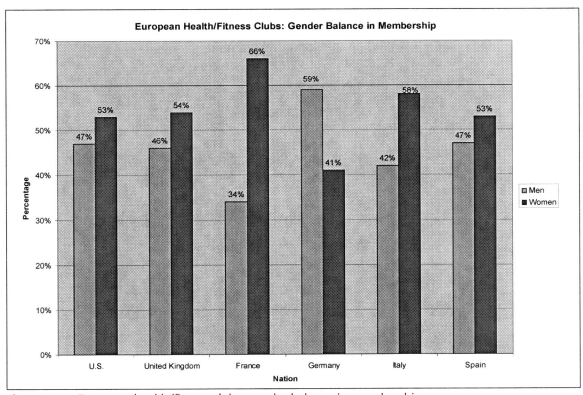

Figure 26-6. European health/fitness clubs: gender balance in membership

gender, with men and women almost equally involved in cardiovascular training (50 percent men and women), men more inclined toward strength training than women (56 percent men and 44 percent women), and women significantly more involved in group fitness than men (27 percent men and 73 percent women). Figure 26-7 provides a sampling of European participation preferences, based on data from the *2007 IHRSA European Market Report.*

In Europe, the largest demographic segment of club membership is driven by adults 18 to 34 years old (36.5 percent), with the second largest population of members coming from those 35 to 54 (34.9 percent). This age demographic is considerably different than the current U.S. club mix, in which 31 percent of members come from the 18 to 34 age group, and 36 percent come from the 35 to 54 age group. Interestingly enough, Europe has a larger portion of its members come from the over-55 population than the U.S., with Germany and Italy having the oldest demographics in Western Europe. (Figure 26-8 provides an overview of the age demographics for select European nations, based on 2006 data.) The aforementioned described age demographics vary considerably, when the data for some of the European nations is examined closely. For example, in Germany, 53 percent of memberships are driven by the 18-to-34 age demographic, while in Italy only 11 percent of memberships are derived from this same demographic category. Although no specific rationale was put forth in IHRSA's data on these varying demographic swings in membership penetration, it is quite possible that some of the following factors might come into play:

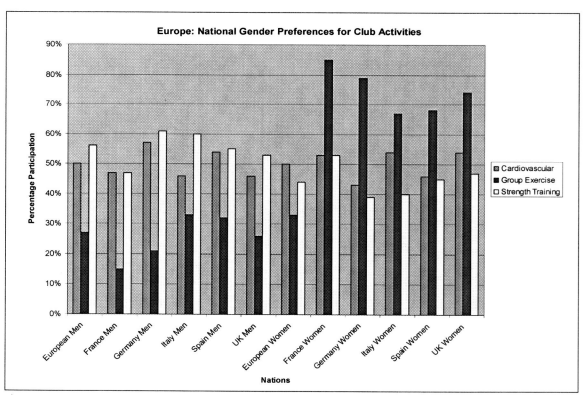

Figure 26-7. Europe: national gender preferences for club activities

- The nearly equal penetration of the 55-plus demographic in both Europe and the U.S. possibly speaks to the fact that for baby boomers, regularly scheduled exercise is still a new lifestyle phenomena. In many Eastern European nations, penetration into this demographic category is further impacted by the fact that this generation of Europeans has not had an equal opportunity to exploit the financial rewards of a free-market economy.

- The high penetration of the 18 to 34 age demographic in Europe parallels what the U.S. experienced back in the 1980s when having an exercise and club membership was primarily the domain of the younger population (in the U.S., it's moving back in that direction). In Europe, this phenomenon might exist for a couple of reasons. First, this is an age in which younger individuals are likely to be most interested in a person's physical appearance and athletic accomplishments. Second, this generation, which is very technologically savvy, has been exposed through the World Wide Web to the trends in fitness, something that their parents were not afforded.

- Penetration of the 35 to 54 age demographic, on the other hand, is less in Europe than in the U.S., with the exception of Italy, where it is much higher (refer to Figure 26-8). This difference of approximately 10 percent between the involvement of 35- to 54-year-olds in Europe and the U.S. might be a byproduct of several factors, including household incomes, access to information, and traditional cultural values.

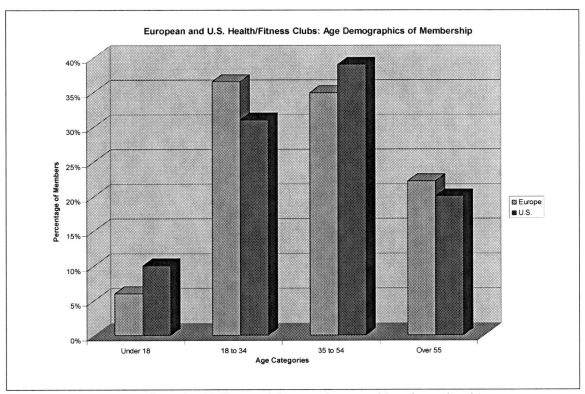

Figure 26-8. European and U.S. health/fitness clubs: age demographics of membership

The Leading Players in the European Health/Fitness Club Market

The European health/fitness club market, particularly in those nations represented by the European Union, has similar parallels to the U.S. market, when it comes to the role of leading health/fitness club operators. While the European industry is still the domain of the independent, entrepreneurial club operator, significant changes have occurred over the past 10 years that reflect a growing trend for commoditization and consolidation among club operators. According to the *2010 IHRSA European Health Club Report*, the top five club operators (based on the number of health/fitness clubs) in each of the European nations represent anywhere from 1 percent of the market (Italy) to 26 percent of the market (Norway). Figure 26-9 provides an overview of the market share of the top five companies in several European markets for the years 2006 and 2009. In fact, if the dollar value of the top five market-share companies was used as the basis for comparison, the relative importance of the top operators would be much larger. Over the next 5 to 10 years, this trend will continue, as equity capital continues to find its way into the European club market, and many of the leading club operators pursue a consolidation strategy aimed at leveraging core strengths in specific markets.

What may be more significant than the influence of the top five operators in each nation is the influence of the top six companies in Europe. This group of six companies manages approximately 2 percent of the total clubs in Europe and represents over 8 percent of the total club members in Europe (refer to Figure 26-10 for a breakdown of the top seven European operators). It should

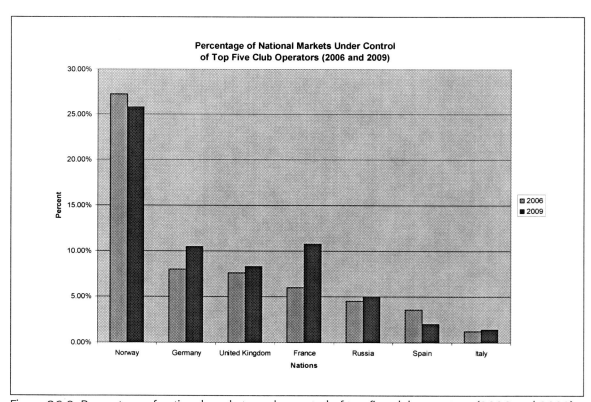

Figure 26-9. Percentage of national markets under control of top five club operators (2006 and 2009)

be noted that the United Kingdom and Germany are home to six of the top 10 companies in Europe. The largest player in terms of the number of clubs it operates, the club members it represents, and the revenue it generates is Fitness First, based in the United Kingdom. On a global basis, Fitness First operates more clubs (over 500 globally) and generates more revenue (approximately $1 billion in 2009) than all but one company—U.S. club operator 24 Hour Fitness. In the next few years, Virgin Active may surpass Fitness First as the largest operator in Europe, at least from a revenue perspective, given its acquisition of Holmes Place several years ago, as well as its 2010 purchase of Esporta, which have pushed its revenues close to $800 million on an annual basis.

The consolidation and commoditization of the European market has been driven primarily through an influx of private equity and large-scale mergers. Several companies, such as Elixia and SATS in Norway and Finland, Health City in the Netherlands and Belgium, McFit of Germany, World Class Fitness of Russia, Virgin Active in the United Kingdom, and David Lloyd Leisure of the United Kingdom, have all benefited from either a merger with another club company that was funded by private equity or an acquisition by a non-industry player with significant capital to invest. For example, Virgin Active, over the past several years, has been pursing an aggressive acquisition strategy, as evidenced by its purchase of two leading U.K. players.

Another company that has been particularly active in the acquisition and consolidation arena is Health City, which is based in the Netherlands. In the last two years, it has purchased over 100 clubs in various European markets, most

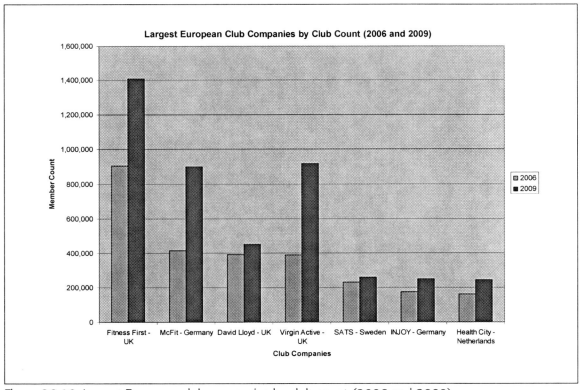

Figure 26-10. Largest European club companies by club count (2006 and 2009)

of which it acquired from Fitness First. In recent years, Fitness First has sold over 100 clubs in its non-core markets and has used those funds to pursue acquisitions and growth in its strongest markets (e.g., England and Germany). To augment those funds, Fitness First has also announced plans to pursue an IPO on the Singapore Exchange.

The acquisition of a club business by a non-industry player with a desire to grow their investment can fuel significant organic club growth.

The outcome and advantages of these various mergers and acquisitions is at least three-fold. First, many of the mergers have brought together the top players in their respective market niches, thus giving the purchaser significant advantages in cost efficiencies, market pricing, and possibly more importantly, in market presence and top-of-mind awareness with the consumer (for example, McFit's purchase of a portion of Fit24, Health City's purchase of over 100 Fitness First clubs, and Virgin Active's acquisition of 55 Esporta clubs). Second, many of the mergers have enabled the purchaser to enter new market niches, thus allowing it to assume a leading position in more than one market segment (for example, Virgin Active's purchase of Holmes Place and Esporta has enabled it to be a player in the premium and high-end premium segments). Third, the acquisition of a club business by a non-industry player with a desire to grow their investment can fuel significant organic club growth (e.g., David Lloyd Leisure, U.K., and Healthy City of the Netherlands).

While the primary outcome of consolidation and commoditization in the European club market is larger and more powerful players that can influence industry-pricing activities and consumer perceptions of the industry (for example, in the U.S., big-box players, such as 24 Hour Fitness, LA Fitness, Planet Fitness, and Lifetime Fitness, have a substantial impact on both consumer perceptions and club pricing), there are other valuable outcomes that can occur for the industry, particularly the development of key market niches, such as the following:

- *Creation of budget-club brands.* In Germany, McFit has carved out a very successful niche as a convenient and inexpensive brand. At under 18 Euros a month and with over 140 locations throughout Germany, it has become the darling of the club industry. McFit's model, which involves having limited staffing (usually one or two staff members per club), leveraging technology (members join on-line or through club kiosks, providing all club information through in-club kiosks and the Internet, facilitating exercise advice and member communication through the Internet, and gaining entry through the use of imbedded chip cards), offering limited amenities (members actually have to pay to take a shower and have to purchase drink and food through vending machines), and renting space in secondary locations, has allowed the company to generate, on average, 7,500 members per club and achieve EBITDA margins of over 35 percent. Building on the business model established by McFit, other operators in Germany (e.g., Jumpers, Pure Fitness, Clever Fit, etc.), as well as in the U.K. (e.g., The Gym Group and Fitspace), and most recently, in Spain, have entered the budget segment. This emerging segment of the club market in Europe has placed strong pricing and service pressure on operators, such as Fitness First and LA Fitness, which at one time, were the leading operators of convenient and affordable fitness.

Kiosks, McFit, Munich, Germany

- *Creation and expansion of premium brands.* In the U.K., Virgin Active's acquisition of Holmes Place, a premium brand in the United Kingdom, and most recently Esporta, has allowed Virgin Active to expand and broaden its brand's presence in the premium segment. For example, many of the Holmes Place and Esporta clubs have been repositioned as Virgin Active Classic clubs, which operate in the premium- and luxury-market segments. Fitness First has also used acquisitions, particularly in Germany, to move into the premium segment. By acquiring several premium clubs, Fitness First has established the Black Label brand of Fitness First clubs that targets a more affluent membership audience than the standard Fitness First club.

- *Expansion across national borders.* In the past, many European operators have found it difficult to take their brand to another European nation and operate clubs successfully and profitably. The merger-and-acquisition approach enables club operators to reach across borders and leverage the local talent of an acquired organization to expand their brand's market reach in new national markets. Fitness First, for example, while selling its clubs in the Netherlands and Spain, has expanded its presence in Germany. Health City, which formerly dedicated itself to serving its core markets in the Netherlands, has currently expanded into other markets, such as Spain, through its purchase of Fitness First clubs in those markets. Virgin Active has recently used an acquisition strategy to expand its presence in England, as well as in other European markets, such as Italy.

Opportunities and Challenges for the European Health/Fitness Club Industry

❏ *Opportunities*
*   *Market penetration.* The overall European market has a membership penetration rate that currently runs at approximately 5 percent of the population. While some countries, such as the Netherlands, Spain, and the United Kingdom, have achieved membership penetration rates that approach or even exceed those that exist in the U.S., as a continent overall, a huge opportunity for membership growth exists in Europe. According to the *IHRSA 2010 European Health Club Report*, if those nations within the EU whose penetration percentages are below the EU average were able to bring their market-penetration levels up to the average, it would entail nearly 4,500,000 new members and generate new revenues of nearly 2.3 billion Euros. For operators and investors, this situation is an enormous opportunity.

*   *VAT.* The value added tax (VAT) is a significant issue in many, if not most, of the European nations. The cost impact of VAT to club members in Europe is far greater than sales taxes on club memberships in the U.S. In some countries, the VAT runs over 20 percent. Through the newly formed Brussels-based European Health and Fitness Association (EHFA) and IHRSA Europe, club owners have a unique opportunity to leverage their combined voice with the political leaders of the EU to reduce the VAT burden on the health/fitness club industry. If this goal can be achieved, then the result will be a more affordable club experience for the members, which, in turn, would help increase market penetration and grow industry revenues.

Fitness floor, Jumpers, Munich, Germany

Stephen Tharrett

Portugal provides a great example of how VAT can positively and negatively impact the club industry. A few years back, club operators in Portugal were able to get the VAT on club dues reduced to 5 percent, a significant reduction from the former VAT rate. When the VAT tax reduction was put in place, clubs did not reduce their pricing, and as a result, a greater portion of revenue flowed to the bottom line of each club business. Just this past year, the government pushed the VAT on membership up to 23 percent. Since most club operators could not increase their prices that significantly, the portion of revenues flowing to their bottom line dropped significantly. In those cases where an operator tried to increase the membership price to offset the increased VAT, consumers responded by not purchasing as many memberships. One operator indicated that the added VAT tax could drive as much as 30 percent of the clubs out of business. This example shows both the challenge and the opportunity inherent in VAT policy. If club operators, through the efforts of their European and national associations can get governments to reduce the VAT load, it can have a significant impact on the profitability and growth of the industry.

• *Obesity pandemic.* Unfortunately, the obesity epidemic that has occurred in the U.S. has also "spread" across Europe. Similar to the U.S., the growing trend in obesity among both adults and children is fueling an increase in lifestyle diseases throughout the continent of Europe. This obesity pandemic represents an outstanding opportunity for European club operators to take the lead in their respective communities and serve as facilitators of obesity-prevention and weight-reduction programs. If club operators are able to establish greater credibility as resources and destinations for fighting the obesity pandemic, a surge in club membership growth is quite likely.

Relaxation area, Pfitzenmeier, Schwetzingen, Germany

Stephen Tharrett

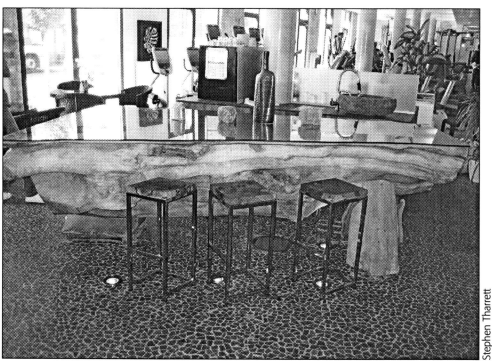

Front Desk, Intenso, Darmstadt, Germany

- *Staff professionalism.* One of the most important steps that European club operators can undertake to enhance their standards and the quality of their services is to employ educated and certified staff. In that regard, EHFA has introduced the very successful REPS program in the U.K. and in the rest of Europe under the name EREPS, which is a web-based, European-wide register for certified fitness professionals. In the past two years, EHFA has released standards that address the competencies and education of fitness instructors and personal trainers. Furthermore, the European Commission has created a think tank called the "EU Platform on Diet, Physical Activity and Health," which is charged with working with private industry to develop specific action-plans to combat lifestyle diseases. Representing the fitness industry on this Platform, EHFA is committed to promoting a healthier Europe.

- *Healthcare.* European operators, like their counterparts in the U.S., have the same opportunity to establish a strong presence in the healthcare continuum. In England, the Fitness Industry Association (FIA) has already made inroads interacting with the healthcare industry by working with one of the country's primary healthcare insurers. Similar efforts are now occurring in other countries in Europe. If the industry is able to make significant inroads in this arena, it will have a huge impact on the health/fitness club industry's growth in Europe. For instance in the Netherlands, one of the leading groups is ACHMEA, a healthcare-insurance company that owns a national chain of 32 health clubs. In Scandinavia, SATS (the leading operator) was purchased in late 2006 by the largest health-insurance company (Trygg) in the region. In the U.K., Cannons (65 clubs) was acquired by Nuffield Hospitals in late 2007, and as a result, a new club brand, called Nuffield Health, was introduced. Nuffield clubs have positioned themselves as a "wellness" and health-promotion group, rather than just a chain of fitness clubs. It is also interesting to note that in Switzerland, about half of the members in the health/fitness club industry receive a subsidy from their health-insurance company. As such, the industry is able to make significant inroads in this arena it will have a huge impact on the industry's growth in Europe.

❑ *Challenges*

• *Commoditization.* The club industry, particularly in the EU, is experiencing incredible merger and acquisition activity. While this situation offers some outstanding opportunities, it also presents the industry with some potentially critical challenges. As clubs continue to merge or be acquired, the tendency is to move more and more toward a commodity-business model and further away from a personalized business offering. Club memberships are different than most retail and service sector experiences. Often, they are unique to a particular geographic region. As such, club operators will need to be cognizant of these subtle but important factors. If the industry moves too fast or too heavily into the commoditization arena, it will potentially sacrifice its ability to create personalized-business models that will enable it to reach into untapped markets. European operators need only look at the U.S. market to see the basic challenge that is inherent in this model.

• *Pricing.* As the top players in the European health/fitness industry continue to expand their reach and influence, the challenge of pricing will raise its ugly head. Larger companies will begin to leverage their operating efficiencies and marketing clout by using price discounts to wage war on their competitors. Furthermore, with the recent advent and rapid growth of budget clubs that have price points that are typically less than 20 Euros a month, pricing pressure on the market has increased. The impact of budget clubs, as well as the pricing power of the very large operators, could be devastating to clubs, both small and large. Already in the U.K., pricing, which was not an issue a decade ago, has become a topic of serious discussion among club

Gym floor, Gym Group, London, England

operators. Again, European operators should learn from the experiences of the U.S. market to find an approach to deal with this potential challenge to their profitability in future years.

- *Talent availability.* One of the biggest challenges any industry faces is finding the appropriate amount and blend of staff talent, especially when it is experiencing exponential growth. As the number of clubs grows, so will the demand for appropriately educated and trained personnel. In the U.S., the health/fitness club industry faces a significant challenge in finding the appropriate leadership and management talent that will allow it to continue experiencing significant profitable growth. Similarly, club operators in many European markets are already beginning to face this challenge. The key to overcoming this challenge is to develop industry-based systems and practices to fuel the internal growth of leadership and management talent.

- *Industry representation.* Unlike the USA, where the commercial health/ fitness club industry is represented by one national association (IHRSA) as well as numerous regional associations, Europe remains fragmented. In fact, many countries do not have a national association (e.g., Russia), or in some instances, the industry associations are operated under a profit umbrella. Perhaps, more importantly, the industry has only recently obtained the needed representation at the political level in Europe, with the formation of EHFA (the European Health and Fitness Association). EHFA's offices in Brussels have given the European industry a boost in its efforts to navigate the political landscape and to gain traction on several agenda items that are important to the continuing success of the industry. Beyond EHFA, only a few countries have managed to establish organizations that can provide assistance in tackling the political and governmental hurdles that face the industry (for example the FIA in the U.K., which has been around for over 15 years, has done an outstanding job representing the interests of the club industry in the U.K.).

Concluding Thoughts

The European health/fitness club industry is possibly the most unique club-related industry in the world. On one end of the spectrum, the European industry is at a level of maturity that rivals and possibly exceeds that of the U.S., with large, professionally run organizations that continue to attract members and investors. On the other end of the spectrum is an industry in its infancy, one trying to establish itself in emerging economies that are still in the process of defining their economic models. What is known, however, is that as a whole, Europe has more clubs, an almost an equal number of club members, and generates greater revenue than the North American market. Over the next 10 years, the health/fitness club industry in Europe will pass the North American market in all of the aforementioned categories. It is also quite possible that Europe's largest club operators will pursue acquisitions in North America.

As a whole, Europe has more clubs, an almost an equal number of club members, and generates greater revenue than the North American market.

27

The Latin American Health/Fitness Club Market

Chapter Objectives

This chapter provides an overview of the Latin American market and the implications that this information holds for the health/fitness club industry in Latin America and throughout the world. The chapter then takes a closer look at the dynamics of the Latin American health/fitness club industry, including some of the differences that exist between this particular club market and other global club markets. Finally, the chapter reviews the opportunities and challenges that may arise for Latin American health/fitness club operators over the next decade.

Overview of the Latin American Market

The Latin American market is comprised of three distinct segments—Central America, South America, and the Caribbean. In total, Latin America is home to approximately 597,283,165 people, with approximately 10 percent of the entire population of the world. Latin America is the third largest global market after Asia and Europe. Population-wise, Latin America is 27 percent smaller than the European market and approximately 70 percent larger than the North American market.

Central America has approximately 156 million residents, while South America has an estimated 441 million residents. Brazil, with nearly 198 million residents, is the largest nation in Latin America and is home to just over 38 percent of the total population of Latin America, and 43 percent of the South American population. Mexico, with an estimated population of just over 112 million residents, is the second largest nation in Latin America and is home to nearly 22 percent of Latin American residents and approximately 72 percent of the population of Central America.

According to the publication, the *IHRSA 2010 Global Report*, which looked at four South American markets (i.e., Argentina, Brazil, Chile, and Uruguay),

Population-wise, Latin America is 27 percent smaller than the European market and approximately 70 percent larger than the North American market.

there were an estimated 21,442 clubs in South America. This data indicates, based on club count, that the South American health/fitness club market is approximately 27 percent larger than the Asian health/fitness club market, approximately 56 percent the size of the North American health/fitness club market, and 46 percent the size of the European health/fitness club market. It should be noted that the 2010 IHRSA report did not include health/fitness club statistics from a number of South American nations and Latin American nations. As a result, the total club count for both South America and Latin America is not an accurate portrayal of the entire Latin American health/fitness club market. It is interesting to note that Brazil, with an estimated 15,551 clubs, has the second largest health/fitness club market in the world. In fact, only the U.S. club market (29,750 clubs) is larger. Brazil, based on the *IHRSA 2010 Global Report*, has 73 percent of the total club count in South America, and is second only to the U.S., with regard to a single nation's dominance of a regional market.

The 15,551 health/fitness clubs in South America serve an estimated population of 6.4 million members or approximately 2.4 percent of the entire population (based on the four South American countries studied). In contrast, the Asian health/fitness club market serves less than 1 percent of its population, the European health/fitness club market serves approximately 5 percent of its population, and the North America health/fitness club market serves approximately 15 percent of its population. The *IHRSA 2008 Global Report* detailed data on one Central American country—Mexico. According to this data, Mexico has approximately 4.6 million members, which means that Mexican club operators have attracted 4 percent of its population for membership. As such, a strong argument can be made that Latin America is a fertile territory for the further development of the health/fitness club industry.

Overview of the Health/Fitness Club Industry in Latin America

The Latin American health/fitness club market, when compared to the club markets in Europe and North America, is still in its infancy (e.g., based on total club count and membership-penetration levels).

❏ *Clubs, Members, and Penetration.* As indicated previously, the South American health/fitness club market, based on data from the four countries studied, is comprised of approximately 15,551 clubs, and approximately 6.4 million members, which generates annual revenues estimated at 1.85 billion (U.S.) annually. Figures 27-1 and 27-2, based on data from the *IHRSA 2008 and 2010 Global Reports*, provide a visual overview of the number of clubs and the club members for several Latin American nations. The data demonstrates that the Latin American health/fitness club market, when compared to the club markets in Europe and North America, is still in its infancy (e.g., based on total club count and membership-penetration levels). At the same time, the health/fitness club market in nations, such as Argentina, Mexico, and Brazil, more closely approximate the level of industry maturity (e.g., based on club counts and membership levels), as seen in markets, such as Germany, Japan, Italy, and the United Kingdom. The health/fitness club market in a few of the urban centers of Latin America, such as Buenos Aires, Argentina; Mexico City, Mexico; and Rio de Janeiro and Sao Paulo in Brazil, rival the sophistication and maturity of health/fitness club markets, such as London, Tokyo, and New York.

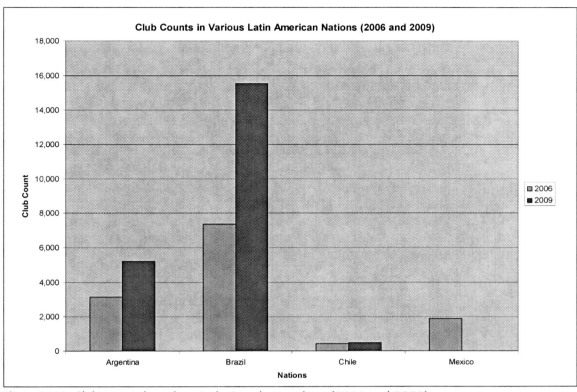

Figure 27-1. Club counts in various Latin American nations (2006 and 2009)

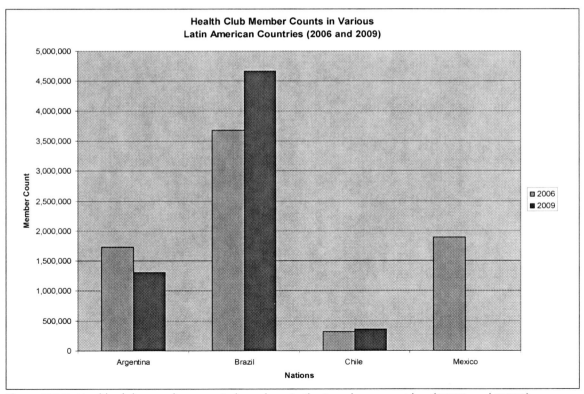

Figure 27-2. Health club member counts in various Latin American countries (2006 and 2009)

Brazil accounts for approximately 73 percent of the number of health/fitness clubs in South America as reported in the *IHRSA 2010 Global Report*, while Argentina accounts for another 24 percent of the market. When industry revenue contributions are considered, Brazil contributes 61 percent of the total revenue generated by South American health/fitness club operators, as reported in the 2010 IHRSA data. In contrast, the revenue generated by clubs in Argentina represents slightly less than 18 percent of the measured market. The metrics of Mexico were not presented in the 2010 report, but were shared in the *IHRSA 2008 Global Report*. These statistics show that Mexico has approximately 2,000 clubs, serving 4.6 million members, generating approximately 1.3 billion in revenue. Based on revenue data, Mexico would be the largest market in Latin America (approximately the same revenues as Brazil), the second largest with regard to the number of members (Brazil is the largest), and the third largest, based on club count (smaller than Brazil and Argentina).

When estimating the health/fitness club industry's growth potential in a market like Latin America, it is critical to look at data on market penetration. The Latin American health/fitness club industry has penetrated less than 3 percent (refer to Figure 27-3 for penetration percentages for the various nations in Latin America) of the eligible population (e.g., based on the nations included in the *IHRSA 2008 and 2010 Global Reports*). When compared to Europe's market penetration of 5 percent and North America's at slightly over 15 percent, these statistics indicate that a large upside for growth exists

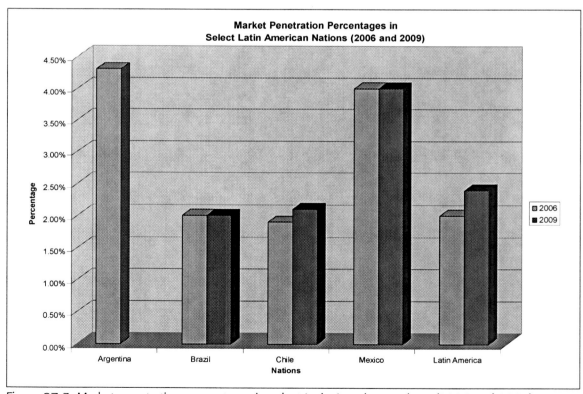

Figure 27-3. Market penetration percentages in select Latin American nations (2006 and 2009)

in Latin America. It should be noted that Mexico, which ranks third in the number of clubs and a close second in revenue generation, ranks first in the region for market penetration, having enrolled approximately 4 percent of the country's population (data from the *IHRSA 2010 Global Report*) in the health/fitness club experience.

In comparison, the other four Latin American nations appearing in IHRSA's 2008 and 2010 reports have achieved membership penetration percentages that are one to two points less than Mexico (e.g., Argentina, 3 percent; Brazil 2 percent; Chile 2.1 percent; and Uruguay 1.6 percent). These market-penetration levels fall considerably below most European nations, and just above most of the Asian nations. Mexico, as the leader in this region, with a market penetration of approximately 4 percent, still falls well below the leading penetration rates that exist in the other regional markets (19 percent by Australia in the Asian Pacific region, 19 percent by Spain in Europe, and 16 percent for the U.S. in North America). Interestingly enough, Brazil, which operates 73 percent of the clubs in the South America nations tracked by IHRSA, and generates 61 percent of the market's total revenue, has only been able to reach 2 percent of its population, similar in many respects to the levels achieved by the Japanese in the Asian market.

IHRSA has accumulated statistical data on the average monthly dues rates in Asia, Europe, and North America, but not for the Latin American market. As a result, specific statistical metrics on dues pricing are unavailable for the various Latin American countries. On the other hand, the authors are familiar with the dues-pricing structure of many of the health/fitness clubs in Brazil, particularly those in Sao Paulo. In clubs, such as those operated by Companhia Athletica and Bio Ritmo Academia, as well as independently run clubs, such as Eco Fit and the Pele Club, monthly dues range from just under $100 to upwards of $125 (U.S.) a month. At first glance, these numbers might seem high when contrasted with the average per-capita income of Brazil (such dues levels represent a staggering 10 percent to 15 percent of the average per-capita income). What must be understood, however, is that many of the premier Brazilian health/fitness clubs serve an affluent audience, whose actual per-capita earnings either equal or frequently exceed the demographic earnings profile of many European and North American club members. In fact, in many smaller markets in Brazil, the dues pricing is considerably lower than in the aforementioned levels.

Many of the premier Brazilian health/fitness clubs serve an affluent audience, whose actual per-capita earnings either equal or frequently exceed the demographic earnings profile of many European and North American club members.

Among the possible reasons to explain why the Latin American health/fitness club market achieves lower levels of market penetration than club operators in Europe or North America are the following:

• *Disposable income of the populace*. The average per-capita earnings across Latin America is $7,500 (U.S.), with the five nations detailed in the *IHRSA 2008 and 2010 Global Reports* having average per-capita incomes in U.S. dollars as follows: Brazil approximately $10,800 annually, Argentina approximately $14,200, Chile approximately $15,400, and Mexico approximately $13,900. According to the Organization of Economic Cooperation and Development (OECD), Latin America has one of the most unequal distributions of income in the world, with

> Since per-capita incomes are so low and income distribution is quite unbalanced, it is somewhat easy to understand why Latin American operators have had less success than their North American and European counterparts penetrating the populace.

the lower 40 percent holding 15 percent of the income and the top 20 percent holding approximately 55 percent. Forty percent of Latin American's live below the poverty line (e.g., $3,000 per-capita income). In contrast, most of Europe and North America have average per-capita incomes of $30,000 and over. Since per-capita incomes are so low and income distribution is quite unbalanced, it is somewhat easy to understand why Latin American operators have had less success than their North American and European counterparts penetrating the populace. In essence, these operators are limited to an audience that represents closer to 20 percent of the total population. If viewed from this perspective, the membership-penetration levels of the health/fitness club industry in the five Latin American nations that are highlighted in the *IHRSA 2008 and 2010 Global Reports* would be closer to 10 percent, and very similar to the penetration levels seen in many European nations and North America.

- *Education levels.* According to global statistics, Latin America has a lower than average level of education among its populace. While the region boasts some outstanding institutions of higher learning, the general population is not as well educated as the residents of either Europe or North America. According to industry statistics provided in the publication, the *IHRSA 2010 Profiles of Success* and other industry-based studies, one of the best predictors of health/fitness club membership is education level (in the U.S., a college education or higher is an excellent predictive demographic for club membership). As a rule, the higher a nation's educational attainment, the higher the level of market penetration for club membership. All factors considered, the educational demographics of the Latin American market are not as suitable for attracting club memberships, when compared to the education demographics of regions such as North America and Europe.

- *Industry longevity.* The Latin American market is relatively new when compared to the markets in either Europe or North America. The Brazilian health/fitness club market has been in existence since the mid-1980s, with Companhia Athletica opening in 1985 and Runner S/A beginning operations in 1983. In Mexico, the industry has been in existence for just over 40 years, with Organizacion Britania opening its doors to the public in 1970. While industry players, such as Companhia Athletica, Runner S/A, and Organizacion Britania, have been in business for nearly as long as the leading club operators in Europe, Japan, and North America, the majority of club operators in Latin America have been in business for less than 15 years, and, in many cases, for less than a decade. As a result, health/fitness clubs are still a relatively new industry in Latin America. As industry longevity increases, the public's awareness of it will also increase, thus fueling the industry's growth.

❑ *Membership Characteristics.* Data pertaining to the general membership characteristics of the Latin American club market are not as readily available as they are for North America and Europe. While the age, gender, and general-usage demographics of club members in Europe and the U.S. have been published by IHRSA in various reports (e.g., the *IHRSA 2008 and*

2010 European Market Reports and the *IHRSA 2010 Profiles of Success*), no such data has been released with regard to Latin America. Based on personal observations on visits by the author to the Latin American market and conversations with a few of the leading club operators in the respective markets during those visits, the following points can be made about the membership characteristics and activities of the Latin American club market:

- In Brazil, as well as in Argentina and Mexico, the typical health/fitness club member has a higher per-capita income and household income than his counterparts in Europe or North America. This situation is, in part, the result of a dues-pricing policy that is affordable to only a certain market demographic. Based on the region's market demographics, most health/fitness club members in Latin America come from the top 20 percent of household incomes.

- It appears that the general age demographics of a Latin American health fitness club member more closely parallels the age statistics reflected in Europe and North America than those of Asia. In North America, the 35 to 54 age demographic is the largest, while the 18 to 34 age demographic is slightly larger in Europe. It could be argued that the 35 to 54 age demographic in Latin America may be slightly larger than the 18 to 34 age demographic because of financial considerations.

- Similar to other global geographic regions, a larger percentage of health/fitness club members in Latin America are women. It appears that the percentage of Latin American health/fitness club members who are women is comparable to the percentages seen in North America and many European nations (which range from 50 percent to 60 percent).

- Group-exercise classes are extremely popular. One indicator of this high popularity of group exercise is the level of market penetration achieved by the Les Mills group-exercise programs. For example, Les Mills has over twice the number of licensed programs in Brazil, as it does in the U.S., and yet, Brazil has only approximately half the numbers of clubs as the U.S. The range of group-exercise programs offered in Latin America easily rivals the selection of classes available in either Europe or the U.S.

- Cardiovascular training, resistance training, and free-weight training are all popular activities, and compare favorably with the usage levels seen in Europe and the U.S.

*Additional information about the membership characteristics of the Latin American market can be obtained by contacting the International Health, Racquet & Sportsclub Association, based in Boston, MA.

Similar to other global geographic regions, a larger percentage of health/fitness club members in Latin America are women.

The Leading Players in the Latin American Health/Fitness Club Market

The Latin American market differs considerably from the Asian, European, and North American markets, with regard to the role that the key industry players have in influencing the overall health/fitness club market. In Latin America, the largest industry players own and operate between one dozen and two dozen clubs, with the exception of Organizacion Britania in Mexico, which oversees approximately 51 clubs that have revenues approaching $40 million (U.S.). It should be noted that a significant portion of the company's clubs are licensed operations. Another leading operator in Mexico is Sport City, which operates five distinct brands and over 35 clubs. In Brazil, Companhia Athletica operates 13 clubs, with revenues of approximately $42 million (U.S.), and Bio Ritmo Academia, which operates approximately 20 clubs, has revenues approximating $29 million (U.S.). In Argentina, Megatlon operates 23 clubs and reports annual revenues of around $25 million (U.S.). While these statistics are impressive, they pale in comparison to the leading club companies in Asia, Europe, and the U.S., where companies such as Fitness First of the U.K., 24 Hour Fitness of the U.S., and Konami of Japan all operate well in excess of 250 clubs, and all have revenues approaching one billion $U.S. In these other global regional markets, especially in Europe and North America, numerous club companies either operate in excess of 50 clubs and/or generate club-based revenue exceeding $100 million (U.S.) annually.

When the Latin American market is viewed on a nation-by-nation basis, it is evident that each of these national markets has yet to be dominated by one single player, a situation that has occurred in Asia, Europe, and North America. The Latin American market seems to consist primarily of some small, yet dominant, brands—such as Compania Athletica, Brazil; Bio Ritmo, Brazil, Runner/SA, Brazil; Megatlon, Argentina; Organizacion Britania, Mexico; Sport City, Mexico; and BodyTech, Columbia—who operate between two and four dozen clubs, and then a host of smaller and less-recognizable brands that operate from one to a half-dozen clubs. In only one instance does a Latin American health/fitness club company own or operate more than 2 percent of the clubs in its nation—Organizacion Britania of Mexico. In comparison, in Asia, Europe, and North America, several club companies have greater than 2 percent penetration of their national market. Another interesting point that can be made about health/fitness club operators in Latin America is that the leading club brands have stayed within their own national markets and have not attempted to expand their operations into adjacent national markets, such as has occurred in Europe and some of the Asian nations.

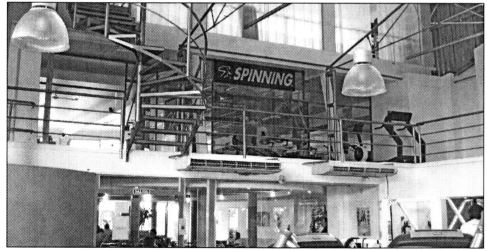

Interior, Megatlon, Argentina

The Latin American market has not experienced the merger and acquisition activity that has occurred among its European counterparts, or the large influx of private equity that has fueled the incredible growth of some club operations in Europe and North America. The environment for mergers or acquisitions does not seem as opportunistic, at least at this point in time, as they are in Europe and North America. As of yet, private equity firms have not taken the big leap into the Latin American market, as witnessed in the European and North American markets.

Opportunities and Challenges for the Latin American Market

❑ *Opportunities*
  • *Increased market penetration.* As an industry in its infancy, the health/
    fitness club industry in Latin America has an incredible future ahead of it.
    As the statistics show, with approximately 2 percent market penetration in
    the leading Latin American markets (e.g., Argentina, Brazil, Chile, Mexico,
    and Uruguay) served by health/fitness clubs and less than 1 percent
    in the other national markets of Latin America, the opportunity for new
    business development is immense. Brazil and Mexico, both with well-
    developed health/fitness club markets, are only penetrating between 2
    and 4 percent of a combined population, approximating 310 million
    people. If the market penetration of just these two markets increases to
    the average level of the European market (e.g., 5 percent penetration),
    the total membership base in Latin America would increase by nearly 11
    million members. Imagine the opportunities for club operators if market
    penetration in these countries, as well as the other Latin American
    nations, were to approach 3 to 5 percent penetration levels.

> As an industry in its infancy, the health/fitness club industry in Latin America has an incredible future ahead of it.

  • *Consolidation.* The Latin American market, possibly more than any
    other global regional market, is ripe for consolidation. With the leading
    companies only operating between a dozen and two dozen clubs, the
    right consolidation of industry leaders could lead to a global industry
    leader, as well as efficiencies that might lead to further growth within the
    various domestic markets. Consolidation is a by-product of merger and
    acquisition activity, which, in turn, is driven by the influx of private equity
    into the market. As a result, attracting private-equity investment is also a
    great opportunity for the Latin American market.

❑ *Challenges*
  • *Economic clout.* The most significant hurdle for the Latin American
    market involves the economic conditions and earning power of its
    citizens. As discussed previously, the majority of Latin American citizens
    don't have the financial resources to make club membership a part
    of their day-to-day routine. Until a larger segment of the population
    achieves the economic equivalency of middle-class status, the health/
    fitness club industry in Latin America will have a difficult time achieving
    rapid growth. Over the past few years, Brazil has emerged as a growing
    global economic power, and as a result, it may lead the rest of Latin
    America into a more prosperous economic environment.

- *Education*. As detailed previously, the overall education level of many Latin Americans is below that of their counterparts in markets of other regions, such as Europe and North America. Health/fitness club membership penetration parallels the education level of the market, and as a result, one of the challenges that operators in Latin America face is finding a means to bring fitness education to the market.

- *Talent availability*. Finding, identifying, and hiring talented staff is a global challenge, not just a challenge for Latin America. Nonetheless, in order for the industry to achieve significant growth, health/fitness club operators in Latin America will have to establish results-driven strategies to quickly develop fitness professionals, who can step in and manage their clubs.

Concluding Thoughts

While Latin America is the third largest geographic populace in the world, this continent encompasses only approximately 10 percent of the world's population. Brazil, the largest nation in Latin America and currently the most dominant economically, is recognized as one of the three emerging global economic giants, along with China and India. This combination of populace size and growing economic clout suggest a market that may in the next 20 years be one of the leading health/fitness club markets in the world. The Latin American health/ fitness club market is an emerging and dynamic one that is being fueled by the efforts of several excellent operators, including Bio Ritmo, BodyTech, Companhia Athletica, Megatlon, Organizacion Britania, and Runner S/A, among others.

In Argentina, Brazil, and Mexico, the club industry is well established and serves as a template for entrepreneurs in other Latin American markets who wish to build successful and profitable club companies. In addition, the growth of industry publications, such as *Mercado Fitness*, based in Argentina, and *Fitness Business Brazil*, and the continuing development of large industry meetings directed toward health/fitness professionals, such as those organized by Fitness Brazil and Mercado Fitness, are two of the factors helping to spur the spread of the health/fitness club industry across the Latin American continent.

Pool lobby, Ecofit, Sao Paulo, Brazil

THE FUTURE OF THE HEALTH/FITNESS CLUB INDUSTRY

Medioimages/Photodisc

Part Nine

28

The Future of the Health/Fitness Club Industry

Chapter Objectives

The health/fitness club industry is an evolving entity, both domestically and internationally. While it is more of an accepted part of the American culture and lifestyle than it was 40 years ago or even a decade ago, the industry remains somewhat susceptible to the whims of changing demographics and trendy popular culture. Several factors involving these demographics and the popular culture may have a significant impact on the club industry over the next two to three decades. The more clubs are aware of those factors and respond accordingly, the more the industry will be able to sustain continued growth and profitability. This chapter details seven important demographic and cultural trends and the potential impact these trends will have on the future of the health/fitness club market.

Seven Important Demographic and Cultural Trends That Will Shape the Future of the Health/Fitness Club Market

1. The Age Wave: Baby Boomers and Echo Boomers

The initial decades of the 21st century will be impacted significantly by two age-related demographic trends. The first factor is the aging of the "baby boomers," 78 million U.S. adults and over 600 million global adults who were born after 1946 and who, collectively, are the wealthiest population in the world. Baby boomers represent an aging and affluent generation of "me"-oriented adults, seeking the fountain of youth. This population is willing and able to spend the money necessary to strive for their goals. This demographic wave also represents the largest population segment in several nations, such as England, Germany, Italy, and Japan. According to global statistics, it is estimated that by 2050 there will be approximately two billion people age 60 and older.

The second factor is a population referred to by demographers as the "echo boomers," or "millennial generation," a group of individuals who were born after 1981. Seventy-seven million strong, the echo boomers are the second

> The initial decades of the 21st century will be impacted significantly by two age-related demographic trends.

largest demographic population in the U.S. This group grew up in the era of technology, social media, and multi-tasking. Echo boomers are attuned to the environment, are computer savvy, socially connected via the Internet, and possibly more significantly, are rebelling against many of the institutions created by the baby boomers.

According to global demographers, nations can be classified into one of four core age profiles, based on the percentage of their population that is under the age of 30 (echo boomers): very young (66 percent of the population under age 30), youthful (60 percent of the population under age 30), transitional (between 45 percent and 60 percent of the population under age 30), or mature (less than 45 percent of the population under age 30). To a degree, these classifications indicate that the very young, youthful, and even transitional markets are very strongly influenced by the echo-boomer wave, while nations that have substantial transitional and mature markets are more heavily influenced by baby boomers. It is interesting to note that all of North America, Europe (including Russia), and Australia have substantial mature populations, in which baby boomers have a significant influence with regard to purchasing behavior and other trends. On the flip side, most of Asia, Latin America, and Africa feature markets that can be defined as being very young, youthful, and in a few cases, transitional. In those markets, the echo boomers are the dominant demographic influence.

The potential business implications for the health/fitness club industry of serving two diverse demographic populations, such as baby boomers and echo boomers, may include:

❏ Implications Driven by the Baby Boomer Population:
  • Exercise for health and well-being will take center stage. While baby boomers want to extend their lifespan, more importantly, they want to enjoy life as long as they can. As the saying goes, 60 is the new 40!
  • Programming will need to focus on creating results for those with growing physical limitations and increased disease states.
  • Health/fitness professionals will need to be educated in working with individuals who have special conditions, with a focus on creating exercise progressions that accommodate the interests, needs, and goals of those with health-related problems.
  • Member service will become essential to the overall member experience, as aging and affluent members seek more personalized encounters.

❏ Implications Driven by the Echo Boomers:
  • Clubs will need to incorporate new programs and services that encompass virtual platforms. Member blogs, virtual personal-training sites, and virtual communication will become necessary in attracting this generation. Social media sites, such as Facebook and YouTube, will become essential tools in reaching out to the echo boomers.
  • Entertainment will take on greater importance, since echo boomers need and want to be entertained when they exercise. As a result, clubs will need to redefine entertainment, since echo boomers connect entertainment to technology in many instances.

Health/fitness professionals will need to be educated in working with individuals who have special conditions, with a focus on creating exercise progressions that accommodate the interests, needs, and goals of those with health-related problems.

- Clubs will need to re-think how they deliver the club experience, because echo boomers prefer to be involved in the service-delivery process.
- Coaching skills will become a critical part of management's arsenal, since employees from this generation respond less favorably to baby-boomer management techniques, such as, "do it or else."

2. The State of Health: A Shifting Paradigm

In just the past decade, the world has seen an exponential increase in obesity and the many negative health conditions that are attendant to obesity. According to researchers, it is believed that for the first time in the history of mankind, children will die at a younger age than their parents. The increasing role of technology in the world has created a generation of adults who move less, eat more, and as a result, experience significantly higher rates of obesity and obesity-related disorders, such as diabetes, heart disease, and cancer. The fact that the healthcare system is broken only exacerbates the situation. Built on a model of expensive treatment, rather than inexpensive prevention, the healthcare system is overtaxed, and in many cases, not within the financial reach of the average person. These factors present both a challenge and an opportunity for the health/fitness club industry. The potential business implications of a changing state of health in the health/fitness industry may include:

- Fitness providers must establish greater credibility with the healthcare industry in an effort to be perceived as an essential provider of preventative health services.
- Fitness programming will need to evolve into specialized niches for various special populations, such as arthritic, obese, diabetic, and COPD, among others.
- Fitness professionals will need to expand their educational horizons and become better educated in subject matter related to healthcare. Basic fitness certifications will become an outdated notion of the past, as the credentials of fitness professionals will align more with those of other healthcare professionals, such as physical therapists and nurses.
- Alternative and complimentary medicine will slowly emerge as an entirely new and profitable programming segment for many health/fitness clubs.

Fitness providers must establish greater credibility with the healthcare industry in an effort to be perceived as an essential provider of preventative health services.

3. The Wealth Gap and Income Inequality

According to researchers, approximately 1 percent of adults hold 40 percent of the world's wealth, while another 50 percent of the population have another 1 percent of the world's wealth. In addition, approximately 10 percent of adults hold 85 percent of the world's wealth, which means that the remaining 90 percent hold only 15 percent of the globe's wealth. Regionally, the U.S., Japan, China, England, and Germany hold over 50 percent of the world's net worth. Since the mid-90s, the disparity between those who have money and those who don't has continued to grow. This trend of wealth inequality is not limited to the U.S., rather it is an international trend. According to recent government data, over 100 million Americans are classified as being below the poverty line. This growing disparity represents a significant challenge to those in the health/fitness club industry. On one hand, the industry must balance between the desire to appeal to a larger audience of prospective members, many of whom have little disposable income, while on the other hand, it must operate profitably and compete with multiple new competitors for a small fragment of the population that has enough wealth to spend liberally on its services. The potential business implications of wealth disparity in the health/fitness club industry may include:

- Owners and operators will need to create new business models that will provide an appealing and results-oriented environment for those individuals with relatively low levels of discretionary income. While the emergence of budget clubs may be one answer to this situation, it is not likely the only one.

- Clubs may have to adapt their current business model to accommodate a new delivery model that focuses on providing club-like experiences over the Internet and through less expensive virtual environments. Because the use of virtual-training environments will continue to evolve, club operators will need to find a way to employ these non-traditional training platforms to reach out to new audiences.

- Clubs may need to adapt to becoming resource centers that provide fitness and physical activity outside their physical facilities. Appealing to the less-affluent will require a less asset-oriented approach.

- Owners who understand how to deliver transformational experiences that have been built on a foundation of authenticity will be able to create niche business models that are appealing to the most affluent, and thus generate significant profitability by serving a relatively small, but affluent, audience.

4. Globalization: The World Is Now One

The 21st century is an era of cultural fusion, one in which physical borders alone no longer allow individuals to be protective of their independent cultures. Technology has shrunk the world and, in many cases, erased many of the cultural borders and protections of the past decades. At the present time, countries and cultures have fused together in a mesh of economic and popular culture. As indicated by the title of Thomas L. Friedman's landmark book, *The World is Flat*, the globe has become significantly more fused, and as a result, most business and cultural phenomena can literally impact the entire world within minutes. This fusion of cultures means that the communities served by health/fitness clubs are no longer represented by a singular audience, but instead consist of multiple audiences—each with its own set of unique preferences and traditions.

> Technology has shrunk the world and, in many cases, erased many of the cultural borders and protections of the past decades.

According to the *IHRSA 2010 Global Report*, less than 30 percent of all health/fitness club members reside in the U.S. While the U.S. still has the largest number of clubs and members, its domination of the industry is slowly losing out to a global encroachment of outstanding club operators and a global market that is more aware of the value of fitness. The potential business implications for a global health/fitness industry may include:

- Industry best practices will continue to emerge from several markets, such as Asia, Europe, and Latin America. Industry trends will no longer be the

The Future of the Health/Fitness Club Industry

sole domain of U.S. clubs, but instead will represent a blend of fused ideas from many nations (for example, the explosion of Zumba).

- Individual communities served by health/fitness facilities will continue to see a more diverse membership, made up of people who speak different languages and, more importantly, have different values and interests. Clubs will need to expand programming and find niche programs that appeal to various global audiences. Already in parts of the U.S. (California, Texas, and Wisconsin, for example), club operators are finding they have to introduce new programs to satisfy the cultural needs of its contingency.

- Clubs will begin considering niche markets, based on cultural background. As a result, new social communities will be created around physical activity. In turn, a club targeted toward specific ethnic and cultural communities will not be far behind.

- Fitness professionals will seek opportunities around the globe, thus changing the dynamics of employee recruitment. Global players will be forced to compete for the best talent in the health/fitness club industry.

5. Green: Reconnecting With Nature

The 21st century has evolved into a time of environmental consciousness. Individuals and businesses have become more conscious of the need to protect the world's natural resources. Global warming and dwindling energy sources have created a sense of urgency in the global mindset to think and act in a manner that protects, rather than scavenges, the environment. Automakers are building and selling hybrid vehicles with lower emissions and greater energy efficiency. Developers are creating more "green" buildings—buildings that are constructed with sustainable and renewable products and that are more energy efficient. Suddenly, it is "cool" to think and even act "green." Corporations now speak a mantra of environmental consciousness in the hopes of appealing to the ever-growing consumer audience who wants all things "green." The potential business implications for going "green" in the health/fitness club industry may include:

Global warming and dwindling energy sources have created a sense of urgency in the global mindset to think and act in a manner that protects, rather than scavenges, the environment.

- Clubs will need to consider the use of environmentally friendly products for cleaning their facilities, as consumers demand less use of environmentally unfriendly, cleaning products.

- Clubs will need to incorporate sustainable products in their new construction and renovation. Renewable woods, bamboo, cork, recycled glass, solar power, recycled rubber, and reclaimed rain water will become essential elements in the design and construction of health/fitness clubs. At Ecofit in Brazil, the club harnesses both reclaimed rain water and solar energy to power its club.

- Clubs will need to be seen as supporters of the "green" push in their communities. At Ecofit in Sao Paulo, Brazil, the club provides recycling containers, in which members can deposit paper, glass, metal, and even technology equipment will later be recycled.

- Clubs will need to provide programming that helps their members connect with the environment in a manner that allows them to feel they are one with nature, and just as importantly, doing something to help the environment.

- Clubs will need to move away from equipment that is energy inefficient and move toward equipment that places fewer demands on the environment.

6. Narcissistic Capitalism and Karaoke Innovation

Narcissistic capitalism refers to a highly selfish and self-serving form of capitalism that is all about "me," or in the case of global economics, a small clan of investment bankers, private-equity houses, and private investors. In narcissistic capitalism, making money is both the end and the means. It is also a situation in which ethics take a back seat to integrity. The global economic meltdown of 2008, 2009, and 2010 was, in large part, due to this narcissistic approach to generating wealth in an ethically challenged manner. It would appear that the lessons of the recession have not had much of an influence on this highly evolved form of autocratic-style capitalism.

An excellent example of the aforementioned narcissistic phenomena is the acquisitions of several health/fitness club firms during the middle of the last decade. During the first five to six years of the 21st century, PE firms purchased club companies for large multiples (equivalent to 8 to 12 times EBITDA), and funded the purchases with high levels of debt (i.e., interest-coverage ratios that were less than 1.5). These highly leveraged deals resulted in some businesses declaring bankruptcy, others selling for a loss, many dramatically restructuring their debt and organizational structures, and, in some cases, the purchaser holding on to the investment longer than desired because they could not sell the business for at least the purchase price.

In their book, *Karaoke Capitalism*, the authors, Jonas Ridderstrale and Kjell A. Nordstrom, speak about a business environment in which innovation has given way to replication. Rather than create new business models, business leaders are recycling and putting a new skin on old ideas. The authors claim that this karaoke mindset is slowly creating a commoditized world, one in which businesses are becoming more like physical commodities than unique business models that focus on the needs of consumers. In the past 5 to 10 years, the health/fitness club industry has seen an influx of highly leveraged venture capital enter the industry. This influx of highly leveraged capital has resulted in the creation of numerous large and successful club models that essentially all lookalike (e.g., LA Fitness, 24 Hour Fitness, Urban Active, Fitness First, etc.). The demand for high returns and rapid growth from investors has helped the industry become more commoditized, rather than more unique. Among the potential business implications for the club industry of this growing commoditization are the following:

> The demand for high returns and rapid growth from investors has helped the industry become more commoditized, rather than more unique.

- Well-capitalized and well-leveraged club companies will bring about further consolidation of the industry, both domestically and globally. Like Walmart in the retail sector, one of these well-capitalized club companies could further drive the pricing wars in the years to come. In England, Virgin Active was able to purchase two other club operators, as a result of Virgin Active's capitalization and the overleveraged position of the companies that they purchased.
- Over leveraged companies will either be sold at well below initial shareholder value or declare bankruptcy, in order to alleviate much of their debt.

- Entrepreneurs will seek out new niche markets by creating unique business models that hold little value to the large commodity players. Entrepreneurs will perish if they are unable to create unique business models that target markets that are less appealing to the commodity players.
- Fitness professionals will need to become fluent in the culture and language of business. Fitness professionals will need to become as well-versed in business as they are in fitness.
- The industry will need to find a balance between growing the bottom line and creating an environment that provides clients with a transformational and results-oriented experience.

7. Technology: The Antithesis of Activity

Over the past decade, technological advances have evolved so rapidly that the world seems to change as fast as technology innovates. The growth in portable electronic communications (e.g., smart phones, hand-held computers and tablets, satellite-based broadband networks, etc.), the evolution of virtual worlds and social networking sites, and the continued growth in virtual games that enable individuals to do more by physically doing less is creating an entirely new business and operational framework for the health/fitness club industry. While technology has given the world many wonderful and helpful tools, it has also created a society that is less inclined to be physically active and interpersonally engaging. As technology continues to evolve at lightening speed, people will have less reason to be active and even less reason to interact with others in a face-to-face environment. As a result, individuals will be able to travel across nations virtually, but may not be able to walk across the street without the help of an AED. Among the potential implications of the technological boom for the health/fitness club industry are the following:

While technology has given the world many wonderful and helpful tools, it has also created a society that is less inclined to be physically active and interpersonally engaging.

- Clubs may need to create virtual environments to supplement their physical environments. Marketing and even basic programming may begin in the virtual world in an effort to draw interest in the physical world. Facebook, Twitter, and YouTube will be a part of every club's lexicon, and in a few years, operators will ask how they ever operated without them.
- Web-based exercise programming may become as important as in-club personal training is currently. Getting members started through virtual personal training may lead to new clients for in-club personal training and programming. In reality, members can currently leverage great personal training and nutritional tools on their computer or smart phone.
- The use of technology to monitor and communicate with members will free up staff to work more directly with those members who need personal attention and instruction. Eye scans and facial recognition for member check-in, fingerprint or chip entry to lockers, web-based scheduling for programs, and real-time communication with members may become essential to the successful club of the future.
- Entertainment, especially for the echo boomers, will require the creative use of technology.

No one can accurately predict the future, including that of the health/fitness club industry. The real key to success for club owners and operators over the

"It appears that when we first gaze into our past, we elongate our future."

next two decades will come from understanding the demographic and cultural forces driving the world, understanding the rich history of the industry, and creating innovative solutions that build on that understanding. A quote from an unknown author may have summed it up best by saying, "It appears that when we first gaze into our past, we elongate our future." This chapter has attempted to view the recent past through a discussion of current and emerging trends, with the hope that the information presented can be utilized to elongate the future of the health/fitness club industry.

CASE STUDIES IN THE HEALTH/FITNESS CLUB INDUSTRY

Jupiterimages

Part Ten

The only way to really learn management and leadership is by dealing with the unique and unexpected situations that often transpire when working with members and employees.

My first manager called it, "baptism by fire." He was referring to the leadership and management scenarios that occur in the health/fitness club industry that are not taught in textbooks. Later in my career, I decided that his primary point was that the only way to really learn management and leadership is by dealing with the unique and unexpected situations that often transpire when working with members and employees. Most first-time managers and leaders enter their new roles armed with a rudimentary understanding of the basic principles of financial management, leadership, programming, sales and marketing, member/customer relations, and employee relations. In reality, such basic competencies will only carry a person so far in business. Individuals who want to operate a great club—one that is known for its outstanding member/customer service—must be prepared to lead and manage during challenging and unexpected circumstances. Addressing these events in an appropriate manner is an ever-evolving process that can benefit from continual nurturing. Among the steps that can be undertaken in this regard is to study and learn from the problem-solving efforts of others in particular situations.

This part of the book presents a recap of several of the most demanding and challenging situations that actually occurred in the club business and how seasoned and not-so-seasoned leaders and managers dealt with them. Information about these scenarios has been provided by some of the industry's most seasoned professionals. Collectively, the individuals who shared their experiences and the actions they took to address them have over 300 years experience in the health/fitness club industry. It is important to note that each of the scenarios recounted in Chapters 29 to 31 represents events that actually occurred. The individuals involved are actual people, either club members or employees (although for privacy reasons, no names are used in the chronicles, and the locale of each story has been changed). The chronicles presented in this part are grouped into three basic scenarios. Chapter 29 addresses scenarios that involved customers and members of clubs. Chapter 30 deals with employee scenarios, while Chapter 31 features a series of synopses involving business scenarios.

Each management scenario is defined in three parts. The first part describes the event or scenario; the second summarizes the solution or response of management; and the third discusses the event and solution.

The primary objective of Part X is to provide an opportunity to consider and examine selected leadership/managerial-related scenarios that typically are not addressed in either formal schooling programs or company-sponsored managerial training efforts. Equally important is seeing and reflecting on how experienced professionals dealt with each set of circumstances. All factors considered, studying these unique business scenarios can help individuals to be better prepared to lead through the most challenging of situations.

29

Customer and Member Chronicles

Chapter Objectives

The situations recounted in this chapter focus on events and experiences involving the customers and members of health/fitness clubs. Each of these stories represents a unique situation that required extraordinary leadership and management.

Sun Wars

❏ *Scenario.* In the mid-80s, a high-end club located in the northeast had just completed an extensive renovation. Serving approximately 2,000 memberships with an average household income in excess of $200,000 annually, the club had a fitness center, group-exercise studios, locker rooms, dining area, pool, and sun deck.

The new fitness director had just been hired. One of the first stories he heard from his colleagues concerned the "sun wars" that were occurring on the club's sun deck, which was located eight stories above street level. He was told that over the past few summers, members had hit each other, stole others items from the sun deck, and thrown lifeguards in the pool— all in an effort to get one of the 30 lounge chairs that were located on the sun deck. Rather than take these stories at face value, the new fitness director decided to observe the actions of the club's members and staff. Since the sun deck did not officially open until Memorial Day, the fitness director felt that by observing events in the spring, he might be able to gain a better idea of what was really happening. After a couple of sunny weekends, the fitness director observed a litany of troubling events, including one of the facility's lifeguards being hit and thrown into the pool, member's clothes that were hanging on lounge chairs being thrown off the deck, members pulling each other's hair as they pulled each other off lounge chairs, members yelling at each other when they thought it was time for them to have a lounge chair, and verbal and physical threats being made against staff by members.

> Rather than take these stories at face value, the new fitness director decided to observe the actions of the club's members and staff.

The fitness director met with his senior-level department heads and a few members to try to identify a possible solution that would eliminate the dangerous situation and, hopefully, produce a mutually satisfactory outcome for all involved.

❏ *The Solution.* The fitness director met with his senior-level department heads and a few members to try to identify a possible solution that would eliminate the dangerous situation and, hopefully, produce a mutually satisfactory outcome for all involved. After considerable discussion, a solution was proposed that included the following elements:

• A reservation system for lounge chairs was developed that would allow members to reserve a specific chair up to seven days in advance.

• Each lounge chair would be marked with a number and a corresponding reservation card, and a chair-reservation book would be prepared for the summer and kept at the front desk.

• A sun deck map was devised that showed the location of the lounge chairs.

• A ten-dollar charge to reserve a chair for a two-hour time period would be implemented.

• A cancellation and no-show policy would be instituted. If someone failed to cancel their chair reservation at least 24-hours in advance or if they did not show to claim their reservation, they would be charged the full amount for their lounge chair.

• The reservation, which had to be made in person or over the phone, could be made no earlier than seven days in advance.

• A concierge would be provided for the deck and would circulate every couple of hours with the reservation sheet to verify reservations and to pass out complimentary beverages.

• Details about the chair-reservation program would be communicated to the members, approximately two months before it was set to begin. Such efforts would include such steps as sending a personal letter to each member, placing posters up in conspicuous locations in the facility, putting notices in the club's member newsletter, and having the staff speak to the members they know.

When the chair-reservation program was first introduced to the members, the club received considerable feedback from the membership, most of which was not very flattering. And yet, one week before Memorial Day, all of the lounge chairs had been reserved, and a waiting list had been created. Over the course of the first summer, the chairs were 100 percent booked each weekend in two-hour time slots, with a waiting list of at least 10 people each weekend. By the July 4th weekend, the club had introduced food-and-drink service. During the first summer of the program, only one argument ensued. As a result, the club's members and staff did not have to deal with all of the fights and disorder that had previously existed. Another positive by-product of the new policy was the fact that the club generated approximately $1,000 to $1,500 in revenue each weekend.

❏ *Discussion.* The aforementioned scenario is an example of a club not listening to its membership and understanding that a membership need existed that was not being addressed with an appropriate service-delivery process. The members wanted to see and feel the sun, a goal that was not so easily attained in this northeastern market. The members also needed to know that once they had a spot on the sun deck, that someone could not just walk up and take it. In essence, it was a basic supply-and-demand situation that had evolved into a member/customer relations headache for the club and, in the end, had led to a considerable degree of member/customer outrage. The proposed solution worked for the following reasons:

- The staff took the time to talk with members and staff, as well as observe the situation before attempting to identify a solution. Because the club got everyone involved in the situation in its efforts to understand the attendant circumstances, those individuals took ownership of the subsequent solution.
- The solution leveraged the supply-and-demand issue and provided the facility's customers and members with the opportunity to get what they wanted on a relatively exclusive basis.
- Value was created where it did not exist before. By putting a time limit on the use of a chair, setting a price for the service, and requiring reservations, the club had established a value for the sun deck.
- The club communicated its intentions sufficiently in advance so that it could address any concerns that might arise well before the program went into place.
- The club took a dynamic approach to the solution by continually offering new services to the members.

In reality, other possible solutions to the situation existed, including closing the deck, incorporating a reservation system but not charging for it, selling the chairs for the season, etc. Ultimately, the solution that was implemented achieved its desired goal of preventing more fights. It also resulted in an unexpected benefit—additional revenue and cash for the club.

Odor Eaters

❑ *Scenario.* This situation occurred in the mid-90s and involved a high-end club that was located on the west coast. The club had 2,500 memberships and provided full-service amenities. One of the unique services of this club was that all of the members rented lockers ($25 a month), which included access to such amenities as laundry service and shoeshines. Each individual paid an initiation fee of $1,000 to join this facility and $100 monthly dues to maintain their individual membership.

The fitness director, who had responsibility for the locker rooms and the fitness areas of the club, was approached by several members complaining about one of the club's most prominent constituents. Their grievance involved the fact that this particular individual had a very distinct aroma about him, both when he exercised and in the locker room. In fact, several of the complaining members stated that they would resign their membership if the offensive odor problem was not resolved. These members made it clear who the offending member was and that they did not want it to be known that they had complained. His pungent aroma made it difficult not only for other people to be on the exercise floor at the same time with him, but also (and possibly worse) to be in the locker room area around his locker.

The solution leveraged the supply-and-demand issue and provided the facility's customers and members with the opportunity to get what they wanted on a relatively exclusive basis.

❏ *The Solution*. Understandably, the fitness director was very concerned. He was fully aware of the fact that the offending individual was an important member who spent a considerable amount of money in the club. He also knew that the club could not afford to lose the other members. The effort to identify a possible solution to this problem involved the following steps:

- He talked privately with the members who had complained in an attempt to get a better handle on the issues. He also told them that he would be taking action on their concerns.
- He spoke with his staff to get additional information on the situation. In addition, he checked out the offending member's locker during after-hours.
- He subsequently contacted the offending member by phone and asked if there was a time that they could meet. A meeting was set up in one of the private offices of the club. During the meeting, the fitness director told the individual about the other club members' concerns. The fitness director then asked the individual to express his feelings about the issue. The member was upset and wanted to know who was complaining. The fitness director replied that he understood the member's hurt feelings and that he would like to work with him to resolve the issue.
- The member and fitness director agreed to take several steps, including the club would provide the member with free laundry service for his clothes and provide him with his own soap solution that he could keep in his locker. Furthermore, the club agreed that they would always check to make sure that the member's laundry was done, even if he did not leave it out for laundering.
- The fitness director got in contact with the members who had complained and informed them that he had talked with the member who had the odor problem and that a solution had been reached. He told them that he appreciated their bringing this matter to his attention and asked that they let him know if the proposed solution did not work to their satisfaction.

❏ *Discussion*. This scenario is one that will likely occur at some point in every health/fitness club, especially if the facility provides rental lockers. When a facility has a diverse membership that extensively utilizes the club's services during the hours that it is open, it can expect situations such as this to occur. While no "perfect" solution to this kind of situation and problem exists, the club in this scenario handled the circumstances in a professional manner. The aforementioned solution worked for several reasons, including:

- The manager took the time to gather information about the situation by talking to members and staff and by personally observing what was occurring.
- The manager made sure to let the members who were complaining know that he would address the situation and get back to them.
- The manager set up a private appointment with the offending member. During that meeting, as professionally as he could, he discussed the situation that had been brought to his attention. Furthermore, he asked

> **The member and fitness director agreed to take several steps, including the club would provide the member with free laundry service for his clothes and provide him with his own soap solution that he could keep in his locker.**

the member how he felt about the issue and made sure that the member had the opportunity to express his feelings about the situation.

- The manager worked with the offending member to identify a solution that would be appropriate for everyone involved.
- The manager made sure to follow-up with those individuals who had complained to thank them and let them know what actions had been taken. He also asked these members to feel free to contact him if the proposed solution did not seem to be working.

It is always difficult to share unfavorable news with members, especially when it is unflattering. Whether it is odor or any other difficult issue, it is important to remember that the privacy and feelings of everyone involved should always be accorded an appropriate degree of attention and respect. When dealing with such a situation, the manager should communicate openly, but with a sense of empathy. Managers who are open-minded, are good listeners, and demonstrate that they can be trusted, will likely elicit favorable responses from the members.

Naked Man on the Loose

❑ *Scenario*. This scenario took place in an urban fitness club that was located along the northeast corridor. Open for just over 10 years, the club served a rather upscale market of business professionals who lived in the area.

The club had just hired a new operations manager, who was experiencing his first week on the job. At the time, he was going through his initial training with the club's staff. On this particular day, he was training with one of the facility's sales directors. This particular sales director was giving a tour to a couple in their 40s. The operations director was tagging along to learn more about how to conduct a tour of the club.

As the tour proceeded towards the locker-room areas (the men's and women's locker rooms were located across the hall from each other), a man suddenly ran out of the locker room completely naked and confronted the sales director. The member jumped up and down in front of the sales person, prospects, and operations manager, shouting that someone was in the locker room rifling through lockers. He demanded that the situation be taken care of immediately, thinking nothing of the fact he was standing naked in front of a group of people—several of whom were complete strangers to him.

> He demanded that the situation be taken care of immediately, thinking nothing of the fact he was standing naked in front of a group of people—several of whom were complete strangers to him.

❑ *The Solution*. Within seconds of the man appearing naked and screaming at the sales director, the following actions took place:

- The first step that the sales director took was to tell the member that the club's operations manager would be right in to address the situation.
- The sales director then turned to the prospects and apologized to them for the member's behavior. She attempted to diffuse the awkwardness of the moment by casually mentioning that in this city anything was possible. The sales director affirmed that having a member of the club stroll the hallways in the nude was not a normal part of the sales tour.

She added that the operations manager would address the member's issues and invited everyone to proceed with the tour.

- The operations manager immediately escorted the member into the locker room, and then contacted security to let them know that a stranger was in the club who was stealing from member's lockers.

- After making the call to security, the operations manager continued through the locker room and found the culprit. He tried to retain him, but he escaped to the freight elevator.

- Subsequently, security personnel captured the would-be thief as he left the freight elevator and contacted the operations manager to give him an update about the situation.

- The operations manager then met with the member who had originally seen the thief and let him know how the situation had turned out. Furthermore, he informed him that, in the future, it would be more appropriate if he would at least wrap a towel around himself before leaving the confines of the locker room.

- The operations manager then let the sales director know what had occurred so that she could communicate it to the prospects.

❑ *Discussion.* While having a naked member run out in front of everyone when a tour is being conducted is not likely to happen often, it does represent a situation that can be embarrassing for everyone involved. As such, it requires quick thinking on the manager's part. The staff involved in this situation handled it professionally. Their response and solution were effective because of several factors, including:

- The sales director maintained her calm and responded to the member's concerns at once by indicating that immediate action to address the situation would be taken.

- Exhibiting a professional presence, the sales director immediately apologized to the prospects. Her efforts to apologize also included a touch of humor that helped diffuse any tension that was present.

- The operations manager escorted the member back into the locker room and then immediately contacted security.

- The operations manager, after contacting security, searched for the thief and attempted to retain him until security personnel arrived.

- After the thief was apprehended, the operations manager contacted the sales director and gave her an update on the actions that had been taken. He also made sure to inform the member who had originally brought the matter to the club's attention.

Paying attention (listening), apologizing, taking action, and finally, following-up are all critical steps in dealing with any member or customer issue that arises in the club.

Paying attention (listening), apologizing, taking action, and finally, following-up are all critical steps in dealing with any member or customer issue that arises in the club. Furthermore, by maintaining a calm, professional presence, the team was able to put the member and prospects at greater ease.

Peace and Harmony During the Holiday Season

❑ *Scenario.* This scenario occurred in a small suburban fitness club in the southwest. The club was a fitness-only facility that served a corporate market. The club had been in business for several years at the time of the event.

It was the holiday season, and the club was brightly decorated. The club, as was its usual practice each holiday season, was filled with the sounds of joyful holiday music. While most of the club's members enjoyed the holiday music, one particular member felt that it was inappropriate music to listen to while working out. All of a sudden, one member of the club started arguing with another member over the music that was being played. The manager noticed that these two individuals were arguing over the music and asked them to separate. The two members then retreated to the men's locker room. Subsequently, the manager heard from yet a third member of the club that the two men were now in a fistfight.

❑ *The Solution.* The manager immediately got hold of one of the male personal trainers and had him go into the locker room. The personal trainer separated the men and broke up the fight. The manager told the trainer to communicate to both of the individuals that the manager would like to meet with them. Subsequently, one of the combatants met with the manager, who explained to him that his behavior was completely unacceptable. Indignant, the member offered a series of excuses. Eventually, he was asked to leave the club by the manager and did. The other member was so angered that he just left the club without talking to the manager. Later on, the manager met with him the next time he was in the club.

❑ *Discussion.* In reality, disputes over music are not that rare. It is relatively amazing how something as simple as the choice of music can cause grown men to get into a fistfight. In this particular scenario, the manager handled the situation very well by taking the following steps:

- Terminating the argument on the exercise floor, and when it continued in another area of the club, having a personal trainer of the same gender enter the locker room and break it up.
- Talking with both of the combatants to let them know that their behavior was unacceptable.
- Requesting that the one recalcitrant member immediately leave the club.

> In almost every situation when a fight breaks out between members, the manager's best course of action is to break it up, ask the members to leave the facility, and schedule time to talk with each of the members at a later date about their behavior.

In almost every situation when a fight breaks out between members, the manager's best course of action is to break it up, ask the members to leave the facility, and schedule time to talk with each of the members at a later date about their behavior. In some instances, suspending a member from the club might be necessary.

With regard to music selection—a factor that causes problems more frequently than most would like to believe—clubs should establish a music policy that is made known to the members. By having a clearly communicated music policy, members are aware of what they can expect and are less likely to behave in an antisocial manner.

Beware of the Nose

❑ *Scenario*. This scenario took place in a fitness club that was located in an urban market in the deep south. The facility served a reasonably high-end corporate membership. At the time of the incident, the club had been in business for over 20 years.

The situation involved a member of the club who ran on a treadmill a few times each week. Several of the club's members and employees complained about the member's behavior while he was using the treadmill. Their complaint involved the fact that every time the member ran on the treadmill, he would perform a "farmer's blow" (i.e., blowing his nose into his hands) and then would touch the treadmill. The fitness director was informed by both the staff and several members that they found the exerciser's disgusting behavior repulsive, to a point where no one wanted to work out in the same area of the club when this member was on the treadmill.

❑ *The Solution*. The fitness director decided to contact the member in question by letter. He felt that if he initially met with the member in person, he might embarrass that individual if the conversation was overheard by others. He sent the letter to the member's home. The letter detailed the member's unacceptable conduct and emphasized how important it was to keep the club clean and hygienic for all of the members. The letter indicated that his actions were insulting to other members and impacted the club's overall cleanliness. The member responded to the letter by contacting the fitness director personally and thanking him for sharing what he did and doing so in a confidential manner. Going forward, the member did not exhibit the offensive behavior any more.

❑ *Discussion*. It is not uncommon for some members to be disrespectful of the club and other members when it comes to hygiene. In this particular scenario, the fitness director handled the circumstances appropriately. As a result, the behavior came to a halt. Among the steps that enabled this situation to be dealt with successfully were:

- The fitness director contacted the member confidentially, thus helping to limit any possible embarrassment.
- The fitness director focused his efforts on addressing the offending behavior, not the member. He ensured that the member knew that his behavior was causing a problem for other members of the club. In essence, he "de-personalized" the issue.

When an individual does something that results in unhygienic conditions and impacts the ability of other members to enjoy the club, it is the responsibility of management to address the issue with that member. To the extent possible, this effort should always be kept private to help prevent

> When an individual does something that results in unhygienic conditions and impacts the ability of other members to enjoy the club, it is the responsibility of management to address the issue with that member.

any embarrassment for the member. Furthermore, the endeavor should focus on the behavior of the offending individual and its impact on other members and staff, rather than making it a personal issue.

Clubs can help head off situations similar to these by having house rules that clarify how members should respect the club, other members, and employees and what behaviors are unacceptable. These rules can be very simple and shared with each individual through a member's handbook, a notice on the website, or other appropriate forms of media (e.g., signage, mailings, etc.).

To the Rescue

❑ *Scenario*. This scenario occurred in the mid-Atlantic region of the U.S. in a facility that was a well-operated multipurpose club serving a family market. In this particular set of circumstances, club management had become aware of a young woman who they believed had an eating and exercise disorder. Management had noticed that this individual, who was in the club almost every day, had become ever-increasingly emaciated over the last several weeks. Management believed that it had an obligation to become involved in the situation, but was not sure how to do so without overstepping its expertise or abusing the privacy and feelings of the member involved.

❑ *The Solution*. After considerable discussion among the senior leaders of the club, an intervention was identified that everyone agreed upon. As such, management decided to take the following actions:

- They identified the club's resident registered nurse as the most appropriate staff person to open a dialogue with the young woman.
- Management asked the nurse to open a dialogue with the young woman and request that she obtain a medical clearance from her physician before continuing with her use of the club.
- Management decided that because they were asking the young woman to seek medical clearance, the club had to be prepared to provide emotional and financial assistance if it was determined to be warranted.
- The nurse set up a private meeting with the member involved in the situation and informed her that the club would require her to obtain medical clearance before she would be allowed to continue using the club's facilities. At first, the young woman was defensive, but then became offended by the club's request.
- After informing the young woman of the club's position, the nurse told her that the club was willing to lend her assistance, both financially and emotionally. Upon hearing this, the young woman's attitude changed dramatically, and she expressed her thanks. Subsequently, the young woman indicated that she was aware that she had a problem and had been struggling to identify a clinic or program that could meet her needs (note: her parents had previously washed their hands of the situation).
- Upon hearing the young woman's comments, the staff nurse researched the clinical options until she found a facility that seemed to offer what the young woman needed. Once the clinic was identified, the nurse and

> Management decided that because they were asking the young woman to seek medical clearance, the club had to be prepared to provide emotional and financial assistance if it was determined to be warranted.

staff worked with the young woman to help her get accepted into the clinic's eating disorder program. Subsequently, after the young woman had been admitted to the program, she reported that she had a fear of travel since losing one of her favorite travel companions a few years earlier (e.g., a stuffed animal).

- The nurse proceeded to purchase a special travel companion for the young woman, which she presented to her prior to her departure to the clinic for the first time.

- The young woman made a commitment to the club to successfully complete her treatment program and to come back healthy.

❑ *Discussion.* This set of circumstances is one of the most challenging situations that management can face. The dilemma facing management involved several interrelated factors: the privacy of a member, the medical diagnosis (which is not the club's role), the endangerment of the member's health, and the self-esteem of the member. By any reasonable standard, determining an appropriate solution to this particular situation could have been very difficult. In this situation, however, management took several steps that led to a successful resolution of the problem, including:

- The staff met as a team and identified the steps that would be taken. Subsequently, the measures were perceived as a team solution, which is the best basis for attempting to resolve any situation.

- The staff person most qualified to deal with this particular issue (e.g., a registered nurse) was identified.

- The nurse spoke privately with the young woman and asked her to obtain medical clearance.

- The club expressed its willingness to provide assistance—both financially and emotionally—to the young woman.

- The club followed through on its commitment.

Collectively, the net effect of management's actions was a young woman who opened up about her problems and was able to make a commitment to pursue much-needed therapy.

Several points should be emphasized to anyone in a leadership position in a club who may be confronted by a situation like this in the future. First, clubs are not (and should not be) in the business of making medical diagnoses and must not assume that a member has a particular health problem unless the individual informs them or provides them with a note from a physician that informs them of that fact. Second, a club is obligated to seek medical clearance from any member or prospective member who has known risk factors that would increase that person's likelihood of experiencing a health or medical problem as a result of exercising. The key for a club, in this regard, is to make sure that it is consistent in how it applies the use of medical clearance to all of its members. Third, all factors considered, the facility should seek advice from its legal council before proceeding in situations like this. Fourth, when the club initiates dialogue with the member, it is best if it involves someone who already has a positive, trusting relationship with the member. Finally, the club should be prepared

> The dilemma facing management involved several interrelated factors: the privacy of a member, the medical diagnosis (which is not the club's role), the endangerment of the member's health, and the self-esteem of the member.

for the likely responses in such circumstances (e.g., denial of any problem, an expression of anger and hurt, and a refusal to obtain medial clearance).

I had two experiences with a member whom we believed had anorexia. In both instances, steps similar to the ones undertaken by the club in this scenario were initiated, with the exception that we talked with our attorney, and we had a physician (rather than a registered nurse) from our medical-advisory committee talk with the member. In both cases, the member was hurt and angered, and we ended up having to remove their membership.

The solution developed and successfully implemented by the club in this scenario is an excellent example of a management team that, through empathy and a commitment to its members, was able to turn a potentially perilous situation into a life-changing one for the member involved.

Cell-Phone Enforcer

❑ *Scenario*. This scenario took place in a mid-western multipurpose club that served a relatively affluent membership base of approximately 4,000 individuals. This particular club had a policy that disallowed camera phones in the locker rooms. One member of this facility was convinced that any individual using a cell phone in the locker room was actually taking pictures of him. Over a period of time, this particular member had become obsessed about cell-phone usage in the locker room and had decided to take it upon himself to be the club's enforcer with regard to camera phones and cell phones. The club's policy concerning this issue was clear. If a member notices that a camera phone is in use in the locker room, that person should contact management and allow staff to deal with the situation. Disregarding the club's policy, this member had begun accosting other members and verbally abusing any individual he saw with a cell phone in the locker room. When this member was approached by the manager on duty about his behavior, the abusive member verbally assaulted him.

> The operations manager contacted the member by phone to rationally discuss the concerns of other members and of club management in an attempt to reach a reasonable solution to the problem.

❑ *The Solution*. The club management took the following steps to resolve the situation to the satisfaction of everyone involved:

- The operations manager contacted the member by phone to rationally discuss the concerns of other members and of club management in an attempt to reach a reasonable solution to the problem. The member responded by saying that the club should ban all cell phones from the club and that furthermore, he would physically accost any individuals whom he found with a cell phone.

- The executive director of the club then contacted the member and explained to him that his behavior was unacceptable. The executive director also informed the member that the club could not ban all cell phones (even if it wanted to), because several of the members were physicians who might need to be reached. On the other hand, he indicated to the member that the club's policy did ban the use of camera phones and that if he noticed another member with one, he should please contact a member of the staff, and management would address the situation.

Cell phones (camera phones in particular) have become a big issue in the club industry.

- Finally, the executive director informed the member that if he continued his verbal attacks on members that he would face expulsion from the club and possible criminal action.

❏ *Discussion.* Cell phones (camera phones in particular) have become a big issue in the club industry. Most clubs have instituted policies that ban the use of camera phones in their facilities. This particular situation arose possibly out of a member's safety concerns and his inability to clearly understand the club's policies. The member's subsequent actions were totally inexcusable and caused serious problems with the other members. The response of management in this situation was effective because of several reasons, including:

- The club had a senior manager talk directly with the member in a manner that did not embarrass him.
- When the member did not respond appropriately to the club's initial efforts to resolve the situation, a senior-level manager spoke with him in a private setting.
- That manager reinforced the club's policies concerning the use of both cell and camera phones and detailed the member's options involving situations that warranted attention. The senior-level manager also communicated his displeasure with the member's actions and informed him that if he continued, that the club would consider banishing him from the club.

When dealing with situations similar to this one, the club should do the following:

- Develop house rules and policies that address such issues and take steps to ensure that each member is aware of these rules and policies. Not only should these policies address the use of cell phones, they should also deal with other issues that are important to maintaining the club's atmosphere and sense of privacy. These rules should also detail guidelines concerning what actions management can take in the event that the policies are violated. For example, the club should have a policy that states that management maintains the right to expel any member of the facility if that individual blatantly ignores the policies and rules of the club.
- Consider having the most noteworthy policies, such as camera-phone rules, posted in the locker rooms and even inside the lockers. Ensuring that the members are fully aware of all key policies and rules of the club is important.
- Establish a hierarchy of management for responding to these types of situations.
- Ensure that all conversations with members concerning the possible violation of the club's rules and policies are conducted in private.
- Document the member's activities and the resulting actions of management concerning those activities and place the report in the member's file.

While prohibiting camera phones in the locker room is a good rule, this policy should apply throughout the club. Prohibiting the use of these phones in only one area of the facility can cause problems. All factors considered, it is better to preclude their use anywhere in the club. It should be emphasized that it is always advisable for a club to get its legal council's advice before establishing any policy concerning the use of camera phones in the facility.

While prohibiting camera phones in the locker room is a good rule, this policy should apply throughout the club.

30

Employee Chronicles

Chapter Objectives

The scenarios related in this chapter involve situations that entail employee experiences in health/fitness clubs. Resolving them required both insight and thoughtful managerial acumen.

Health Hearsay

❑ *Scenario*. This scenario took place in a large upscale club during the mid to late 1980s, which was located in an affluent residential neighborhood on the east coast. At the time, the club had approximately 3,000 memberships, for which it charged approximately $120 a month for dues for a single membership. The club offered approximately 150 to 200 personal training sessions a week at an average cost of $40 each. These workouts were supervised by a group of eight personal trainers, two of whom conducted about 35 to 40 sessions each week.

> In only a few short days, over 100 complaints about this individual had been received, all based on a similar rumor.

One of the most popular trainers was a gentleman who had been in the personal training business for a considerable time period and had a reputation as being one of the best in his field. Subsequently, several female members approached the fitness director with their concerns about the trainer. They indicated that they thought the trainer had AIDS (because of a quite noticeable skin condition) and that he should not be allowed in the club. Within days, over 40 members had come to the fitness director and indicated that they had heard this particular employee had AIDS and asked what the club was going to do about it. Eventually, a number of the club's employees went to the fitness director and reported that they believed that this personal trainer had AIDS and should be dismissed from the club. In only a few short days, over 100 complaints about this individual had been received, all based on a similar rumor.

❑ *The Solution.* The fitness director decided to investigate the situation. His first step was to speak with the other employees and members, each in private. During his talks with these individuals, he informed them that he wanted to initially determine whether a problem existed. If and when he discovered an issue that needed attention, he would address it as appropriately as possible. Subsequently, he took the following steps:

- He met with the manager of the facility to share with him what was occurring and asking for his guidance. The manager replied that he would talk with the club's legal counsel.

- The fitness director then had a private meeting with the personal trainer in question and informed him that some of the club's employees and members had expressed their concern that he might have a contagious virus. Although he was slightly offended, he assured the fitness director that he was fine and that he had a minor illness that was being treated, which posed no problem to others.

- The fitness director, taking the trainer at his word, went back to the manager and detailed their conversation. In addition, the fitness director met privately with the members and staff who had expressed their concern and told them that he had met with the personal trainer, that they had discussed the person's health, and that the rumor was false.

- Subsequently, the manager informed the fitness director that he wanted the trainer to see a physician and be screened for AIDS. The fitness director replied that although he personally felt that such a request was inappropriate, he would reluctantly ask the trainer to do as the manager wanted and get a note saying that he was healthy and not contagious. The manager then announced that the fitness director had no choice; either get the individual screened for AIDS or else.

- Consequently, the fitness director met privately with the physical trainer and told him that the club was willing to pay for him to visit a local physician, undergo a physical, and get a clearance note. Furthermore, he informed the trainer that this step would put the concerns of the members and management to rest. No mention was made of AIDS testing. The personal trainer consented and a physician's appointment was made for him.

- On the day of the appointment, the trainer was accompanied to the doctor's office by his direct supervisor at the club. When the trainer got to the physician's office, he received a physical, but was then asked to sign a sheet regarding undergoing a blood test for AIDS, a request that angered him a lot. He took the blood test, but immediately returned to the club.

- The fitness director then met with the personal trainer and his supervisor and discussed the events that had occurred. The fitness director apologized to the trainer for not telling him about the AIDS test beforehand. In reality, he said that he was very uncomfortable about the situation and wanted to avoid that issue if he could, but felt that there was no other way for him to handle it.

The fitness director then had a private meeting with the personal trainer in question and informed him that some of the club's employees and members had expressed their concern that he might have a contagious virus.

- After considerable discussion, the personal trainer and fitness director came to a mutually agreed upon resolution. The trainer would not come to work for a few days, so he could gather himself. Subsequently, however, the trainer would return for full duty.
- The blood tests indicated no evidence of AIDS, but did show a treatable virus that was affecting his skin. Medicine was provided to him, and his virus was successfully treated.
- The fitness director met with both the members and the employees who had lodged a complaint about the trainer's perceived medical condition. He informed them that the issue had been addressed and that the rumors were blatantly untrue.

❏ *Discussion.* This situation involved a very challenging employee issue that required total privacy. Unfortunately, the situation was not handled as well as it should have been. As a result, the trust of an employee was lost, and the integrity of a leader was negatively impacted. While eventually the matter was addressed to the satisfaction of those who were concerned with the medical condition of the personal trainer, it was not handled in an appropriate manner from the employee's perspective. In fact, the staff's actions could have exposed the club and fitness director to a lawsuit. Several key observations could be made regarding the situation and how it was handled, including:

The fitness director should never have sent the employee to see a physician under false pretenses, no matter how much pressure was applied by senior management.

- The fitness director responded appropriately at first by talking with his manager and collecting information from the concerned members and staff.
- The fitness director also acted in a responsible manner by speaking with the personal trainer in question and soliciting feedback from him.
- On the other hand, the fitness director should never have sent the employee to see a physician under false pretenses, no matter how much pressure was applied by senior management. Because his integrity and character were at stake, the fitness director should have taken a firmer position with senior management.
- Failing that, the fitness director should have been up-front (honest) with the trainer and should have asked him to please bring in a note from his physician that confirmed that he was not contagious. The fitness director should not have recommended a physician, unless asked to do so by the trainer. The choice of which physician to utilize should have been left to the trainer.
- Much earlier in the sequence of events, the fitness director should have informed the members that he had addressed the situation with the personal trainer and that it had been safely resolved. Furthermore, the matter (including the members' concerns, complaints, and accusations) should have been dropped at that point.

It cannot be overemphasized how important it is for managers to respect their employees and be truthful with them at all times, no matter how challenging or difficult the situation. Furthermore, managers must always respect the privacy of both employees and members and never do anything that might compromise their privacy. In addition, managers should address issues truthfully. Parsing the facts or their words is never the right approach for dealing with any situation. Managers should also remember that making the right decision is the proper course of action, even when doing so might cause them to lose their job. Finally, when dealing with members, managers should inform them that they have addressed the issue in a manner that they feel is appropriate. If the members don't feel comfortable with that, it is their problem. Managers should let the members deal with it, rather then try to go too far in appeasing them. A fine line always exists that managers should not cross when attempting to address issues that arise between members and employees.

A Lover's Quarrel

❑ *Scenario.* This scenario occurred in an urban racquet club that was located along the northeast corridor during the early part of the 1990s. Serving an upscale membership base, this facility provided fitness and racquet-sport services for its members.

The situation involved a female assistant general manager with four years experience who was on duty at the time of the incident. This employee started her career at the front desk and, through hard work and stellar performance, had been promoted to her current position. Also on duty during the same shift was the front-desk concierge, who had been with the club for six months and had been, to that point, an exemplary employee. As happens with matters of the heart, both employees had recently begun seeing each other on a personal level.

About 5:00 p.m. that day, during the club's prime time, the front desk was very busy. The desk was manned by the assistant general manager, the front-desk concierge, and two other staff personnel. In addition, at least ten members where checking in at the desk at the time. All of a sudden, without any warning, the assistant general manager and the front-desk concierge began screaming at each other, a situation which quickly escalated into a full-scale battle. Subsequently, the front-desk concierge slapped the assistant general manager, who then punched the front-desk concierge in the head. The fight continued to escalate, with swearing, hissing, and the further threat of physical violence.

> All of a sudden, without any warning, the assistant general manager and the front-desk concierge began screaming at each other, a situation which quickly escalated into a full-scale battle.

❑ *The Solution.* The manager and owner of the club almost immediately became aware of the situation and responded as follows:
- The manager immediately separated the two employees and brought them into his office. He then scheduled meetings with each of them for the next day and sent both home for the rest of the day.
- The manager first met with the assistant general manager and informed her of his dissatisfaction with the behavior that had occurred the prior evening and reiterated with her the type of behavior that was expected. He then suspended her for two weeks without pay.
- The manager next met with the front-desk employee and conveyed his displeasure with the actions that had occurred the prior evening and shared with that individual the type of behavior that was expected of all

club employees. The manager then told the front-desk employee what action had been taken against the assistant manager. The front desk employee got angry, indicated that this was not the end of the situation, and then proceeded to quit.

❑ *Discussion*. Situations such as this one can happen in any business, including the club industry. When employees work together for extended periods of time, the possibility of romantic relationships occurring will increase. While most clubs have policies against employees having relationships with each other, it is still difficult, if not almost impossible, to prevent personal relationships from transpiring. In this particular set of circumstances, the manager handled the situation well by doing the following:

• Immediately separating the two employees and getting them into his office. The manager also did the right thing in sending both employees home separately, but only after scheduling meetings with each of them for the next day. It is important that after such an emotional event, both parties involved be given a cool-down period before meeting with each of them privately.

• Holding private meetings or counseling sessions with each employee was an appropriate next step. In the case of the assistant general manager, the two-week suspension provided a clear message as to the serious nature of the violation. On the other hand, it let the employee know that the manager valued her (she could have also been fired). The other employee quit before further disciplinary action could be taken.

To prevent instances such as this one from occurring, clubs should establish policies and practices that clearly communicate the expectations of the facility with regard to personal relationships between employees. Once instituted, those policies and practices should be enforced on a consistent basis. When it involves personal relationships between supervisors and employees, those policies and practices must be particularly explicit and straightforward. It is never a good idea for supervisors to have a romantic relationship with an employee who reports to them. If and when management becomes aware of a personal relationship between employees, especially those between a supervisor and employee, they should reiterate and reinforce the club's policy concerning such associations with each participant in the relationship. In most instances, when a relationship between a supervisor and an employee happens and management counsels these individuals, one of the following actions should occur:

• The supervisor and subordinate must agree not to see each other anymore.

• One of the two employees should be asked to leave; in most cases it will be the employee with less tenure and perceived value to the club.

By undertaking the necessary steps, a situation such as the one detailed in this scenario can be prevented. However, in the event it does, the actions taken by this manager provide an excellent template to follow.

> To prevent instances such as this one from occurring, clubs should establish policies and practices that clearly communicate the expectations of the facility with regard to personal relationships between employees.

Anyone Up for a Dip?

❏ *Scenario.* This scenario took place in a high-end club that was located in the southwest part of the country. The club offered a variety of sports and recreation-related programs. One of the club's most valued features was its outdoor swimming pool. During the outdoor season, the outdoor pool had a staff of six lifeguards, all between the ages of 18 and 20, and one head lifeguard, who was female. The manager of this operation had had great success with this team for the entire outdoor season. The pool closed each evening around 9:00 p.m.

Near the end of the outdoor season, the manager was returning from a dinner meeting with one of the members, at approximately 10:30 p.m. The manager was walking to his car in the lot when he heard some strange noises coming from the pool. Since the pool supposedly closed over an hour earlier, the manager decided to take a look. As he approached the pool, he heard laughing and loud noises, including some emanating from the club's head lifeguard. When he got up to the edge of the pool, his head lifeguard had swum up to the edge to greet him. There was a moment of silence, until the manager explained to her that everyone must get out of the pool. The head lifeguard did not move. Puzzled, the manager again asked the lifeguards to get out of the pool. All the lifeguards, with the exception of the head lifeguard, proceeded to get out at the other end of the pool. It was then that the manager noticed that his entire staff had been "skinny dipping." Dismayed, he turned away so the head lifeguard could leave the pool.

❏ *Solution.* Once the pool had emptied and the lifeguards had gotten dressed, the manager had them depart, but only after scheduling meetings with each of them for the next day. He then proceeded to clean up and close the pool area.

The next day, he met with each of the lifeguards. He explained to them how disappointed he was with them and how inappropriate their behavior was. Because the club still had to serve the members, the option of dismissing the entire staff was not one that could be taken. Instead, after meeting with each individual, he wrote each one up for behavior unbecoming of staff. In addition, he spent extra time in counseling the head lifeguard. Finally, he spent the remainder of the outdoor pool season working evenings to make sure no further problems occurred.

❏ *Discussion.* It is not uncommon when dealing with a young staff (a common circumstance in the fitness industry), especially when the supervisors are young themselves, for foolish and inappropriate behavior to occur. In this situation, the staff demonstrated a lack of maturity, disregard for leadership, and disrespect to the membership. The manager dealt with the situation in a professional and satisfactory manner by performing the following steps:

- Clearing the pool upon noticing what was occurring
- Respecting the employees by not making a spectacle of them at that time

It is not uncommon when dealing with a young staff (a common circumstance in the fitness industry), especially when the supervisors are young themselves, for foolish and inappropriate behavior to occur.

- Scheduling time to meet the next day with each individual and counseling them on their behavior
- Providing the employees with written warnings concerning their behavior that would go on their employee records
- Monitoring the actions of the staff after the event to ensure that such behavior did not occur in the future

Had a need not existed to have the lifeguards on duty for the remainder of the outdoor pool season, the manager indicated that he would most likely have dismissed all of the employees. From a professional perspective, it would have been wise to suspend the head lifeguard immediately. This step would have sent a relatively strong message to the other lifeguards. While it would have undoubtedly subjected the manager to a heavier workload, the end result of suspending the head lifeguard would have sent the message that the other lifeguards needed to hear.

> **As individuals in a position of leadership, managers sometimes need to make a strong statement about values, respect, and trust.**

As individuals in a position of leadership, managers sometimes need to make a strong statement about values, respect, and trust. Suspending or dismissing a supervisor who has demonstrated behavior that is totally inappropriate can be a necessary step in order to maintain long-term stability and respect among the rest of the team.

A Little Affair

❑ *Scenario.* This scenario took place in a suburban club that was located in the southwest. Designed to serve an affluent family market, the club provided a host of networking and social activities for the members. The facility's membership roster was small, and most of the members knew each other.

Late in the evening one day, the club was nearing the end of another successful member social event. Many of the members and employees in attendance decided to continue the party at a local pub. The manager decided to attend the after-hours event to make sure that nothing inappropriate occurred. The manager noticed that a senior member of the staff was receiving some flirtatious looks from one of the club's female members. The manager thought about the situation for a moment, but figured this employee was a top supervisor and the member was a married woman with children. He felt that he could go home and nothing would happen.

The manager arrived home around midnight and was immediately told by his wife that the security company had called and that an alarm had gone off at the club. The manager immediately returned to the club. When he arrived, he noticed two cars in the lot, one of which was the supervisor's car. The manager then went into the club and kept calling out to see if anyone was there. Hearing no response, he searched the entire club and found nothing. Just before departing, he decided to go to his office. Upon opening the door, he found his employee and the member in a very compromising position, both with blank stares on their face.

❑ *The Solution*. Once the manager had entered the room, the member pleaded with him not to tell anyone. The manager asked the member to leave and told her that he would meet with her the next day. The manager then had the employee get dressed, after which he read the employee the riot act. He told the employee he would meet with him the next morning.

> **The manager decided that it was in the best interest of everyone involved to keep this situation under wraps.**

The manager met with the member first. The member told her side of the story and pleaded for confidentiality. She promised not to place the club or the manager in that situation again. She did not want this to get out and end her marriage. The manager decided that it was in the best interest of everyone involved to keep this situation under wraps. The manager then met with the employee and explained to him that this event was to remain confidential and that he would not be dismissed because it would bring unwanted attention to the situation. On the other hand, the manager did share with him that if word did leak out, he would be immediately terminated. The manager took the time to explain the member's request for confidentiality to the employee. The employee apologized to the member and the manager.

While the manager indicated that he was not sure he did the right thing, he did feel, at the time, that it was important to protect the member. As a result, he did not punish the employee to the degree he might otherwise have.

❑ *Discussion*. As hard as it may be for some individuals to believe, employees and members occasionally enter into inappropriate relationships. When employees work closely with members and begin seeing each other in a social context, situations such as this scenario can arise. In this particular instance, the employee and the member both showed poor judgment—not just by having an affair, but consummating it on club property. The manager, in this instance, handled the situation as best he felt he could, given the fact that he faced a dual dilemma of having to discipline an employee and maintain the privacy of the member, both of which were critical factors. The manager's response dealt satisfactorily with the situation, particularly from the member's perspective, because he undertook the following steps:

- Once he came upon the employee and member together, he separated them and sent the member home.
- He immediately talked with the offending employee to make sure that he knew the gravity of the situation.
- He met privately with the member and kept the situation in total confidence. He maintained the level of trust that is essential in a situation of this magnitude.
- He met privately the next day with the employee and recounted the details of the meeting with the member. He further counseled the employee and gave him a warning that any leak of the information involving the situation would result in his immediate termination.

While the situation seemed to end reasonably well, the manager should have written the employee up and suspended him. While cause certainly existed to dismiss the employee, which would have been a perfectly

Club managers
should be aware of
the fact that member-
and-employee
relationships can
and will occur.
Accordingly, it is
important for clubs to
have policies in place
that make it clear
that such behavior
is unacceptable and
inappropriate for
employees.

appropriate response, a suspension would have worked just as well. With regard to the member, he could have suspended her from the club and asked her not to return. Since this member was married and had a family, the manager decided to focus his efforts to resolve the situation on the member's circumstances, rather than doing something that might cause further damage to her. Considering the social nature of the club and the family situation, this was a good decision. Had the member been single, the more appropriate option might have been to suspend her from the club.

Club managers should be aware of the fact that member-and-employee relationships can and will occur. Accordingly, it is important for clubs to have policies in place that make it clear that such behavior is unacceptable and inappropriate for employees. A club should also have house rules that address this type of situation from a member's perspective as well. Such policies should be reinforced regularly. If and when these policies are violated, the proper discipline should be administered.

31

Business Chronicles

Chapter Objectives

The situations detailed in this chapter encompass stories involving business-related circumstances. Resolving them required sound leadership and managerial skills.

Closing a Club and Gaining Fans

❏ *Scenario*. This scenario took place in a large multipurpose club that was located in the south. Approaching its 10th anniversary, the facility was recognized as the number one adult club in the marketplace and served a membership base of over 2,000 individuals. The building in which the club was located had been sold to new owners in the past year. The new owner had a reputation for demanding premium leases.

The club, which was part of a chain, had not funded all of the necessary capital improvements that it needed over the past several years. As a result, during its 10th anniversary year, the indoor pool experienced problems, causing it to empty into the tenant's space below it. In order to get the pool up and running, the club manager and regional manager sought a capital infusion of a couple of hundred thousand dollars to repair the pool. Concurrently, the new building owner was seeking to ignore the club's request for a lease extension and increase the club's base rent by 200 percent.

The manager and regional manager went before senior management asking for capital to repair the pool and for help with negotiating with the new landlord. While the club had contributed significant cash flow to the company in the past, the prospect of investing a couple of hundred thousand dollars and having the cost of the lease at least double caused senior management to make the difficult decision to close the club. Senior management informed the regional manager and manager that they had decided to close the club.

> While the club had contributed significant cash flow to the company in the past, the prospect of investing a couple of hundred thousand dollars and having the cost of the lease at least double caused senior management to make the difficult decision to close the club.

Once the decision to close the club had been communicated to the regional manager and club manager, they went into action.

Unable to change the minds of senior management, the regional manager and manager received permission to have a 90-day window in which to close the facility.

❑ *The Solution.* Once the decision to close the club had been communicated to the regional manager and club manager, they went into action. Among the steps that they took to address the club's closing were the following:

- The regional manager and manager initially decided that the best course of action was to develop a strategy for closing the club that they would review with the senior staff before settling on a final plan.

- The regional manager and manager met with the senior staff in a private setting and informed them that senior management had decided that the best course of action for the club was to close its doors. In this meeting, the regional manager and manager encouraged the senior staff to share their feelings concerning the situation. As a team, they then identified the best strategy for going forward.

- Before communicating further with either the staff or members, the manager and regional manager determined the steps that would be undertaken to help ensure that both the members and employees ended up in the best possible situation, including:

  ✓ The manager and regional manager would get each employee a severance package that paid that individual all accrued vacation and sick time, as well as one week's pay for every year worked for hourly employees and two week's pay for every year worked for salaried employees.

  ✓ The regional manager would arrange job opportunities with other clubs within the company for the supervisory staff.

  ✓ The manager would contact other local clubs to make special membership arrangements that would allow the club's members to transfer to these other clubs with full privileges and not have to pay for them for a specified period of time (the club would pay the dues for those members for that time period).

  ✓ The manager and regional manager would arrange to sell the equipment in the club to help offset the costs of closing the facility.

  ✓ The senior staff would take responsibility for developing a closing party and would designate a charity that would be the recipient of any funds that would be raised at the party.

- Next, the regional manager and manager met with the entire staff. At this meeting, the regional manager shared the news about senior management's decision and stated the reason for closing the facility. At the meeting, all of the arrangements regarding compensation payments, new jobs, etc. were discussed. In addition, the plans for handling the membership were reviewed. Employees were given the opportunity to go to their new jobs immediately or remain with the club until it closed. Everyone chose to stay and get new jobs after the closing.

- The regional manager and manager then met with a group of vocal and influential members of the club to share the news and seek their ideas on how best to communicate the closing to the entire membership. At that time, management told the group about plans for a closing party and the arrangements made with the other local clubs.

- Management then informed the entire membership about the closing and what was going to occur. Initially, this communication was accomplished through personal letters that were sent to each member and signed by the manager. Once the letters went out, special message boards were put up around the club for member viewing. In addition, the manager and the facility's senior staff met personally with each of the members that they knew. Their dialogue with these individuals included the following information:

  ✓ That there would be a special closing party on the final day. That they could bring a guest, and that all entry fees ($20 a person) would go to a local charity.

  ✓ That the party would include a cash bar and a live band.

  ✓ That the club had made arrangements with other local clubs, and that representatives of those clubs would be available for the members to meet with and sign them up for memberships in those clubs.

  ✓ That the staff would do whatever they could to help members with the transition.

- Management, including the regional manager, kept their doors opened over the next 60 days for anyone who wanted help with a closing-related issue, assisting members with the transition, supporting employees with any problem that they might have, and preparing for the final closing.

- On the final day, the closing party was the highlight event. The staff worked the party so that members and guests could enjoy the party. A total of 2,000 individuals attended the party. In the process, over $10,000 was raised for charity. The party lasted for over five hours, and closed with a special funeral procession.

- The event featured celebrations and storytelling. A local TV station covered the event and collected stories from members. The next day, the by-line of the local station's nightly newscast was "local landmark closes."

- After the party, members called and stopped by to say how much they appreciated how the closing was handled and that they hoped that someday the club would return.

❑ *Discussion.* Closing a club is one of the most challenging tasks that leadership will ever face. Members and employees who have been involved with a facility for any period of time take a sense of ownership in the club. As a result, they often feel an incredible loss when a club closes. Accordingly, club owners and operators need to realize that closing a facility can be traumatic for both members and employees. How the club closes not only impacts the facility's relationship with its members and employees, but also the community. In this particular instance, the facility had been a great club for almost 10 years. The closing, although lamentable, was handled in such a way that the employees, members, and community all retained their sense of pride about the club. Among the keys to this particular closing's success were the following:

Closing a club is one of the most challenging tasks that leadership will ever face.

Management informed members at various levels about the closing and made the process as personal as possible.

- Management took the time to initially communicate and discuss the event with the facility's senior staff. Concurrently, they solicited feedback from the staff regarding what would be the right way to close the club.
- Management informed members at various levels about the closing and made the process as personal as possible.
- Before meeting with the club's employees and members, management made sure that they would be able to answer any important questions that might come up during the meeting.
- Management made the closing a celebration and made it an event that demonstrated that the club was still an important part of the community by contributing proceeds from the closing party to a local charity.
- Management made arrangements for members and employees before the meeting in an effort to help lessen the shock of the closing.
- Management, staff, and members worked together until the end, instead of becoming adversaries.
- Until the very last moment, management's approach was to be upbeat and positive, to view the process of closing the club as a change, instead of an end point.
- If staff or members wanted to talk about the closing on a personal level, the manager and regional manager made themselves available, rather than hiding behind their doors.

While closing a club is not a frequent experience for managers, nonetheless, it is an experience that many managers will have. The ability to close a club, while maintaining the relationships and integrity of the club in the eyes of employees, members, and community, is a sign of exceptional leadership. One key lesson that can be learned from this particular scenario is that managers should never burn a bridge; instead, they should continue to build, since they never know when they might return.

Drive-In Fitness Anyone?

❑ *Scenario.* This scenario occurred in a suburban fitness club in the southwest. Located along a major thoroughfare, the club leased space in a corporate business park. The facility served a corporate market and had approximately 800 memberships. The club opened at 5:30 a.m. and closed at 9:00 p.m. on weekdays.

One night at approximately 1:00 a.m., the manager received a phone call from the building's landlord who informed him that a car had just driven through the exterior window of the club and was lodged in the fitness center. The manager immediately came to the club to find a car situated inside the club, with shattered glass everywhere. Not only had the car broken a significant portion of the exterior window, it had destroyed two offices and part of the fitness floor. Glass was strewn throughout the entire fitness area. Subsequently, the police arrived and had the vehicle towed out of the club.

❑ *The Solution.* Upon surveying the situation, the manager proceeded to take the following actions:

- The manager immediately contacted the staff who were scheduled to open the club the next morning at 5:30 a.m. to let them know what happened and discuss a plan of action.
- The manager showed up at the club prior to 5:30 a.m. the next day and met with the staff. The staff then made signs that explained what happened and what actions would take place.
- Subsequently, the manager and employees greeted the club's members as they arrived at the facility and directed them over to another club for their morning workouts (the manager contacted that club upon arriving to make arrangements for his club's members to use that facility at no cost to them).
- During the course of the day, members were greeted by the facility's staff and manager who informed them of the club's closing and let them know that they would have access to and privileges at another club during the clean-up period.
- The manager brought the entire staff into the club later in the morning, and everyone worked all day cleaning up the space. The building landlord also sent staff down to help clean up.
- The manager also contacted the club's insurance agent to get that process activated.
- The club was cleaned and open to members the next afternoon.
- For a couple of weeks, the club operated with plywood on several of its windows. Within 30 days, however, the window, carpet, and broken equipment were replaced.
- No members left the club as a result of the incident.

❑ *Discussion.* A car driving through the club is not a normal event. Obviously, had it occurred during the club's normal operating hours, serious harm could have resulted. The real challenges in this particular scenario were having to address the members' needs the next morning, get the club repaired, and make sure that staff was completely informed about the situation. Furthermore, an event such as this could have resulted in the loss of members. The club manager did an excellent job on short notice of ensuring that the members were taken care of in an appropriate manner. Among the key actions that helped resolve this situation were:

- The manager visited the site right away and surveyed the situation.
- The manager immediately contacted the club's opening staff to inform them of what happened and made sure that they had a plan upon arriving in the morning.
- The manager and staff got to the club early and greeted the members as they arrived, explained the situation to them, and got them access to another club.
- The manager made arrangements for the members to use another club at no cost to them.

> The real challenges in this particular scenario were having to address the members' needs the next morning, get the club repaired, and make sure that staff was completely informed about the situation.

- The staff, with assistance from the landlord, was able to get the club cleaned up and open within one day.
- The manager made sure that the club maintained communication with the members throughout the period of the incident.

Situations such as the one recounted in this particular scenario cannot be predicted. If they arise, however, the critical factor is the ability of management to communicate with the members to lessen the shock and confusion that can accompany such an event and provide every possible opportunity for the members to pursue their fitness activities, with as minimal a level of disturbance as possible.

Now, Where Did You Say the Fitness Area Was?

❑ *Scenario.* The club involved in this scenario was located along the northeast corridor in a dense urban market. The club had been open for several years and had a membership of approximately 1,600. Recently, the club had decided to go through a three-million dollar renovation that would take approximately 12 months to complete. During the renovation, the facility's goal was to grow membership by at least 500. The club had also decided that during the course of the 12-month renovation, it would remain open for the members and keep its dues pricing unchanged.

❑ *The Solution.* Once the decision to renovate the facility and remain open during the renovation was made, the club's leadership team developed a game plan to tackle the process. In that regard, some of the most important actions that took place included:

- The club had models and color floor plans of the renovation produced that could be used to share information with the members about the renovation process.
- The club created a renovation calendar that provided approximate timelines for each phase of the renovation, including what areas of the club would be under construction, when these spaces would be worked on, and what changes in the facilities would occur during each stage.
- The renovation calendar and pictures were included with a letter that was forwarded to each member. In addition, a notice on the club's plans for renovation was put in the newsletter. These communication efforts occurred approximately 90 days in advance of the start of the project and again at 60 days and 30 days prior to work beginning.
- The club set up a renovation hub in the club that members could refer to every day regarding the status of the project. This hub had a model of the new club, pictures of the new equipment, copies of the renovation calendar, and a daily update poster that showed what was happening each day.
- The staff had daily meetings and updates so they could communicate effectively with the club's members.
- The locker rooms had to be switched on four occasions, with the women utilizing the men's lockers on one occasion, and during another period, the men and women using the locker rooms on alternate days. A special

The club created a renovation calendar that provided approximate timelines for each phase of the renovation, including what areas of the club would be under construction, when these spaces would be worked on, and what changes in the facilities would occur during each stage.

area for lockers was set up so that even during the time that radical changes were occurring in the location of locker rooms, the members always had a locker in which to store their items.

- The club provided special treats and drinks each day to help ease any pain caused by the renovation efforts.
- When the exercise studios were closed, the club provided members with hard hats and held classes in the construction areas after hours. This step was facilitated by using special flooring that the staff could roll out on the concrete floors after the construction workers had left for the day.
- Special classes and programs were offered that provided members with the opportunity to exercise at times they might not otherwise have worked out.
- The manager and department heads made themselves available to the members in 12-hour shifts to address the members' complaints and deal with any other issues that they might have.
- Each time a phase of work was completed, the club held a relatively small celebration party.
- Each of these parties provided an opportunity for special instructors and celebrities to visit the club during those days on which the festivities were held in order to further enhance the experience.

After 12 months of renovation, the club's membership had increased from approximately 1,600, when construction began, to 2,400 at the time of completion. Furthermore, the member retention rate remained at the same level as it was prior to the renovation work.

❑ *Discussion.* One of the most challenging experiences that managers will encounter in the club business is operating a facility and serving the members during a period of major renovation. Clubs cannot afford to just close their doors during renovation, or they would lose their revenue stream from dues. Clubs have to find ways to continue operating at full bore and provide the same (or better) service during periods of renovation. Because the health/fitness club industry changes frequently, clubs will be challenged at one time or another with having to make a facelift— sometimes a major facelift. The key to successfully meeting such a challenge is whether the club can continue to operate and drive revenues during a period when members will be inconvenienced.

Club owners and operators who are involved with facilities that will be undergoing renovation must find a way to succeed at delivering their club experience under times of high duress. Without question, members will complain during renovation. At the beginning of the renovation efforts, most members will be excited about the changes that are occurring and tolerate the inconveniences that are being caused by the construction. As the construction wears on, however, usually at about six months, members will begin to complain and will become less accepting of any inconveniences that might arise. Concurrently, the staff will be challenged to have to provide satisfactory service under the most trying of circumstances. As members

One of the most challenging experiences that managers will encounter in the club business is operating a facility and serving the members during a period of major renovation.

begin to complain more, the employees will be subjected to additional stress.

The aforementioned circumstances require extraordinary leadership if the club's renovation efforts are to proceed smoothly, with minimal disruption to the membership. In this particular scenario, club management did an outstanding job of turning a long renovation into a successful operation. Among the most critical steps that allowed management to be successful in this situation were the following:

- Management created an entire game plan around the renovation that addressed the concerns of both members and staff.
- Management informed the membership well in advance what was going to occur and repeated efforts to communicate with the members throughout the process.
- Management created a communication center that provided daily updates concerning the renovation efforts.
- Management developed a series of newly created experiences that were designed to help take the members' and employees' minds off the actual renovation process.
- Management and staff undertook several activities (e.g., parties, social events, and special classes) that helped lend a measure of excitement to the renovation process.
- The employees pulled together under a common cause to help make the situation better for the members.
- Management provided additional support to the employees so that they, in turn, could take better care of the members during the renovation process.
- A club can do a number of things to help make a renovation, such as this one, relatively palatable to everyone involved. The key point that should be emphasized is that if the management and employees are able and willing to plan and act in an appropriate manner, the entire renovation experience can be somewhat rewarding for members and employees alike, rather than an unnerving, strife-filled struggle.

> The key point that should be emphasized is that if the management and employees are able and willing to plan and act in an appropriate manner, the entire renovation experience can be somewhat rewarding for members and employees alike, rather than an unnerving, strife-filled struggle.

A. Leading Health/Fitness Industry Associations and Organizations
B. Leading Health/Fitness Industry Trade Publications
C. Profiles of Leading Global Health/Fitness Club Companies
D Profiles of Regional U.S. Club Companies
E. Sample Marketing Materials From Leading Global Health/Fitness Clubs
F. Profiles of Leading U.S. Health/Fitness Club Equipment Manufacturers
G. Sample Job Descriptions
H. Sample Compensation Agreements
I. Sample Job Offering Letter
J. Sample Structured Interview Questioning Format for a Fitness Director Applicant
K. Sample Strategic Planning Forms
L. Selected Front-of-the-House Operational Forms
M. Selected Heart-of-the-House Operational Forms
N. Sample Design and Construction Checklist
O. Sample Construction Project Budget
P. Sample Member Satisfaction Survey
Q. Sample Corporate Sales Checklist
R. Selected Health/Fitness Industry Programming Practices
S. Program Best Practices Benchmark Form
T. Selected Risk Management Forms
U. Suggested References

Appendices

Appendix A
Leading Health/Fitness Industry Associations and Organizations

American College of Sports Medicine 401 West Michigan Indianapolis, Indiana 46202 317-637-9200 www.acsm.org	Research, education, and certification for fitness professionals, physicians, and individuals in related sports medicine fields
American Council on Exercise 4851 Paramount Drive San Diego, California 92123 800-825-3636 www.acefitness.org	Education and certification for fitness professionals
Aerobic and Fitness Association of America 15250 Ventura Blvd. Suite 200 Sherman Oaks, California 91403 877-968-7263 www.afaa.com	Education and certification for fitness professionals
European Health & Fitness Association Rue Washington 40, B-1050 Bruxelles Belgium +32–(02) 649 90 44 www.ehfa.ud	Association involved in public policy, education, standard development, and public relations for the European club industry
IDEA Health and Fitness Association 10455 Pacific Center Court San Diego, California 92121-4339 800-999-4332 www.ideafit.com	Education for fitness professionals
International Health, Racquet & Sportsclub Association Seaport Center, 70 Fargo Street Boston, Massachusetts 02210 800-228-4772 www.ihrsa.org	International trade association involved in providing public policy, education, industry benchmarking, and networking services for health/fitness, racquet, and sports clubs
International Spa Association 2365 Harrodsburg Road, Suite A325 Lexington, Kentucky 40504 888-651-4772 www.experienceispa.com	Trade association for the spa industry; education for the spa industry
National Academy of Sports Medicine 123 Hodencamp Road, Suite 204 Thousand Oaks, California 91360 800-460-6276 www.nasm.org	Education and certification for fitness professionals
National Strength and Conditioning Association 1885 Bob Johnson Drive Colorado Springs, Colorado 80906 800-815-6826 www.nsca-lift.org	Education and certification for fitness professionals
National Wellness Institute 1300 College Ct., P.O. Box 827 Stevens Point, Wisconsin 54481-0827 800-244-8922 www.nationalwellness.org	Association involved in delivering education, resources, and communication for professionals with an interest in wellness and health promotion

Appendix B
Leading Health/Fitness Industry Trade Publications

ACSM's Health and Fitness Journal Published by Lippincott Williams & Wilkins 16522 Hunters Green Parkway Hagerstown, Maryland 21740 800-638-3030	Publication for fitness professionals; can be obtained by non-ACSM members; published six times a year
ACE Certified News 4851 Paramount Drive San Diego, CA 92123 800-825-3636	Publication of ACE; published six times a year for certified members of ACE; covers a wide array of health and fitness-related topics
ACE Fitness Matters 4851 Paramount Drive San Diego, CA 92123 800-825-3636	Bimonthly publication that is geared to the consumer; provides information on health, wellness, and exercise
Aquatics International Hanley Woods LLC 6222 Wilshire Blvd Los Angeles, California 90048-5100 888-269-8410	Monthly publication for aquatic professionals serving in all market segments
Athletic Business 4130 Lien Road Madison, Wisconsin 53704 800-869-6882	Monthly publication for athletic, fitness, and recreational professionals; focuses on issues concerning recreation centers, universities, military, and commercial health/fitness clubs
Club Business International Magazine of IHRSA Seaport Center, 70 Fargo Street Boston, Massachusetts 02210 800-228-4772	Monthly publication for members of IHRSA; focus is on the commercial club industry
Club Industry Penton Media 9800 Metcalf Avenue Overland Park, Kansas 66212 913-341-1300	Monthly publication serving various segments of the health/fitness and recreational industry, including commercial facilities, community centers, not-for-profits, and university-based facilities
Club Insider News Box 681241 Marietta, Georgia 30068 770-850-8506	Monthly publication for anyone involved in the health/fitness club industry; offers inside news typically not provided by other publications

Club Solutions Magazine Peake Media 211 Townpark Circle Suite 200 Louisville, Kentucky 40243 877-254-7021	Monthly publication that serves as a business resource for the health/fitness club industry; focus is on new product offerings from suppliers
DaySpa Magazine Creative Age Communications 7628 Densmore Avenue Van Nuys, California 91406 1-800-624-4196	Monthly publication that is dedicated to serving day spa operators, with practical information about the spa industry
Exercise Standards and Malpractice Reporter PRC Publishing 3976 Fulton Drive, N.W. Canton, Ohio 44718 330-492-6063	Monthly publication targeted at professionals in the fitness industry; focus is on legal and risk management issues
IDEA Fitness Journal 10455 Pacific Center Court San Diego, California 92121 800-999-IDEA	Monthly publication for personal trainers and group-exercise instructors
Pulse A publication of ISPA 2365 Harrodsburg Road, Suite A325 Lexington, Kentucky 40504 888-651-4772	Monthly publication targeted at professionals who own and operate spas
Recreation Management CAB Communications 50 North Brockway Street, Suite 4-11 Palatine, Illinois 60067 847-963-8740	Monthly publication targeted at recreation professionals
Strength and Conditioning Journal Professional Journal of NSCA 1885 Bob Johnson Drive Colorado Springs, Colorado 80906 800-815-6826	Bimonthly publication targeted at NSCA members

Appendix C

Profiles of Leading Global Health/Fitness Club Companies

This section provides examples of some of the leading global players in the health/fitness industry.

❏ *24 Hour Fitness, San Ramon, California* (www.24hourfitness.com). 24 hour Fitness was originally founded in 1983 in Northern California. It emerged as an industry leader in the 90s after bringing on a private equity firm and purchasing Ray Wilson's Family Fitness Centers of California. Since the 1990s, it has been able to acquire regionally based club groups, as well as drive organic growth through a combination of debt and equity. In 2005, the company was sold to Forstmann Little, a New-York based private equity firm, for a reported $1.6 billion. Currently, the company operates over 440 clubs in the U.S. and overseas, serving approximately 3.5 million members. The company has several different types of club offerings, including active and express clubs (fitness-only clubs), sport clubs, super sport clubs, and ultra sport clubs (a level of club based on types of facilities and amenities offered). The company also offers a unique group of celebrity-branded clubs, such as Andre Agassi, Jackie Chan, Magic Johnson, and Derek Jeter. Depending on the type of club and market served, dues for an individual could range from under $30 a month to around $70 a month in its branded urban clubs. The company reported revenues of around $1.2 billion in 2010, making it one of the two largest global companies by revenues.

❏ *Equinox Clubs, New York, New York* (www.equinox.com). Equinox is based in New York. As of January 2011, it operated 50 clubs in several markets, including New York, Chicago, Northern California, Southern California, Florida, and Texas. Equinox clubs are premium gyms that serve an affluent, middle-age, urban market. The Equinox brand slogan is, "It's not fitness. It's Life". The brand is built on trendy modern facilities, innovative programs and services, and association with the "star wannabes" in their respective communities. While the clubs range in size, most are in the neighborhood of 25,000 to 45,000 square feet. Some facilities offer pools, and most have a spa. The clubs have between 4,000 and 6,000 memberships per club. Although pricing varies by market, in all instances, an individual membership costs between $120 and $150, with additional fees for gaining full access to other Equinox clubs either in the region or nationally. Equinox is known for its innovative group-exercise and excellent personal-training services, with an estimated 15 percent to 20 percent of members enrolled in personal training. In late 2011, Equinox purchased four Sports Club/LA clubs for approximately $130 million. Equinox leads the U.S. club industry with regard to leveraging technology. It also has one of the most dynamic websites in the industry. The company generates an estimated $350 million in revenues.

❑ *Fitness First, United Kingdom* (www.fitnessfirst.com). Fitness First was founded in 1993 by Mike Balfour. The company was originally founded on a brand promise of affordable and convenient fitness. In its early years, the company grew rapidly through organic development, fueled by private equity and debt. In the late 90s, the company went public on the London exchange, only to return to the private sector in the early part of the 21st century. Currently, the company operates over 500 clubs across the globe (U.K., Germany, Australia, India, Asia, etc.). The company's clubs currently serve a membership base of 1.4 million. In 2009 the company reported revenues of slightly over $1 billion, making it, at the time, one of the two largest global companies by revenues (24 Hour Fitness generates a similar level of revenues). In 2010 and 2011, the company sold off clubs in several European markets, while concurrently acquiring clubs in Germany, which is one of its strongest markets (behind only England and Australia). The company has been active in developing master franchise agreements in Asia and the Middle East over the past few years.

❑ *Konami Sports, Tokyo, Japan* (www.konamisportsclub.jp). Konami Sports was founded in 1973. Originally, the clubs were operated under the People Company banner, but later, after being sold, were rebranded as Konami Sports. The company is public. The company currently operates 327 clubs in Japan, of which 212 are owned and 115 are managed. In 2008, the company reported serving a membership base of nearly 980,000. In 2009, the company reported revenues of $950 million, which when measured by revenues, indicates that it is in the top five globally.

❑ *LA Fitness, U.S.* LA Fitness currently operates over 360 clubs throughout the U.S. The company, which was founded in the 1980s, really took off in the early part of the 21st century, when it acquired considerable private equity and debt financing. The company model was to build large, suburban multipurpose clubs that offered limited amenities and service at a very low price ($29 to $59 a month, depending on the regional market).While the company keeps its metrics private, it is estimated that their clubs serve over two million members and that company revenues exceed $1 billion annually. Some financial people have estimated their enterprise value at well over $3 billion. In late 2011, LA Fitness purchased 171 Bally Total Fitness clubs. As measured by the number of clubs that an organization has, that acquisition made LA Fitness the largest club company in the world.

❑ *Lifetime Fitness, Minneapolis, Minnesota* (www.lifetimefitness.com). Lifetime Fitness was founded in 1992 by Bahram Akradi. The company revolutionized the suburban club market by introducing the first family-oriented, high-volume sales club in the U.S. market. The company's clubs range in size from 80,000 square feet to as large as 140,000 square feet. The company was privately held until 2004, when it went public. The company's growth has primarily been through organic development. Only in the past few years, has it looked at acquisitions to fuel growth. Currently, the company owns and operates over 90 clubs in 21 states. The company has approximately 19,000 employees, who serve a membership base of over 750,000 members (approximately 8,000 to 10,000 members per club). In 2010, the company reported revenues of close to $1 billion, with an EBITDA margin of over 25 percent. As of 2011, it is one of the three or four largest club companies in the world.

❑ *McFit, Germany.* McFit was founded in the late 1990s. The company established the benchmark for budget clubs in Europe. The company model revolves around fitness-only clubs, offering 24-hour access, limited staffing (usually one staff person during staffed hours), no amenities (members actually pay for showers), lots of equipment, and self-directed exercise programming. One of its unique selling propositions is its technology platform, which may be among the best in the industry. Currently, it owns and operates over 120 clubs in Germany and, at the present time, is expanding into other European markets. As of 2010, it served close to one million members and reported revenues of approximately $200 million. It also reports an EBITDA margin in excess of 30 percent.

❑ *Virgin Active, United Kingdom* (www.virginactive.com). Virgin Active was founded in 1998, with the acquisition of the assets of the former Healthland chain of clubs in South Africa. Since its founding, the company has expanded into England, as well as into mainland Europe. In the middle of the 21st century, it purchased Holmes Place, an operator of premium and luxury clubs in the U.K. By the end of 2009, the company owned and operated close to 190 clubs and had over 900,000 members. The Virgin Active chain includes both Virgin Active and Virgin Active Classic clubs (premium and luxury). In 2011, it completed the acquisition of Esporta, a chain of 55 urban and suburban premium clubs in the U.K. With this acquisition, its portfolio of clubs has increased to over 225 clubs. Prior to acquiring Esporta in 2011, Virgin Active reported 2010 revenues of approximately $600 million. With the acquisition of Esporta completed, however, the company's revenues for 2011 should exceed $800 million, making it one of the five largest club companies in the world.

Appendix D
Profiles of Regional U.S. Club Companies

This appendix provides an overview of several leading club companies in the U.S., each of which is a leader in local, regional, or several regional markets.

❑ *Club One, San Francisco, California* (www.clubone.com). Club One was founded in 1991. Currently, it owns and operates 90 clubs (14 owned and 76 managed). In addition to operating commercial clubs in Northern and Southern California, it also manages community recreation centers and sports clubs for local municipalities and non-profit associations, as well as on-site corporate fitness centers for some of the nation's largest corporations. The company serves a member base of over 250,000 and reported approximately $80 million in revenue for 2010.

❑ *DMB Sports Clubs-Village Sports, Scottsdale, Arizona* (www.villageclubs.com). DMB is a chain of four clubs, based in Scottsdale, Arizona. Its clubs are high-end, sport resort-type clubs, serving an affluent family market. Its facilities are multipurpose clubs that range from 50,000 to over 100,000 square feet. Its brand is built on family offerings and a service level that have a resort-feel to them. Its clubs have between 2,000 and 4,000 memberships per club. Overall, the company has a membership base of 14,000. While pricing varies, individual dues at each of their respective clubs may range between $75 and $100 a month. The company's clubs are known for their family programs and customer service.

❑ *Fitness Formula, Chicago, Illinois* (www.ffc.com). Fitness Formula owns and operates 12 clubs in the Chicago market that collectively have over 30,000 members. Its clubs are located primarily in an urban setting, although it does have suburban clubs. Fitness Formula facilities are premium clubs that serve an upper-middle class audience, composed of individuals and families. Its brand promise is to enrich people's lives and deliver results. Its clubs are primarily multipurpose and include gymnasiums and pools. Each facility ranges in size from 30,000 to 100,000 square feet. Its clubs offer group exercise, personal training, physical therapy services, spa services, and cafes. The company offers all members the opportunity for reciprocal privileges in all of its clubs. Pricing ranges from $70 to just over $100 a month for an individual. Its clubs market in the local media. In 2009, the company had estimated revenues to be $32.5 million.

❑ *Healthworks Fitness Centers for Women, Boston, Massachusetts* (www.healthworksfitness.com). Healthworks is a women's-only group of five clubs in the Boston area that has distinguished itself as one of the best women's-only club operations in the industry. Healthworks serves both an urban residential and a corporate market, as well as a suburban market of women. Its target market is middle income-to-affluent women. The company has also established a separate foundation, Healthworks Foundation, that serves less-advantaged women and families in the Boston area and provides membership opportunities to those individuals who could not normally afford membership. Its brand is built on the "women's-only" environment and community involvement. It is known, however, for great group exercise (over 100 classes a week in each club), Pilates programs, and customized wellness programs for women. Pricing differs in clubs, but in most instances, an individual membership is over $70 a month. In 2008, the company reported revenues of approximately $22 million.

❑ *Leisure Sports, Pleasanton, California* (www.clubsports.com). Leisure Sports operates seven high-end, multipurpose clubs in California, Oregon, and Nevada that collectively serve a membership base of slightly over 37,000. Leisure Sports focuses on the affluent (over $100,000 HH income) family market by offering a full-service, multipurpose facility. Its brand is distinguished by the connection of a high-end sports club with a high-end hotel, creating what the owners refer to as a sport resort. Its facilities range from 70,000 to over 100,000 square feet, with over 5,000 members on average per club. Monthly dues vary, but in most instances, individual dues will fall between $90 and $120 a month. Its focus is on service and programming. In 2010, the company reported revenue of approximately $80 million.

❑ *Lifestyle Family Fitness Centers (LFF), St. Petersburg, Florida* (www.lff.com). LFFC operates 55 clubs located in Florida, Ohio, and the Carolinas. Originally serving the Tampa and the St. Petersburg markets, LFF has expanded into other major central-Florida markets, such as Orlando and Jacksonville, as well as into areas in other states. LFF clubs serve both the individual and family market and target the middle class market. The company's brand is built on being affordable and convenient and having great facilities and group-exercise programs. Its clubs typically are fitness-only, but some of its facilities are multipurpose. Its facilities are normally under 30,000 square feet per club. Monthly dues for an individual membership are typically under $50. Its clubs undertake considerable advertising in the local media and have a strong leadership team. In 2010, the company served over 225,000 members and reported revenues of approximately $110 million.

❑ *Midtown Athletic Clubs (MAC), Chicago, Illinois* (www.midtownathleticclub. com). The MAC was originally founded in 1969 by Alan Schwartz and his father, when they opened the Mid Town Tennis Club in Chicago. The company currently operates 22 clubs (10 owned and 12 managed), in addition to a corporate-wellness entity that manages wellness and fitness centers for large corporations. The company's owned and managed clubs target an affluent upper-middle class demographic. The company is known for its outstanding tennis programs, high level of customer service, and commitment to employee education. The company reported revenues of approximately $70 million in 2010.

❑ *Western Athletic Clubs (WAC), Northern and Southern California* (www. westernathleticclubs.com). WAC was founded in 1977 by Jim Gerber, who ran the company until 2010 when it was sold to KSL. WAC operates a total of nine clubs, with a collective membership base of approximately 30,000. The company operates premium and luxury sport resorts that range in size from 40,000 square feet to over 100,000 square feet. Their clubs are multipurpose and offer fitness, aquatics, spa services, extensive youth programs, and tennis. Among its most recognized facilities are the Courtside Club, the San Francisco Tennis Club, the San Francisco Bay Club, and its three Pacific Athletic Clubs in Redwood City, Marin, and San Diego. The company reported earnings of approximately $110 million in 2010.

❏ *Wisconsin Athletic Clubs (WAC), Milwaukee, Wisconsin* (www.thewac.com). WAC owns and operates six clubs in the Milwaukee, Wisconsin market. WAC clubs serve primarily a family market, targeting a middle-class demographic. Its clubs vary in size, but most are under 40,000 square feet and offer either a fitness-only experience or, in the case of a few clubs, a multipurpose-club experience. The company's first facility was a racquetball club that opened in the 1970s. The key mission of the company is to make a difference in people's lives. Its brand is based on accessibility in the local market, convenience, good facilities, a focus on service, and programming. Monthly dues for an individual are $55 to $75 a month. Its clubs advertise in the local media.

The statistical and numerical data included in this section are based on information from the *IHRSA 2010 Global Report*. The company overview was generated from observations made through first-hand knowledge of each company.

Appendix E
Sample Marketing Materials From
Leading Global Health/Fitness Clubs

"Switch Your Routine" ad campaign, Companhia Athletica, Brazil

Direct mail piece, Crunch

Direct mail piece, Companhia Athletica, Brazil

"Fat Imprisonment" ad campaign, Companhia Athletica, Brazil

Smart phone application, Planet Fitness

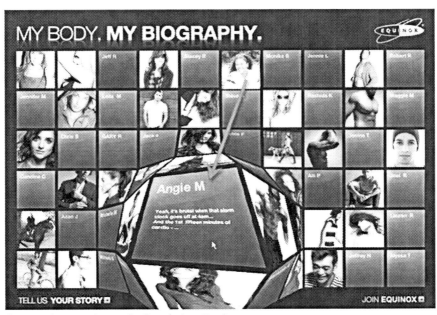

"My Body. My Biography." website, Equinox

Employees ad campaign, World Class, Russia

Member reward program, Club One

Appendix F
Profiles of Leading U.S. Health/Fitness Club Equipment Manufacturers

This appendix provides an overview of several of the leading manufacturers of equipment for health/fitness club facilities in the world.

❑ *Cybex International, Medway, Massachusetts*

Cybex is a full-service equipment manufacturer that offers a complete array of cardiovascular and resistance training equipment. Cybex originated in the 1960s as the Cybex Ergometer Company and was later purchased by Lumex. Originally, Cybex manufactured medically based isokinetic equipment used in rehabilitative medicine. In 1983, Cybex purchased Eagle Resistance Equipment, a step that moved the company into a new manufacturing arena that focused on variable-resistance equipment and free-weight equipment. During its first several years of business, Eagle made significant inroads into the resistance-training equipment market that had been dominated at the time by Nautilus. Subsequently, during the early 1990s, Cybex became the biggest player in the resistance-training arena. Cybex also created a line of isokinetic cardiovascular equipment that was targeted specifically for the fitness/health club industry. At the time, the Cybex Upper-Body Ergometer was considered one of the best, if not the best, of its type in the industry. During the early 1990s, Cybex was known for its quality, service, and its isokinetic cardiovascular equipment. In 1997, Cybex merged with Trotter to form a new company, called Cybex International. In the process, the new company, Cybex International, inherited the treadmills and other cardiovascular equipment that Trotter had developed over the years. In the early part of the 21st century, the company released its most popular piece of equipment—a modified elliptical trainer, appropriately called the Arc Trainer. At the present time, Cybex sells over $120 million in equipment annually. Its line of equipment offerings includes variable-resistance equipment, free-weight benches, plate-loaded equipment, treadmills, bicycles, and the ARC Trainer. Much of Cybex's popularity in the club industry is a result of the variety of its equipment offerings (i.e., it can outfit an entire club), the quality of its resistance-equipment lines, and its ability to provide financing to clubs for the purchase of its equipment. Cybex is a publically held company listed on the New York Stock Exchange.

❑ *Life Fitness, Franklin Park, Illinois*

Life Fitness was founded by Augie Neito, who built the company from the original Lifecycle company that was established by Ray Wilson, when he purchased the rights to market the original Lifecyle, which was invented in 1968 by Keene Dimmick. At the time, Lifecycle became the "band-aid" brand for the fitness industry when it was introduced in 1974. In the process, Life Fitness became the first manufacturer to establish a leadership position in the cardiovascular equipment arena. The Lifecycle later led to the development of the Lifestep and subsequently to a full line of cardiovascular equipment, including treadmills, recumbent bikes, and elliptical trainers. The cardiovascular equipment manufactured by Life Fitness was branded by its unique control panel and the special programming features on each machine, including hill and random programs. Life Fitness became and, to this day, remains the largest manufacturer of cardiovascular equipment in the industry. In the early 1990s, Life Fitness bought a resistance company, called High Tech, and created the Life Fitness strength line. In the later half of the 1990s, Life Fitness purchased Hammer Strength. The merger of the cardiovascular, variable resistance, and Hammer products created the largest equipment company in the industry. Currently, Life Fitness sells over $600 million annually, making it the largest equipment manufacturer in the fitness arena. Life Fitness is known as a leader in several of its product categories. For example, the Hammer line is regarded as the gold standard in the plate-loaded category; its bikes are the top in their category, and its treadmills are among the top three in their category. Life Fitness's strength is based on its ability to completely outfit a club (e.g., treadmills, bikes, stairclimbers, ellipticals, resistance machines, and free weights), the quality of its product from a technical and customer perspective, the innovative nature of its products, the respect that its team of staff garner, and its marketing and sales.

❏ *Precor, Inc., Woodinville, Washington*

Initially, Precor started out by making cardiovascular equipment for the home market. At the time, it was among the leaders in home equipment, such as bikes and treadmills. Precor entered the commercial club market in the 1980s with its treadmills, bikes, and stairclimbers. The Precor treadmill established a unique niche when it was introduced due to its ability to adjust to both positive and negative grades. Precor became an even bigger player in the market when it introduced the EFX Elliptical Trainer in 1995. In the process, the EFX became a landmark for the equipment industry that changed the club industry. By the late 1990s and early 21st century, Precor became one of the top three players in the cardiovascular arena, with the EFX and its treadmills. During this period, Precor also introduced its Stretch Trainer. Over the years, Precor has been renowned for its innovation in equipment design, its equipment esthetics, and its desire to introduce new concepts to the market. In 2004, Precor purchased Icarian, a leading manufacturer of variable-resistance equipment and free-weight benches. In turn, it established its own line of resistance equipment. Precor bought Cardio Theater in 2004, expanding its reach into the entertainment and technology sectors. Currently, Precor, which is owned by Amer Sports, a Finnish company that also owns brands, such as Atomic and Wilson, offers an extensive line of exercise equipment (e.g., treadmills, elliptical trainers, bikes, stairclimbers, and resistance equipment). Not only can the company outfit an entire club, it also has the ability to offer cardio entertainment. It is the third largest player in the industry, with approximately $200 million in annual sales. Precor's strength lies in its approach to innovation, its ability to offer a complete package, the aesthetics of its product offering, and its marketing and sales efforts.

❏ *Star Trac, Irvine, California*

In the early 1980s, Star Trac got its start as a company named Unisen. As Unisen, it produced the electronics for Life Fitness equipment during the early years of Life Fitness. Around 1990, Star Trac entered the market as Star Trac by Unisen, whereupon it positioned itself as a leading producer of commercial treadmills. Star Trac introduced one of the first commercial treadmills in the industry that was customer-friendly, technically sound, and reasonably affordable. Since its inception, Star Trac has subsequently expanded its line of commercial treadmills, as well as added other types of exercise equipment to its inventory, including stationary cycles, stairclimbers, elliptical machines, and group-exercise bikes. Star Trac established itself as a leader in the area of cardiovascular equipment by offering quality equipment that had innovations that served the needs of the end-user. Star Trac's treadmills are the only ones with built-in fans, while its bikes and recumbent bikes are the only ones with an innovative design that includes fans and comfort seating. Star Trac obtained rights to the "Johnny G" line of group-exercise bikes in the early part of the 21st century. In 2005, Star Trac expanded its offerings into the cardio-entertainment arena, as well as the resistance-equipment segment of the market, with its purchase of Flex. The company took the Flex line and created its own line of resistance equipment. In 2010, Star Trac experienced some financial troubles and was sold to a new owner, who renamed the company—Star Trac Health and Fitness. The company continues to provide quality equipment to the global marketplace. Star Trac's strengths lie in its product innovation, its focus on producing user-friendly products, its level of customer service, and its positive relationships with its customer base.

❏ *Technogym USA, Seattle, Washington*

Technogym, an Italian-based firm, is the leading fitness equipment manufacturer in Europe and is second only to Life Fitness in total global sales, with over $250 million in total annual sales worldwide. Technogym released its first product, the isotonic line of resistance training equipment, in 1983, the year that the company was founded. Within five years of launching its isotonic line, the company introduced its first line of cardiovascular equipment. Shortly thereafter, Technogym became the leading manufacturer of exercise equipment in Europe.

Technogym burst on the U.S. scene in the early 1990s after establishing itself as the leading manufacturer of commercial cardiovascular and resistance equipment in the European market. Technogym set itself apart when it entered the domestic U.S. market on two fronts. First, it branded itself as the "wellness" company and provided educational support to the industry. Second, it introduced the technology platform that tied its equipment together through a "key" that contained all of a user's workout information. The "key," which continues to be a benchmark for Technogym, is still offered as an upgrade. Technogym also introduced the flare of contemporary European design to its resistance machines and free-weight benches. In the process, it changed the way that other manufacturers design their resistance-training equipment. Among the factors that Technogym has become a leader in the area of equipment innovation and technology are its built-in LED media systems and its club-based software platform for monitoring member activity. Technogym's various product offerings include treadmills, bikes, stairclimbers, elliptical machines, variable resistance equipment, and free-weight equipment. Technogym's primary strengths lie in the technical quality of its equipment, its innovative design, its focus on wellness, and its ability to equip an entire club.

Appendix G
Sample Job Descriptions

This appendix contains sample job descriptions for various generic positions in the fitness and health club industry.

❏ **Fitness Director**

Position Title: Fitness Director
Position Description Summary:

The position of fitness director is responsible for the overall operations and programming of the fitness facility, with primary oversight of the operating standards, systems and practices as they directly impact the overall operating excellence of the department.

Essential Accountabilities & Functions:

1. To oversee all financial aspects of the fitness department operations, including working with other department heads and supervisors as needed to insure that the financial performance of the fitness department meets budget.

2. To select, hire, coach, mentor and educate fitness department employees in a manner that reinforces the club's values and philosophies and insures the operation of the department meets company standards and provides an environment that promotes membership retention.

3. To oversee all operating practices, policies and systems that are necessary for achieving the department's and club's strategic and business plan goals.

4. To oversee all fitness programming and marketing practices, policies and systems that are necessary for achieving the department's and club's strategic and business plan goals.

Specific Job Accountabilities

1. To select, hire, educate and lead department employees in all work areas, including locker rooms, front desk, childcare, fitness floor, group exercise, massage, racquet sports, etc. This includes managing all aspects of the selection, hiring and education process and providing the leadership for the team on a daily basis.

2. To conduct regular meetings and education sessions for employees, including monthly department meetings and daily line-ups.

3. To oversee the financial success of the fitness department through: correct pricing of services, monitoring and management of employee payroll and lesson payments, daily and monthly audits of sales, forecasting department performance on a monthly basis and whatever other actions must occur for the department to meet its budget and forecast goals.

4. To handle the daily, weekly and period payroll functions for the department, including, but not limited to, collecting and auditing employee commission sheets, doing all payroll activities, managing payroll and commission expense to plan, etc.

5. To create, implement resource and/or execute the necessary actions steps required to successfully meet the fitness operating standards of the club.

6. To create, coordinate, resource, implement, market and sell fitness programs and services. In doing so, to insure proper systems are implemented so as to insure that the club program's meet the needs of membership and drive member participation in such a manner as to create and enhance Member retention.

7. To utilize the available resources of the club in executing the responsibilities of fitness director. This includes incorporating any standards and systems the club has established for operations and programming.

8. To assist in the delivery of department services as required, including providing specific services as qualified to do so by training (examples are working the floor, performing personal training, instructing a class, handling front desk duties, cleaning, etc.)

9. To meet regularly with the manager and other department heads/supervisors to make sure there is complete cooperation between departments in the club and to insure that there is regular communication to other employees in the club regarding the department's services and operation.

10. To assist with any required job activity of the department, as may be needed, so as to insure members are always served in accordance with the club's overall service philosophy.

11. To conduct oneself at all times in a manner of professionalism that aligns with the values, philosophies and standards of the club.

Reporting Relationships:

Reports to:	Club Manager
Directly Supervises:	Front desk staff, locker room staff, childcare staff, fitness floor staff, group exercise staff, massage staff, and racquet sport staff.
Indirectly Supervises:	

Work Experience:

1. Minimum of one year's experience in a supervisory or similar department head role.
2. Minimum of five years experience in the club and/or fitness industry.

Education:

1. College Degree in health, fitness or recreation related field.
2. Master's Degree in related field preferred, but not required.

Certification/License

1. Certification in CPR.
2. Certification from national organization such as ACSM, ACE, NSCA, etc. required..

Working Conditions/Environment

(describe the club's specific facilities and general environment)

Specific Working Conditions

Squatting	Bending	Kneeling
Reaching	Twisting	Crawling
Ladder Climbing	Stair Climbing	Other Climbing
Walking on Rough Ground	Exposure to Temperature Change	Exposure to Dust, Fumes & Gas
Near Moving Machinery	Working from Heights	Cleaning/Scrubbing
Dialing	Collating	Filing
Opening/Closing	Sorting	Stamping
Stapling	Folding/Unfolding	Inserting/Removing

Max. Weight Lifted Occasional	State Weight Lifted if Above 100 lbs.
Max. Weight Lifted Frequently	State Weight Lifted if Above 100 lbs.
Max. Weight Carried Occasionally	State Weight Carried if Above 100 lbs.
Max. Weight Carried Frequently	State Weight Carried if Above 100 lbs.
Max. Weight Pushed Occasionally	State Weight Pushed if Above 100 lbs.
Max. Weight Pushed Frequently	State Weight Pushed if Above 100 lbs.
Max. Weight Pulled Occasionally	State Weight Pulled if Above 100 lbs.
Max Weight Pulled Frequently	State Weight Pulled if Above 100 lbs.
Sit: Hr. Day	Sit: Frequency
Stand: Hr. Day	Stand: Frequency
Walk: Hr. Day	Walk: Frequency
Drive: Hr. Day	Drive: Frequency

❑ **Fitness Instructor**

Position Title: Fitness Instructor/Personal Trainer
Position Description Summary:

The position of fitness instructor/personal trainer is responsible for providing a safe and effective exercise environment for club Members through supervision of Member exercise programs, education of the Members in exercise and a focus on establishing a personalized program of exercise for each Member.

Essential Accountabilities & Functions:
1. To provide supervision of the exercise and fitness areas of the club, including assisting Members with their exercise and fitness program.

2. To evaluate Member fitness needs and provide the appropriate exercise program for meeting those Members needs, including providing personal instruction if necessary.

3. To connect Members to other Members through ongoing contact with the Members and promotion of club activities.

Specific Job Accountabilities

1. Conduct new Member fitness orientations in accordance with club standards.

2. To provide exercise floor supervision, including greeting each Member and servicing their fitness needs.

3. To create personalized exercise/fitness programs for Members, including providing personal coaching and education of the Member in the program.

4. To insure that all exercise areas and equipment are in safe and effective working condition, including cleanliness being maintained to club standards.

5. To assist with any required job activity of the department, as may be needed, so as to insure Members are always served in accordance with the club's overall service philosophy.

6. To conduct oneself at all times in a manner of professionalism that aligns with the values, philosophies and standards of the club. This includes being in club-approved uniform and nametag.

7. To attend all scheduled employee meetings.

Reporting Relationships:
    Reports to: Fitness Director
    Directly Supervises:
    Indirectly Supervises:

Work Experience:
1. Minimum of one year's experience in the fitness or exercise industry.

Education:
1. College Degree in health, fitness or recreation related field.

Certification/License
1. Certification in CPR.
2. Certification from national organization such as ACSM, ACE, NASM, etc. preferred.

Working Conditions/Environment
(describe the club's specific facilities and general environment)

Specific Working Conditions

Squatting	Bending	Kneeling
Reaching	Twisting	Crawling
Ladder Climbing	Stair Climbing	Other Climbing
Walking on Rough Ground	Exposure to Temperature Change	Exposure to Dust, Fumes & Gas
Near Moving Machinery	Working from Heights	Cleaning/Scrubbing
Dialing	Collating	Filing
Opening/Closing	Sorting	Stamping
Stapling	Folding/Unfolding	Inserting/Removing

Max. Weight Lifted Occasional	State Weight Lifted if Above 100 lbs.
Max. Weight Lifted Frequently	State Weight Lifted if Above 100 lbs.
Max. Weight Carried Occasionally	State Weight Carried if Above 100 lbs.
Max. Weight Carried Frequently	State Weight Carried if Above 100 lbs.
Max. Weight Pushed Occasionally	State Weight Pushed if Above 100 lbs.
Max. Weight Pushed Frequently	State Weight Pushed if Above 100 lbs.
Max. Weight Pulled Occasionally	State Weight Pulled if Above 100 lbs.
Max Weight Pulled Frequently	State Weight Pulled if Above 100 lbs.
Sit: Hr. Day	Sit: Frequency
Stand: Hr. Day	Stand: Frequency
Walk: Hr. Day	Walk: Frequency
Drive: Hr. Day	Drive: Frequency

❏ **Group Exercise Instructor**

Position Title: Group Exercise Instructor

Position Description Summary:

The position of group exercise instructor is responsible for providing a safe and effective group exercise environment for club Members by providing instruction, coaching and supervision to the Members during scheduled group exercise activities.

Essential Accountabilities & Functions:

1. To provide group exercise instruction to Members that is safe and effective.

2. To provide a safe and motivating group exercise environment for the Members.

3. To connect Members to other Members through ongoing contact with the Members and promote other club activities.

Specific Job Accountabilities

1. To provide group exercise instruction for Members per the requirements and standards of the Club.

2. To insure that the group exercise studio is prepared to club standards for each class taught, including having the right equipment for the class, insuring that the classroom is properly cleaned, having the right music available and having the correct temperature.

3. To assist with any required job activity of the department, as may be needed, so as to insure Members are always served in accordance with the club's overall service philosophy.

4. To conduct oneself at all times in a manner of professionalism that aligns with the values, philosophies and standards of the club. This includes being in club-approved uniform and nametag and being on time for scheduled classes.

5. To attend all scheduled employee meetings.

Reporting Relationships:

Reports to: Fitness Director or Group Exercise Coordinator

Directly Supervises:

Indirectly Supervises:

Work Experience:
1. Minimum of one year's experience or 200 hours class instruction experience.

Education:
2. College Degree in health, fitness or recreation related field preferred, but not required.

Certification/License

1. Certification in CPR.
2. General group exercise certification from national organization such as AFAA or ACE.
3. For specialty classes such as Yoga, Pilate's, Group Cycling, Resist-a-Ball, etc., then certification from representative organization.

Working Conditions/Environment

(describe the club's specific facilities and general environment)

Specific Working Conditions

Squatting	Bending	Kneeling
Reaching	Twisting	Crawling
Ladder Climbing	Stair Climbing	Other Climbing
Walking on Rough Ground	Exposure to Temperature Change	Exposure to Dust, Fumes & Gas
Near Moving Machinery	Working from Heights	Cleaning/Scrubbing
Dialing	Collating	Filing
Opening/Closing	Sorting	Stamping
Stapling	Folding/Unfolding	Inserting/Removing

Max. Weight Lifted Occasional	State Weight Lifted if Above 100 lbs.
Max. Weight Lifted Frequently	State Weight Lifted if Above 100 lbs.
Max. Weight Carried Occasionally	State Weight Carried if Above 100 lbs.
Max. Weight Carried Frequently	State Weight Carried if Above 100 lbs.
Max. Weight Pushed Occasionally	State Weight Pushed if Above 100 lbs.
Max. Weight Pushed Frequently	State Weight Pushed if Above 100 lbs.
Max. Weight Pulled Occasionally	State Weight Pulled if Above 100 lbs.
Max Weight Pulled Frequently	State Weight Pulled if Above 100 lbs.
Sit: Hr. Day	Sit: Frequency
Stand: Hr. Day	Stand: Frequency
Walk: Hr. Day	Walk: Frequency
Drive: Hr. Day	Drive: Frequency

❏ **Massage Therapist**

Position Title: Massage/Spa Therapist

Position Description Summary:
The position of massage/spa therapist provides relaxing, soothing and effective bodywork treatments for Members and Guests that allows them to connect with themselves.

Essential Accountabilities & Functions:

1. To provide relaxing, soothing and beneficial bodywork treatments.

2. To provide warm greetings and an enriching environment within the context of the massage/spa work area.

3. To connect Members to other Members through ongoing contact with the Members and promotion of club activities.

Specific Job Accountabilities

1. To provide warm greetings and an enriching environment to all Members/Guests who you interact with.

2. To conduct relaxing, soothing, safe and beneficial bodywork treatments for Members and Guests in accordance with club standards.

3. To make sure that the massage/spa workspace is in compliance with standards and ready to be occupied by Member & guests. This includes having all equipment well maintained and cleaned, having the room cleaned and set-up, having all necessary information on the Member/guest that is needed, etc.

4. To assist with any required job activity of the department, as may be needed, so as to insure Members are always served in accordance with the club's overall service philosophy.

5. To conduct oneself at all times in a manner of professionalism that aligns with the values, philosophies and standards of the club. This includes being in club-approved uniform and nametag.

6. To attend all scheduled employee meetings.

Reporting Relationships:

Reports to: Fitness Director and/or Spa Director
Directly Supervises:
Indirectly Supervises:

Work Experience:
Minimum of six month's experience providing massage/spa treatments.

Education:
1. Degree from accredited school of massage therapy if conducting bodywork treatments.
2. Degree from accredited cosmetology school if conducting services such as facials, manicures or pedicures.

Certification/License

1. State licensure in massage if conducting massage and bodywork treatments.
2. State licensure in cosmetology or similar if conducting manicures, pedicures and facials.
3. Certification in CPR.

Working Conditions/Environment

(describe the club's specific facilities and general environment)

Specific Working Conditions

Squatting	Bending	Kneeling
Reaching	Twisting	Crawling
Ladder Climbing	Stair Climbing	Other Climbing
Walking on Rough Ground	Exposure to Temperature Change	Exposure to Dust, Fumes & Gas
Near Moving Machinery	Working from Heights	Cleaning/Scrubbing
Dialing	Collating	Filing
Opening/Closing	Sorting	Stamping
Stapling	Folding/Unfolding	Inserting/Removing

Max. Weight Lifted Occasional	State Weight Lifted if Above 100 lbs.
Max. Weight Lifted Frequently	State Weight Lifted if Above 100 lbs.
Max. Weight Carried Occasionally	State Weight Carried if Above 100 lbs.
Max. Weight Carried Frequently	State Weight Carried if Above 100 lbs.
Max. Weight Pushed Occasionally	State Weight Pushed if Above 100 lbs.
Max. Weight Pushed Frequently	State Weight Pushed if Above 100 lbs.
Max. Weight Pulled Occasionally	State Weight Pulled if Above 100 lbs.
Max Weight Pulled Frequently	State Weight Pulled if Above 100 lbs.
Sit: Hr. Day	Sit: Frequency
Stand: Hr. Day	Stand: Frequency
Walk: Hr. Day	Walk: Frequency
Drive: Hr. Day	Drive: Frequency

❏   Front Desk Attendant

Position Title: Front Desk Attendant

Position Description Summary:
The position of front desk attendant is responsible for creating the first and last impressions of the club experience for Members by providing warm greetings and great service.

Essential Accountabilities & Functions:

1. To provide warm greetings and great service for members and guests..

2. To assist Members with the scheduling of appointments/reservations and the provision of information regarding club services and programs.

3. To connect Members to other Members through ongoing contact with the Members and promotion of club activities.

Specific Job Accountabilities

1. To provide warm greetings and great service to all Members/Guests who enter and leave the club.

2. To provide warm greetings and great service to all Members, guests and others over the telephone through compliance with the club" phone etiquette standards.

3. To assist Members in scheduling appointments and reservations for club programs and services in accordance with club standards.

4. To assist in providing information to club Members about club facilities, programs and services.

5. To assist with any required job activity of the department, as may be needed, so as to insure Members are always served in accordance with the club's overall service philosophy.

6. To conduct oneself at all times in a manner of professionalism that aligns with the values, philosophies and standards of the club. This includes being in club-approved uniform and nametag.

7. To attend all scheduled employee meetings.

Reporting Relationships:

   Reports to: Fitness Director/Front Desk Supervisor
   Directly Supervises:
   Indirectly Supervises:

Work Experience:
Minimum of six month's experience in the club or hospitality business in a similar capacity.

Education:
High School Diploma or Equivalent.

Certification/License
1. Certification in CPR.

Working Conditions/Environment
(describe the club's specific facilities and general environment)

Specific Working Conditions

Squatting	Bending	Kneeling
Reaching	Twisting	Crawling
Ladder Climbing	Stair Climbing	Other Climbing
Walking on Rough Ground	Exposure to Temperature Change	Exposure to Dust, Fumes & Gas
Near Moving Machinery	Working from Heights	Cleaning/Scrubbing
Dialing	Collating	Filing
Opening/Closing	Sorting	Stamping
Stapling	Folding/Unfolding	Inserting/Removing

Max. Weight Lifted Occasional	State Weight Lifted if Above 100 lbs.
Max. Weight Lifted Frequently	State Weight Lifted if Above 100 lbs.
Max. Weight Carried Occasionally	State Weight Carried if Above 100 lbs.
Max. Weight Carried Frequently	State Weight Carried if Above 100 lbs.
Max. Weight Pushed Occasionally	State Weight Pushed if Above 100 lbs.
Max. Weight Pushed Frequently	State Weight Pushed if Above 100 lbs.
Max. Weight Pulled Occasionally	State Weight Pulled if Above 100 lbs.
Max Weight Pulled Frequently	State Weight Pulled if Above 100 lbs.
Sit: Hr. Day	Sit: Frequency
Stand: Hr. Day	Stand: Frequency
Walk: Hr. Day	Walk: Frequency
Drive: Hr. Day	Drive: Frequency

Appendix H
Sample Compensation Agreements

<u>COMPENSATION AGREEMENT</u>
Fitness Director
(Employee)

The undersigned agrees to be employed in the position of Fitness Director ("Employee") of _____ ("Club"), effective _____, and shall continue for so long as Employee and Club both agree. This Compensation Agreement confirms our entire agreement concerning your employment compensation, which shall be based upon and subject to the following:

1. **Definitions**: The terms set forth shall have the following meanings:

    (a) "Fitness Department Net" shall mean the gross receipts from all fitness programs, services and retail merchandising minus any necessary expenses, including but not limited to all department expenses involved in the delivery of those programs, services and retail merchandise, but not limited to, promotional material, operational supplies, staff payroll and payroll costs, incentive items, etc.

    (b) "Membership Net" shall mean the amount of dues added, which is the additional dues from (i) new Members, and (ii) an increase in the amount of dues paid by Members, minus the dues lost from Members leaving the Club.

    (c) "Fitness Department Gross" shall mean the gross receipts from all fitness programs, services and retail merchandising, including but not limited to personal training, locker rental fees, massage, program fees, etc.

2. **Bi-Weekly Base Salary:** You will receive a bi-weekly salary of _____ to be paid out every two weeks in an amount equal to _____ (annualized amount equal to _____)

3. **Biweekly Performance Lesson Fee Rate**

    (a) Personal Training instruction taught by Employee shall earn a lesson fee rate equal to _____ _____ Dollars ($) for each lesson taught, up to a maximum of ten (10) lessons a week. The lesson rate earned will be the total compensation due Employee for each lesson.

    (b) Lesson fees shall be paid to you biweekly.

4. **Monthly Performance Bonus**:

    (a) A bonus of _____ Dollars ($) for meeting or beating budgeted Fitness Department Gross.

    (b) A bonus of _____ Dollars ($) for meeting or beating budgeted Fitness Department Net.

    (c) A bonus of _____ Dollars ($) for meeting or beating budgeted Membership Net.

    (d) Bonuses shall be calculated and paid to you within thirty (30) days following the end of each monthly accounting period.

    Employee must be employed on the last day of each monthly accounting period to receive the applicable period bonus.

Annual Performance Bonus

    (a) A bonus of _____ Dollars ($) for meeting or beating budgeted Fitness Department Net.

(b) Bonuses will be calculated and paid to you within thirty (30) days following the end of each calendar year.

5. **NO CONTRACT OF EMPLOYMENT: NEITHER THIS AGREEMENT NOR ANY OTHER COMMUNICATION SHALL BIND CLUB TO EMPLOY NOW OR HEREAFTER. THE EMPLOYMENT RELATIONSHIP BETWEEN YOU AND THE CLUB IS EMPLOYMENT AT WILL, AND THAT RELATIONSHIP MAY BE TERMINATED BY YOU OR BY CLUB FOR ANY REASON, AT ANY TIME, WITH OR WITHOUT NOTICE, AND WITH OR WITHOUT CAUSE. THE EMPLOYMENT AT WILL NATURE OF THIS RELATIONSHIP CANNOT BE ALTERED BY ANY STATEMENTS, ORAL OR WRITTEN, MADE BY ANYONE. IN THE EVENT OF TERMINATION, WEEKLY BASE SALARY AND COMMISSIONS/BONUSES SHALL BE PRORATED ON A DAILY BASIS TO THE DATE OF TERMINATION.**

6. Exempt Position: Your position as Fitness Director is an exempt position under the overtime provisions of the Fair Labor Standards Act and you are not entitled to overtime compensation. The compensation herein provided to you shall constitute full payment for the services rendered by you to Club.

7. Entire Agreement. This Agreement embodies the entire agreement and understanding of the parties relating to Employee's employment and supersedes all prior representations, agreements, and understandings..

If the foregoing accurately sets forth all of the terms of our agreement concerning your compensation, please indicate your acceptance by signing below.

EXECUTED this _____ day of _____, 20____.

Employee

Signature: _____

Print: _____

Club

Signature: _____

Title: _____

COMPENSATION AGREEMENT
(Personal Trainer/Fitness Instructor)

The undersigned agrees to be employed in the position of Personal Trainer ("Employee") by
_____ ("Club"), effective _____,20____, and shall continue
for so long as Employee and Club both agree. The purpose of this Agreement is to spell out the
compensation for this position.

1.   **Compensation**. The compensation paid to Employee will be comprised of the following:

      1.1 Employee shall earn a wage equal to _____ Dollars ($) for every member/guest paid
      one-hour personal training session that is conducted and appropriately recorded.

      1.2 Employee shall earn a wage equal to _____ Dollars ($) for every member/guest paid
      one-half hour personal training session that is conducted and appropriately recorded.

      1.3 Employee shall earn a wage equal to _____ Dollars ($) per hour for every fitness
      orientation, fitness test or other service that is provided by the Employee at the request of the
      Club.

      1.4 Time and one-half of Employee's Net Regular Rate will be paid to Employee for all hours
      worked over forty (40) in any one workweek.

2. **Duties**. Employee's duties shall include, but not be limited to, those described in Employee's job
description.

3. **Full Compensation**. The compensation provided for Employee by this Agreement shall constitute full
payment for the services rendered to Club. Employee shall not receive any additional compensation
for any services performed unless such services and payment, prior to their rendition, are authorized in
writing by the Club's General Manager. Employee expressly waives, discharges, and releases Club
from any claims for such services performed unless authorized in writing in the manner provided
above.

4. **THIS AGREEMENT IS NOT A CONTRACT FOR EMPLOYMENT FOR A FIXED TERM,
INSTEAD, IT DESCRIBES THE TERMS UPON WHICH EMPLOYEE'S COMPENSATION
IS TO BE BASED. EMPLOYEE UNDERSTANDS EITHER PARTY MAY TERMINATE THE
EMPLOYMENT RELATIONSHIP AT ANY TIME, FOR ANY REASON, WITH OR
WITHOUT CAUSE. THE EMPLOYMENT-AT-WILL NATURE OF THIS RELATIONSHIP
CANNOT BE ALTERED BY ANY STATEMENTS, ORAL OR WRITTEN, MADE BY
ANYONE. EMPLOYEE FURTHER UNDERSTANDS NO COMMISSIONS, BONUSES, OR
OTHER FORM OF COMPENSATION ACCRUE AFTER EMPLOYMENT TERMINATES.**

5. **Entire Agreement**. This Agreement embodies the entire agreement and understanding of the parties
relating to Employee's employment and supersedes all prior representations, agreements, and
understandings, oral or written, relating to Employee's employment.

      EXECUTED this _____ day of _____,20____.

Employee:

Signature: _____

Printed Name: _____

Club:

Signature: _____

Title: _____

<u>COMPENSATION AGREEMENT</u>
SPA DIRECTOR
(Employee)

The undersigned agrees to be employed in the position of Spa Director ("Employee") by _____ ("Club"), effective _____, and shall continue for so long as Employee and Club both agree. This Compensation Agreement confirms our entire agreement concerning your employment compensation, which shall be based upon and subject to the following:

1. **Definitions**: The terms set forth shall have the following meanings:

    (a) "Spa Department Net" shall mean the gross receipts from all spa programs, services and retail merchandising minus any necessary expenses, including but not limited to all department expenses involved in the delivery of those programs, services and retail merchandise, but not limited to, promotional material, operational supplies, staff payroll and payroll costs, incentive items, etc.

    (b) "Spa Department Gross" shall mean the gross receipts from all spa programs, services and retail merchandising, including but not limited to hairstyling, massage, facials, pedicures, manicures, etc.

2. **Bi-Weekly Base Salary:** You will receive a biweekly salary of _____ to be paid out every two weeks in an amount equal to _____ (annualized amount equal to _____).

3. **Biweekly Performance Treatment Fee Rate**

    (a) Any spa service rendered by Employee shall earn a treatment fee rate equal to _____ Dollars ($) for each service rendered, up to a maximum of ten (10) treatments a week. The treatment fee rate earned will be the total compensation due Employee for each treatment performed.

    (b) Treatment Fee rate shall be paid to you biweekly.

4. **Monthly Performance Bonus**:

    (a) A bonus of _____ ($) for meeting or beating budgeted Spa Department Gross.

    (b) A bonus of _____ ($) for meeting or beating budgeted Spa Department Net.

    (c) Bonuses shall be calculated and paid to you within thirty (30) days following the end of each monthly accounting period.

    Employee must be employed on the last day of each monthly accounting period to receive the applicable period bonus.

5. **Annual Performance Bonus**

    (a) A bonus of _____ ($) for meeting or beating budgeted Spa Department Net.

    (b) Bonuses will be calculated and paid to you within thirty (30) days following the end of each calendar year.

6. **NO CONTRACT OF EMPLOYMENT: NEITHER THIS AGREEMENT NOR ANY OTHER COMMUNICATION SHALL BIND CLUB TO EMPLOY YOU NOW OR HEREAFTER. THE EMPLOYMENT RELATIONSHIP BETWEEN YOU AND THE CLUB IS EMPLOYMENT AT WILL, AND THAT RELATIONSHIP MAY BE TERMINATED BY YOU OR BY CLUB FOR ANY REASON, AT ANY TIME, WITH OR WITHOUT NOTICE, AND WITH OR WITHOUT CAUSE. THE EMPLOYMENT AT WILL NATURE OF THIS RELATIONSHIP CANNOT BE ALTERED BY ANY STATEMENTS, ORAL OR WRITTEN, MADE BY ANYONE. IN THE EVENT OF TERMINATION, WEEKLY BASE SALARY AND COMMISSIONS SHALL BE PRORATED ON A DAILY BASIS TO THE DATE OF TERMINATION.**

7. Exempt Position: Your position as Spa Director is an exempt position under the overtime provisions of the Fair Labor Standards Act and you are not entitled to overtime compensation. The compensation herein provided to you shall constitute full payment for the services rendered by you to Club. You shall not receive additional compensation for any services performed unless such services and payment therefor, prior to their rendition, are authorized in writing by, or on behalf of Club. Employee expressly waives, discharges and releases Club from any claims for such services performed unless the same are authorized in writing as provided above.

8. Entire Agreement. This Agreement embodies the entire agreement and understanding of the parties relating to Employee's employment and supersedes all prior representations, agreements, and understandings.

If the foregoing correctly sets forth all of the terms of our agreement concerning your compensation, please indicate your acceptance by signing below.

EXECUTED this _____ day of _____, 20____.

Employee

Signature: _____

Printed
Name:_____

Club:

Signature:_____

Title: _____

Printed
Name: _____

COMPENSATION AGREEMENT
(Group Exercise Instructor)

The undersigned agrees to be employed in the position of Group Exercise Instructor ("Employee") by _____ ("Club"), effective _____,20____, and shall continue for so long as Employee and Club both agree. The purpose of this Agreement is to spell out the compensation for this position.

1. **Compensation**. The compensation paid to Employee will be comprised of the following:

    1.1. Group Exercise Instruction by Employee to Members or Guests shall earn a class rate equal to_____ DOLLARS ($_____) for each class instructed that is forty-five minutes to one – hour in duration. The class rate earned will be the total compensation due Employee for the instruction;

    1.2 Group Exercise Instruction by Employee to members or Guests shall earn a class rate equal to _____ DOLLARS ($_____) for each class instructed that is one – half hour to forty-four minutes in duration. The class rate earned will be the total compensation due Employee for the instruction.

    1.3 A rate of _____ DOLLARS ($_____) per hour for all hours worked when not providing group exercise instruction (base pay). The stated hourly rate will be the total compensation due Employee for all hours worked when not providing group exercise instruction, including holiday, personal and vacation time;

    1.4. Time and one-half of Employee's Net Regular Rate will be paid to Employee for all hours worked over forty (40) in any one workweek.

    1.5 Employee shall be paid every two weeks in an amount equal to what is earned based on 1.1, 1.2, 1.3 and 1.4 above.

2. **Duties**. Employee's duties shall include, but not be limited to, those described in Employee's job description.

3. **Full Compensation**. The compensation provided for Employee by this Agreement shall constitute full payment for the services rendered to Club. Employee shall not receive any additional compensation for any services performed unless such services and payment, prior to their rendition, are authorized in writing by the Club's General Manager. Employee expressly waives, discharges, and releases Club from any claims for such services performed unless authorized in writing in the manner provided above.

4   **THIS AGREEMENT IS NOT A CONTRACT FOR EMPLOYMENT FOR A FIXED TERM, INSTEAD, IT DESCRIBES THE TERMS UPON WHICH EMPLOYEE'S COMPENSATION IS TO BE BASED. EMPLOYEE UNDERSTANDS EITHER PARTY MAY TERMINATE THE EMPLOYMENT RELATIONSHIP AT ANY TIME, FOR ANY REASON, WITH OR WITHOUT CAUSE. THE EMPLOYMENT-AT-WILL NATURE OF THIS RELATIONSHIP CANNOT BE ALTERED BY ANY STATEMENTS, ORAL OR WRITTEN, MADE BY ANYONE. EMPLOYEE FURTHER UNDERSTANDS NO COMMISSIONS, BONUSES, OR OTHER FORM OF COMPENSATION ACCRUE AFTER EMPLOYMENT TERMINATES.**

6. **Entire Agreement**. This Agreement embodies the entire agreement and understanding of the parties relating to Employee's employment and supersedes all prior representations, agreements, and understandings, oral or written, relating to Employee's employment.

EXECUTED this _____ day of _____,20____.

Employee:

Signature:_____

Printed Name: _____

Club:

Signature: _____

Printed Name: _____

Title: _____

<u>COMPENSATION AGREEMENT</u>
(Massage Therapist)

The undersigned agrees to be employed in the position of Massage Therapist ("Employee") by
_____ ("Club"), effective _____,20____, and
shall continue for so long as Employee and Club both agree. The purpose of this Agreement is to spell out
the compensation for this position.

1.   <u>Compensation</u>. The compensation paid to Employee will be comprised of the following:

    1.1.   A rate of _____ DOLLARS ($_____) per forty-five minute to
            one-hour massage/body treatment that is delivered to a Member of Guest.

    1.2   A rate of _____ DOLLARS ($_____) per massage/body
            treatment of less than forty-five minutes duration.

    1.3   A rate of _____ DOLLARS ($_____) per hour for all
            hours worked when not providing massage/body treatments (base rate). The stated
            hourly rate will be the total compensation due Employee for all hours worked when not
            providing body massages. This base rate applies to all vacation, holiday and personal
            time;

    1.4   Time and one-half of Employee's Net Regular Rate will be paid to Employee for all hours
            worked over forty (40) in any one workweek.

    1.5   Employee shall be paid every two weeks in an amount equal to what is earned based on
            1.1, 1.2, 1.3 and 1.4 above.

2.   <u>Duties</u>. Employee's duties shall include, but not be limited to, those described in Employee's job
        description.

3   <u>Full Compensation</u>. The compensation provided for Employee by this Agreement shall constitute full
        payment for the services rendered to Club. Employee shall not receive any additional compensation
        for any services performed unless such services and payment, prior to their rendition, are authorized in
        writing by the Club's General Manager. Employee expressly waives, discharges, and releases Club
        from any claims for such services performed unless authorized in writing in the manner provided
        above.

4   **THIS AGREEMENT IS NOT A CONTRACT FOR EMPLOYMENT FOR A FIXED TERM,
        INSTEAD, IT DESCRIBES THE TERMS UPON WHICH EMPLOYEE'S COMPENSATION
        IS TO BE BASED. EMPLOYEE UNDERSTANDS EITHER PARTY MAY TERMINATE THE
        EMPLOYMENT RELATIONSHIP AT ANY TIME, FOR ANY REASON, WITH OR
        WITHOUT CAUSE. THE EMPLOYMENT-AT-WILL NATURE OF THIS RELATIONSHIP
        CANNOT BE ALTERED BY ANY STATEMENTS, ORAL OR WRITTEN, MADE BY
        ANYONE. EMPLOYEE FURTHER UNDERSTANDS NO COMMISSIONS, BONUSES, OR
        OTHER FORM OF COMPENSATION ACCRUE AFTER EMPLOYMENT TERMINATES.**

5. **Entire Agreement**. This Agreement embodies the entire agreement and understanding of the parties relating to Employee's employment and supersedes all prior representations, agreements, and understandings, oral or written, relating to Employee's employment.

EXECUTED this _____ day of _____,20____ .

Employee:
Signature: _____

Printed Name: _____

Club:
Signature: _____

Title:_____

Printed Name: _____

Appendix I
Sample Job Offering Letter

CLUB LETTERHEAD

[Date]

[Name]
[Address]

Dear [Name]:

We are delighted to have you as the newest addition to our team. This letter outlines the terms of your agreement with [Entity] regarding your employment:

You will begin work at (Location) Club on [Date], as [Position] reporting directly to me. You will be paid at the biweekly Base rate of $[Rate] (annualized $[Base Amount]

You will also have the ability to earn income by giving lessons and/or providing training. The expectation is that those services will provide approximately $_____ in additional income which equates to approximately _____ hours per week/period. The Club and Employee agree that the number of lessons/sessions taught/given on an annual basis will not encumber the Employee's ability to manage all aspects of the golf/tennis/athletic operation, achieve his Performance Objectives and fulfill the requirements of his Job Description.

You will have an additional incentive potential of 30% of eligible base wages for the year _____ based upon the annual Club EBITDA Performance, the Department Financial Performance by period and your annual Individual Performance.

You will receive a Summary Plan Document that will provide detail regarding performance scales and earnings for the incentive potential component of your compensation.

You will be eligible to participate in the companies benefit plans upon completing six months of regular, full-time employment. Medical and dental coverage is also available for your dependents.

It is understood that you will move your personal belongings from
_____ to _____. Please submit receipts on your direct
cost move, including travel expenses (gas, meals and lodging) to my office for
approval prior to reimbursement by _____. (Include the
relocation repayment agreement.)

Enclosed is a copy of the company handbook covering policies, procedures, and
privileges with which you will want to become familiar. Be prepared to ask any
questions you may have concerning the handbook during your orientation. You
will need to bring it with you, as you will be asked to sign the receipt.

It is understood that nothing in this letter or in any previous or future
communications is intended or should be construed to guarantee employment for
any specified period of time. It is understood that either party, with or without
cause may terminate this relationship at any time. It is likewise understood that
the employment-at-will nature of this relationship cannot be altered by any
statements, oral or written, made, or which may be made, contrary to the above.

If this is in agreement with discussions held, please sign and return one copy of
this letter. Also, please complete the enclosed paperwork and be prepared to
return it to the human resources department during your orientation at 9:00 am
on your first day at work.

[Name], congratulations on your new responsibilities. We look forward to our
mutual success.

If you have any questions or would like any assistance, please do not hesitate to
call.

Sincerely,

[Name of Supervisor]
[Title]

Enclosures

Agreed to this_____day of _____, 2005

_____
(Name)

Appendix J
Sample Structured Interview Questioning Format for a Fitness Director Applicant

❑ General Fitness

- Please indicate what steps you would normally take to ensure that prospective exercisers receive a safe and effective exercise program when they first decide to begin exercising.

Key elements of response:

Have the individual complete a pre-activity screening, such as health history, Par Q, or similar tool.

_____ Have the individual obtain medical clearance, if that person is at high risk.

_____ Perform a fitness test to obtain baseline information on the physical abilities and fitness level of the individual.

_____ Complete an exercise prescription, and then lead the individual through the actual prescription.

_____ Follow-up with the individual on a regular basis to ensure that the person is correctly following the program, and make adjustments to the program, if needed.

- A significant portion of the exercising and non-exercising population at this club is over the age of 50. What special precautions might you need to take when programming physical activity for a population of this age?

Key elements of response:

_____ Make sure that the individuals have received the appropriate screening, including medical clearance and screening, when indicated.

_____ Make sure that the staff is familiar with the special physical requirements of this population and provide the necessary training, if needed.

_____ Make sure that the activity programs for this age group are characterized by certain attributes, including the following: lower impact, include lower-intensity activity, are monitored by qualified staff, include all of the basic components of the fitness spectrum (flexibility, muscular fitness, cardiovascular fitness, and body composition), and are programmed to be conducted at a time that is convenient for the exercisers.

_____ Make allowances for more personal attention.

- Please describe the critical elements involved in developing an exercise program for a 45-year-old male who has been diagnosed as having type II diabetes. Assume that he has been cleared to exercise by his physician.

Key elements of response:

_____ Would make sure that he establishes a regular time to exercise each time he visits.

_____ Would make sure that he exercises at a lower-intensity level and for a longer duration, as opposed to at a high-intensity level and for a relatively shorter duration.

_____ Would make sure to monitor performance and check for signs of fatigue, dizziness, etc.

- According to the most recent literature, what are some key steps that can be undertaken to assist exercisers in their efforts to maintain their exercise program?

Key elements of response:

_____ Have each individual complete an interest questionnaire to obtain information about that person's goals, interests, support structure, etc.

_____ Establish realistic short-term and long-term goals (process and outcome) with the individual exerciser.

_____ Develop a behavioral contract that commits the exerciser, as well as the exercise leader, to certain process goals and actions; in addition, establish a self-monitoring or tracking program.

_____ Make the exercise program progressive by starting out easy and gradually increasing the demands (via intensity and duration) placed on systems of the exerciser's body.

_____ Establish a reward system to recognize achievement of process and reward goals.

- What are the top four or five current trends in the fitness/club industry, including group exercise?

Key elements of response:

_____ Group cycling

_____ Pilates

_____ Yoga and related activities

_____ Spa services, such as massage and related activities

_____ Personal training

_____ Sports-performance training

❑   Employee Relations

- You have just been hired as the fitness director. What steps would you take to ensure that the employees under your responsibility are aware of your expectations and are prepared to perform as a team?

Key elements of response:

_____   Would arrange to have a meeting with the entire group to provide an overview of my expectations.

_____   Would meet one-on-one with each of the employees to get to know them and better understand their roles and individual needs.

_____   Would establish some basic ground rules for performance with the team.

_____   Would establish job descriptions and performance models for each employee.

_____   Would communicate with each employee on a regular basis through individual meetings, team meetings, etc.

- You have an employee who is responsible for the group-exercise program. Over the past month, you have noticed that the overall program is not being well-received by the members. In addition, you have had complaints from members and employees about the quality of the program and their feeling that the individual in charge is not concerned about it. What steps would you take to address the perceived problem?

Key elements of response:

_____   Would meet with the employee to gather information about the situation from that individual's perspective and share with that person some of the concerns brought up by the members and fellow employees.

_____   Would set up an action plan for performance, with some 30-, 60-, and 90-day goals. This plan would include expectations and actions that would be undertaken if those expectations were not met.

_____   Would provide additional coaching and training to address specific areas of need.

_____   Would meet with on a regular basis with that employee to review performance, counsel, redirect, and hold accountable.

_____   Would inform all others who have expressed concern about this situation that matters are being addressed and that the situation is being dealt with in a proactive manner.

❑ Financial Management

- Please describe the primary streams of revenue and the largest expense areas for a fitness department in a typical health/fitness and sports club.

Key elements of response:

_____ The primary sources of revenue would be personal training and program fees.

_____ The largest expenses would be payroll, commissions, program supplies, etc.

- Please describe the primary steps that you would take to prepare a budget for your department, including the difference between a zero-based budget and a trend-line budget.

Key elements of response:

_____ Would gather information on existing financial performance and usage patterns.

_____ Would identify opportunities for revenue growth and expense control, including targets for specific revenue and expense areas.

_____ Would create a preliminary budget, based on the historical information and projected targets.

_____ A zero-based budget is when you start from scratch and build budget on projected targets, while a trend-line budget is when you project budget targets off of prior historical trends.

- The net financial performance of your department is 10 percent behind plan after the first six months of the year. Please briefly describe actions that you would take to get back on plan before the year was over.

Key elements of response:

_____ Would gather information on performance, and identify specific strengths and weaknesses.

_____ Would identify revenue opportunities, and set up action plans to achieve.

_____ Would identify expense-control opportunities, particularly in payroll, and then establish action plans for making the necessary changes.

_____ Would monitor the situation each week and make necessary adjustments.

❏ Member Relations

• Please describe, from your perspective, the key elements in creating great service and memorable experiences for members using the club.

Key elements of response:

_____ Make sure that all employees are trained in providing great service.

_____ Make sure that all members are greeted by name.

_____ Make sure that the club provides programs and services that interest the members and address their needs.

_____ Make sure that the club has enough equipment and that it is in good working condition.

_____ Make sure that the programs in which the members participate are monitored and that feedback from members concerning those programs is both elicited and considered.

_____ Listen to the members and try to meet or exceed their expressed expectations.

• A member comes to you complaining that another member is making excessive use of the equipment and not allowing other individuals to use the equipment when they are in the club. Furthermore, the member says the other member has exhibited rude behavior. The member believes that you should remove this other member from the exercise area. Please describe how you would address this member issue.

Key elements of response:

_____ Would listen to the member's concerns and make note of them.

_____ Would let the offended member know that I would address the concern provide a response as soon as feasibly possible.

_____ Would then meet with the other member and gather that person's perspective, without letting that individual know who had brought the issue to my attention.

_____ Would determine the appropriate course of action, and then meet with the offending member and inform that person of the action that I feel needs to be undertaken.

_____ Would meet with the offended member and let that individual know what action was taken.

❏ Marketing and Sales

• Please describe the strategies that you would use to increase personal-training participation and revenue.

Key elements of response:

_____ Would first gather information about current participation and why members either used or did not use personal training.

_____ Might employ a variety of tools to gather information, for example, focus groups, a survey, one-on-one discussion, etc.

_____ Would establish targeted quotas for the department and each of the trainers. Would also monitor these targets on a regular basis.

_____ Would package personal training to appeal to members, including having the right pricing.

_____ Would market, using specific strategies, such as pictures of the trainers with bios, a brochure on personal training, personal training bulletin board, etc.

_____ Would provide personal trainers with sales training.

• What do you consider to be the most critical elements of promoting fitness programs to members so that participation levels are maximized?

Key elements of response:

_____ Making sure to communicate to members in advance the programs that are available, using such tools as an annual program calendar or a monthly program calendar.

_____ Making sure that every employee is aware of the programs in the club and talks it up with the members (i.e., make each employee a salesperson).

_____ Getting members aligned with the programs and have them become spokespersons for the programs (committees, loyal member programs, etc.).

_____ Developing the appropriate mix of promotional materials, such as flyers, posters, statement stuffers, email, etc.

Appendix K
Sample Strategic Planning Forms

Strategic Planning Worksheet

I. Mission (who do you serve, what is your product, how do you deliver it and its value)

II. Vision (what is it that your audience will see in 3 – 5 years)

III. Promise (what is it the member and/or employee will always experience)

IV. Core Values (the roots for every decision and action you take)

1	
2	
3	
4	
5	

V. Objectives & Goals (what is it you want to achieve and target)

Audience	Objectives	Target

VI. Strategies (the guidelines and general actions that will lead to achievement of the objectives)

Objective	Strategies

Strategic Plan
Action Worksheets

Objective:	

Target #:		Timeline:	

Strategy:	

#	Action Steps	Leader

Appendix L
Selected Front-of-the-House Operational Forms

OPENING REPORT

Name:_____   Date:_____

—   Turn on lights

—   Turn on radio; adjust volume. Set Television on desired channel.

—   Turn on computer in fitness testing room and front desk. Type in the club ID, date, and day of the week

—   Set up control desk:

- Pull out appointment book and turn to correct date
- Check on message from previous night
- Sharpen pencils if needed
- Rip day off of small calendar

—   Check out locker rooms and make sure they are clean, and supplies are replenished; roll out shower mats

—   Check out the fitness floor and make sure all equipment is turned on and ready to go (unplug cyclone charger)

—   Put away uniform bags

—   Fold towels

—   Put load in dryer

—   Read MOD log

—   Unlock fruit bar case

—   Check tires on Velodyne

—   Check all offices, aerobic room, and both locker rooms

—   Check free-weight area for footprints and note in MOD book

—   Call time before opening

—   Check all clocks before opening

—   Check temperature throughout club (thermostats on 68 degrees)

—   Make sure no light bulbs are burned out

—   Check ceiling tiles for leaks

—   Walk entire perimeter of the club

—   Check schedule and note activities, special events, and massage appointments

—   Turn on copier

—   Write cleaning inspection notes in log book

DEPARTMENTAL CLOSING REPORT

Date:_____   Day:_____

Shift Supervisor:_____   Signature:_____

Control Desk

1. Report completed and attached _____
2. All tickets completed/correct _____   (control sheet attached)
3. Desk cleaned up _____
4. TV and stereo off _____
5. Lights out _____

Fitness Floor

1. All weights, plates, etc., picked up _____
2. Selectorized equipment set _____
3. All electrical equipment off _____
4. Exercise cards replaced/signed _____
5. Floor cleaned _____
6. Equipment cleaned _____
7. Lights off _____

Exercise Classroom

1. Attendance checked (#_____) _____
2. Stereo off _____
3. Equipment replaced _____
4. Studio cleaned _____
5. Lights off _____

Locker Rooms and Laundry

1. All dirty towels/uniforms emptied _____
2. Clean towels restocked _____
3. All supplies restocked _____
4. All cleaning completed _____
5. Spa amenities checked _____
   Steam temperature _____
   Sauna temperature _____
   Whirlpool temperature _____
   Whirlpool pH _____
   Whirlpool chlorine _____

6. Spa amenities turned off   _____
7. Massage linens emptied   _____
8. Massage room cleaned   _____
9. Laundry cleaned   _____
10. Dryers emptied   _____
11. Lights out   _____

Pool Area

1. Pool report completed and attached   _____
2. Equipment put away   _____
3. Pool area cleaned   _____
4. Pool temperature and chemistry okay   _____

Gym/Racquet Courts

1. Gym equipment away   _____
2. Gym cleaned   _____
3. Racquet courts cleaned   _____
4. Lights out in courts   _____
5. Lights out in gym   _____

Supervisor's Comments

_____

_____

_____

_____

_____

_____

_____

_____

Company Name and Address

Staff Name _____

Club Name _____

Department: _____

Purpose: _____

SS# or TAX ID # _____

DATE	AIR TRAVEL	AUTO EXPENSE MILES	AUTO EXPENSE AMOUNT	RENTAL	TAXI	LODGING	TRAVEL MEALS BRKFST	TRAVEL MEALS LUNCH	TRAVEL MEALS DINNER	TIPS	PARKING /TOLLS	TELEPH.	ENTRTNMNT (SCH.A)	Other Expenses EXPLANATION	Other Expenses AMOUNT	GRAND TOTAL
			$0.00													$0.00
			$0.00													$0.00
			$0.00													$0.00
			$0.00													$0.00
			$0.00													$0.00
			$0.00													$0.00
			$0.00													$0.00
			$0.00													$0.00
			$0.00													$0.00
			$0.00													$0.00
			$0.00													$0.00
			$0.00													$0.00
			$0.00													$0.00
			$0.00													$0.00
			$0.00													$0.00
TOTAL	$0.00	0	$0.00	$0.00	$0.00	$0.00	$0.00	$0.00	$0.00	$0.00	$0.00	$0.00			$0.00	$0.00

TOTAL DUE EMPLOYEE _____

EXPLANATION OF ENTERTAINMENT EXPENSES

DATE	Supplier	BUSINESS PURPOSE	INDIVIDUALS ENTERTAINED	AMOUNT

EXPLANATION OF OTHER EXPENSES

DATE	TYPE OF EXPENSE	DESCRIPTION	AMOUNT

Chart of Account Numbers

	AMOUNT

AUTHORIZATION

Supervisor Approval and Signature

I hereby indicate by my signature below that I have reviewed the expenses indicated in this report and hereby approve them as fully reimbursable.

Approved By _____ Date _____

I hereby indicate by my signature below that the above listed expenses are legitamate expenses related to the performance of my job.

Employee Signature

Employee Signature _____ Date _____

Rev 5/1/98

Group Exercise
Class Attendance Sheet

Month: _____   **Week:** _____

Date/Day	Class Title	Time of Class	Instructor's Name	# of Participants in Class	Instructor Initials

LOST AND FOUND LOG SHEET

Item Found	Date	Day	Time	Staff Person	Member's Name if Known	Put in Closet

Share Your Experience
Member & Guest Comment Card

Date: _____   Time: _____

Experience you would like to share:

```
┌─────────────────────────────────────────────────────────────┐
│                                                               │
│                                                               │
│                                                               │
│                                                               │
│                                                               │
│                                                               │
└─────────────────────────────────────────────────────────────┘
```

Overall how did you feel about your experience in the club today? Please indicate by checking of the appropriate response!

_____ Unsatisfactory (did not meet your expectations)

_____ Satisfactory (meet your expectations and needs)

_____ Delighted (exceeded your expectations, wow)

Would you like us to follow-up directly with you?   _____ Yes   _____ No
If yes, please provide us with your name and contact information.

Name (optional): _____

Contact phone #: _____   Contact email: _____

Thank you for sharing your feelings about your experience today.

ATHLETIC DEPARTMENT
TELEPHONE MESSAGE LOG

20

Period:_____
Week of:_____

Day/Date	Time	Who Called (Name) Who Called For (Name)	Message/Action	Staff Person's Initials

CLOSING REPORT

Name:_____   Date:_____

_____   Check laundry; make sure everything is on schedule

_____   Fill all supplies to the top of the label in both locker rooms and massage shower

(body wash, shampoo, conditioner, deodorant, hand soap, and lotion)

_____   Put away all uniforms

_____   Prop locker room doors open

_____   Restock towels, washcloths, paper towels, toilet paper, feminine napkins,

and hand soap

_____   Make sure boom box and lights are off in massage room

_____   Make sure all curling irons are off in the laudry room(s)

_____   Make sure fans throughout club are off

_____   Release Keiser air pressure

_____   Take half plates off all Cybex machines

_____   Readjust the volume in locker rooms and club

_____   Turn off lights, TV, VCR, DVD, CD and audio tape players

_____   Check stereo in aerobic room

_____   Check all thermostats in club to make sure temperature is correct (68 degrees);

aerobics studio (62 degrees)

_____   Put any problems or reminders for the next day in the MOD log

_____   Make sure exercise cards are signed and put away

_____   Lock fruit bar case

_____   Empty hampers in MLR and WL

_____   Turn computer off in F.Troom and front desk

_____   Complete recap sheet

_____   Lock up the club and recheck to make sure everything is finished

_____   Clean lint traps

_____   Turn off the copier

Day_____Date_____/_____/_____

Time				**APPOINTMENTS**			
6:00							
6:30							
7:00							
7:30							
8:00							
8:30							
9:00							
9:30							
10:00							
10:30							
11:00							
11:30							
NOON							
12:30							
1:00							
1:30							
2:00							
2:30							
3:00							
3:30							
4:00							
4:30							
5:00							
5:30							
6:00							
6:30							
7:00							
7:30							
8:00							
8:30							
9:00							
9:30							

Day_____Date_____/_____/_____

MEMBERSHIP ACTIVITY SHEET

Member Name	Member No.	Time	Pool	Classes	Weights	CV Equip.	RB/SQ	LRS	I-I's	Other

Appendix M
Selected Heart-of-the-House Operational Forms

Club Name

Check/Petty Cash Request Form

Staff person making request: _____

Position/title: _____

Signature: _____

Information Pertaining to Request

1. Requesting: _____ Check _____ Petty Cash

2. Amount being requested: _____

3. What are the funds being requested for (describe what the requested funds are for):

_____

_____

4. If a check is required, please provide the following information:

Check made out to: _____

Fed Tax ID or SS#: _____

Purchase order # (if applicable): _____

Day/date check needed: _____ Time needed: _____

5. If petty cash is being requested, the name of the staff person receiving the petty cash:

Name: _____ Position: _____

6. If petty cash requested, day/date and time needed: _____

Support information

Check Information

Check Number: _____ Amount of Check: _____

Date Check written: _____

Date Check cashed: _____

Receipt/invoice provided: _____ Yes _____ No

If yes, the invoice or receipt number was: _____

Product received: _____ Yes _____ No

Accounting signature: _____ Date: _____

Petty Cash Information

Amount of Petty Cash: _____

Date provided: _____

Receipt/invoice provided: _____ Yes _____ No

If yes, the invoice or receipt number was: _____

Amount of invoice/receipt: _____

Change returned: _____

Product received: _____ Yes _____ No

Staff person providing change and receipt: _____

Accounting signature: _____ Date: _____

Lost & Missing Item Report

Day and Date item reported: _____   Time: _____

I. General Information on Person Reporting Lost/Missing Item

1. Person reporting lost/missing item (e.g. member, guest, employee, etc.)?	Name: Status: _____ member _____ guest _____ employee
2. Address of person reporting?	Street: _____ City/State/Zip: _____
3. Phone and email information on person reporting?	(H) _____ (B) _____ (C) _____ email: _____
4. If a member, provide their membership number:	

II. Information on the Lost/Missing Item

1. Description of lost/missing item:
2. Location it was last seen:
3. Time that it was last seen:

III. Actions and Witness Information

Name: _____ Address: _____ _____ Phone: (B) _____ (H) _____ Email: _____	Name: _____ Address: _____ _____ Phone: (B) _____ (H) _____ Email: _____

IV.   Club Action and Response

Staff person responding: _____

Day/Date responding: _____ Time: _____

Action/response description: _____

_____

_____

Were the police contacted?   _____ Yes   _____ No

Did the police investigate?   _____ Yes   _____ No
If yes, please provide name, title and contact number for the officer.

Name: _____ Title: _____

Contact information: _____

Result of investigation? _____

_____

Did we follow-up with the person reporting the lost/missing item? _____ Yes   _____ No

What was the nature of the club's follow-up? _____

_____

Staff person completing report: _____

Staff person signature: _____

Date completed: _____ Time completed: _____

			Pool and Whirlpool Weekly Report Week of: _____	
Date	**Day**	**Time**	**Pool Chemistry**	**Whirlpool Chemistry**
	Monday		pH level: Chlorine level: Alkalinity level: Temperature: Filter PSI:	pH level: Chlorine level: Alkalinity level: Temperature: Filter PSI:
	Tuesday		pH level: Chlorine level: Alkalinity level: Temperature: Filter PSI:	pH level: Chlorine level: Alkalinity level: Temperature: Filter PSI:
	Wednesday		pH level: Chlorine level: Alkalinity level: Temperature: Filter PSI:	pH level: Chlorine level: Alkalinity level: Temperature: Filter PSI:
	Thursday		pH level: Chlorine level: Alkalinity level: Temperature: Filter PSI:	pH level: Chlorine level: Alkalinity level: Temperature: Filter PSI:
	Friday		pH level: Chlorine level: Alkalinity level: Temperature: Filter PSI:	pH level: Chlorine level: Alkalinity level: Temperature: Filter PSI:

Date	Day	Time	Pool Chemistry	Pool Chemistry
	Saturday		pH level: Chlorine level: Alkalinity level: Temperature: Filter PSI:	pH level: Chlorine level: Alkalinity level: Temperature: Filter PSI:
	Sunday		pH level: Chlorine level: Alkalinity level: Temperature: Filter PSI:	pH level: Chlorine level: Alkalinity level: Temperature: Filter PSI:

Purchase Order Request

Staff completing purchase order request: _____

Day and Date of Request: _____ Time of Request: _____

Signature of staff person making request: _____

Supplier/Vendor Information

Name: _____

Address: _____

_____

Contact person: _____

Phone number: _____ Email: _____

Federal Tax ID #: _____

Have we purchased from this supplier in the past? _____ Yes _____ No

Payment terms: _____

Purchase Order Request Detail (attach any applicable forms from supplier)

Item Being Requested	Amount of Item
1.	
2.	
3.	
4.	
5.	
Sub- total	
Freight	
Taxes	
Total Amount of Purchase Order	

Purchase Order Approval Information

Person approving the purchase order: _____

Signature of person approving: _____

Date of approval: _____Purchase Order # Assigned: _____

Date Purchase order placed: _____

Purchase Order and Invoice Verification

Purchase order #: _____   Purchase order amount: _____

Invoice #: _____   Invoice order amount: _____

Variance between purchase order and invoice: _____

Explanation of variance: _____

_____

Person verifying purchase order to invoice: _____

Signature: _____   Date: _____

Maintenance and Repair Service Request Form

Service Order Request Number: _____ Date of Request: _____

Staff Person Requesting Service: _____ Position/title: _____

Signature of staff person requesting service: _____

I.   Description of Service being Requested (completed by person requesting service):

1. Area of the facility:	
2. Piece of equipment (if applicable):	
3. Description of repair/service/work needed:	
4. When repair/service/work needs to be completed:	Day: _____ Date: _____ Time: _____

Please submit this form to the staff person in charge of facilities and equipment and keep a record for the files.

II.   Results of Request (completed by staff person completing the repair/service/work):

1. Name of staff person completing work:	
2. Day, date and time work completed:	
3. Signature of staff person completing work:	

After work is completed, place form in the appropriate file and return copy to the staff person who originally requested the work.

Appendix N
Sample Design and Construction Checklist

I. FACILITY DESIGN

_____ Select an architect

_____ Complete Agreement with Architect (AIA document B 141 Standard Form of Agreement between Owner and Architect).

_____ Have initial meeting with architect and share strategic conversation and marketing information. Complete architect program questionnaire.

_____ Architect will do Three phases of planning, schematic design, design development and construction documents.

_____ Team should meet with architect once during each of the phases. All plans should be reviewed and signed off on before the next phase begins. Last sign-off is at 90% construction documents.

_____ Identify with architect the need for additional specialists such as landscape architect, civil engineer, acoustical engineer, etc. (Architect provides mechanical, electrical, plumbing, and structural engineers).

_____ Any changes in architect services are to be handled through AIA ASP Form signed by architect and owner.

_____ Architect will work with owner to identify contractors for bidding documents. Bidding should take about three weeks.

_____ Architect and owner should interview each contractor before selecting the final contractor.

_____ Contractor will be selected by owner and architect.

II. CONSTRUCTION

_____ Once the contractor is selected, a pre-construction meeting is held to review and clarify plans, clarify contract terms and responsibilities, establish timelines, etc.

_____ Sign legal agreement with contractor (AIA Document A101 Standard Form of Agreement between Owner and Contractor for where the Basis of Payment is a Stipulated Sum).

_____ Owner and architect should meet with contractor at least once a month. If club/owner has a construction manager, then the construction manager should meet with the contractor weekly. Meetings should focus on work progress, schedules, delays, inspections, change orders, etc.

_____ Contractor will meet with subs on a weekly basis. Owner should get relevant notes and pictures from meetings.

_____ All clarifications on construction documents are done between architect's construction administrator and contractor's construction manager. Often, contractor will issue a request for Information (RFI) as part of the process.

_____ Any changes to project scope, whether a credit or cost is handled through change orders. Only the architect requests a change order after talking with the owner and contractor. A change order, to be completed, must be approved by both architect and owner. Recommend keeping a change order log.

_____ Contractor will submit monthly pay applications (in triplicate) using standard AIA form. To be paid, the pay application must be notarized, signed by contractor and approved by architect.

_____ Contractor will submit partial lien waivers starting with the second pay application. The liens must match up with previous pay application before current pay application is processed.

_____ Each pay application will have retainage taken out, usually equal to 10% until 50% of the project is completed, after which retainage is reduced to 5%.

_____ Final pay application will be for retainage and must be accompanied by final lien waivers.

_____ Contractor must submit letter of substantial completion when to work at 95% to 98% completed and prior to punch list. All warranties are effective this date.

_____ At completion of construction a punch list is done with architect, owner and contractor. The punch list should be done off the approved construction documents.

_____ Contractor, as part of closing project must conduct an HVAC balance report.

_____ Prior to final contract payment, contractor must provide three sets of closing documents. These contain:

     ❏ As-built construction drawings.
     ❏ All subcontractor warranties on work.
     ❏ All equipment manuals.
     ❏ All permits and certificates.
     ❏ All final lien waivers.
     ❏ Signed punch list and balance report.

Appendix O
Sample Construction Project Budget

Project Phase		Budget	%		Actual
General Construction		**$1,632,292**	69.9%		**1,645,400.00**
Construction		$1,522,229			1,522,229.00
Landscape Allowance		$54,825			77,946.00
Contingency/CO's		$55,238			45,225.00
Price per square foot		**$131**			
Fees & Consultants		**$246,048**	10.5%		**223,771.00**
Architect and Engineers		$220,000			177,569.00
Permits & Related		$0			12,919.00
CCF&G Fees		$0			0.00
Consultants		$12,000			20,235.00
Landscape architects		$13,048			13,048.00
Marketing & Membership		$0			0.00
Models and Boards		$1,000			
Soft Costs		**$50,088**	2.1%		**49,821.00**
Reimbursables		$50,088			49,821.00
FF&E		**$373,118**	16.0%		349,277.00
Cardiovascular		$69,656			74,780.00
Resistance Circuit		$24,008			24,008.00
Ground Zero		$10,485			10,485.00
Freeweights		$25,240			10,334.00
Spa Equipment		$7,099			16,308.00
Child Care Areas		$6,706			6,847.00
Group Exercise Equipment		$9,647			13,469.00
Office/Business		$5,336			5,026.00
Café & Kitchen		$26,584			29,118.00
Audiovisual Equipment		$30,800			30,724.00
Spa Lounge/Relax		$0			497.00
Lobby furniture		$1,876			2,130.14
Control Desk		$532			512.00
Teen Center		$750			750.00
Women's Locker Room		$0			478.00
General Fitness		$14,185			32,407.00
Computers/phones		$46,394			49,932.00
Freight		$44,595			30,744.00
Tax		$20,810			14,347.00
Laundry		$18,000			18,000.00
Contingency		$10,415			-21,619.14
Miscellaneous Fees		**$32,091**	1.4%		**26,586.00**
Start-up Supplies		$32,091			26,586.00
Pre-Opening		$0			0.00
Miscellaneous		$0			0.00
Total Phase One Budget		***$2,333,637***			***2,294,855.00***
Balance Remaining					**$38,782**

Appendix P
Sample Member Satisfaction Survey

Please tell us how the following areas of the club are meeting your needs and expectations.
Please rate only those areas that you have experienced personally, otherwise check the "no experience" box.

	Strongly Disagree	Disagree	Neutral	Agree	Strongly Agree	No Experience
Sports Desk						
Greeting is friendly, warm and sincere	1	2	3	4	5	○
Staff is well-trained	1	2	3	4	5	○
Information is readily available	1	2	3	4	5	○
Staff is able to problem solve effectively	1	2	3	4	5	○
Staff is service-oriented	1	2	3	4	5	○
Locker Rooms						
Locker room is kept clean, well-stocked and maintained	1	2	3	4	5	○
Steam room and sauna are kept clean and in working order	1	2	3	4	5	○
Spa is clean and well maintained	1	2	3	4	5	○
Showers are clean and well maintained	1	2	3	4	5	○
Staff is service-oriented	1	2	3	4	5	○
Café						
Quality of food meets expectations	1	2	3	4	5	○
Variety of food meets expectations	1	2	3	4	5	○
Café is kept clean and well maintained	1	2	3	4	5	○
Speed of service meets expectations	1	2	3	4	5	○
Value for your money meets expectations	1	2	3	4	5	○
Staff is service-oriented	1	2	3	4	5	○
Dining Room for Lunch						
Quality of food meets expectations	1	2	3	4	5	○
Variety of food meets expectations	1	2	3	4	5	○
Dining room is kept clean and well maintained	1	2	3	4	5	○
Speed of service meets expectations	1	2	3	4	5	○
Value for your money meets expectations	1	2	3	4	5	○
Staff is service-oriented	1	2	3	4	5	○
Club Activities and Programs						
Club sponsored events are valuable to me	1	2	3	4	5	○
I am satisfied with the parties offered	1	2	3	4	5	○
I am satisfied with the social/athletic outings offered	1	2	3	4	5	○
Programs are effectively promoted	1	2	3	4	5	○
I would like the club to offer more social events	1	2	3	4	5	○

	Strongly Disagree	Disagree	Neutral	Agree	Strongly Agree	No Experience
Business Office						
Staff is professional, knowledgeable and helpful	1	2	3	4	5	○
Staff is able to problem solve effectively	1	2	3	4	5	○
Staff is service-oriented	1	2	3	4	5	○
Tennis						
Tennis courts and surrounding areas are kept clean and well maintained	1	2	3	4	5	○
Pro staff is knowledgeable, enthusiastic and available	1	2	3	4	5	○
I would like the department to offer more social events	1	2	3	4	5	○
The department effectively promotes its programs	1	2	3	4	5	○
I am satisfied with the USTA league structure	1	2	3	4	5	○
I recommend the department to others	1	2	3	4	5	○
Aquatics						
Pool deck and surrounding area are kept clean and well maintained	1	2	3	4	5	○
Water quality in pool and spa meets expectations	1	2	3	4	5	○
I am satisfied with the adult aqua classes	1	2	3	4	5	○
I would like the department to offer more classes, clinics, programs	1	2	3	4	5	○
Staff is service-oriented	1	2	3	4	5	○
Spa						
Massage staff are professional, knowledgeable and helpful	1	2	3	4	5	○
Skin care staff are professional, knowledgeable and helpful	1	2	3	4	5	○
Value for your money meets expectations	1	2	3	4	5	○
Group Exercise Program						
Studios and equipment are kept clean and well maintained	1	2	3	4	5	○
I am satisfied with the variety of classes and programs offered	1	2	3	4	5	○
Staff is knowledgeable, enthusiastic and friendly	1	2	3	4	5	○
The department effectively promotes programs and communicates class changes	1	2	3	4	5	○
Fitness						
The fitness center and equipment are kept clean and well maintained	1	2	3	4	5	○
I am satisfied with the variety of equipment offered	1	2	3	4	5	○
Availability of fitness equipment meets expectations	1	2	3	4	5	○
Staff is knowledgeable, enthusiastic and friendly	1	2	3	4	5	○
Staff is service-oriented	1	2	3	4	5	○
Children's Center						
The center and equipment are kept clean and well maintained	1	2	3	4	5	○
Staff is knowledgeable, enthusiastic and friendly	1	2	3	4	5	○
The security/safety of the center meets expectations	1	2	3	4	5	○
I would like the department to offer more programs	1	2	3	4	5	○

	Strongly Disagree	Disagree	Neutral	Agree	Strongly Agree	No Experience
Squash						
The squash courts and surrounding area are kept clean and well maintained	1	2	3	4	5	○
Pro staff is knowledgeable, enthusiastic and available	1	2	3	4	5	○
I am satisfied with the variety of programs offered	1	2	3	4	5	○
The department effectively promotes its programs	1	2	3	4	5	○
I recommend the department to others	1	2	3	4	5	○
Pro Shop						
Staff is friendly, knowledgeable and enthusiastic	1	2	3	4	5	○
The Pro Shop carries merchandise that meets my needs	1	2	3	4	5	○
Staff is service-oriented	1	2	3	4	5	○
Gymnasium						
The gymnasium is kept clean and well maintained	1	2	3	4	5	○
I am satisfied with the variety of programs offered	1	2	3	4	5	○
Club Overall						
I am satisfied with the overall club appearance	1	2	3	4	5	○
The club is kept clean and well maintained	1	2	3	4	5	○
Repairs and maintenance are completed quickly and efficiently	1	2	3	4	5	○
Staff is knowledgeable, friendly and enthusiastic	1	2	3	4	5	○
Value for your money meets expectations	1	2	3	4	5	○
The club meets my needs and expectations	1	2	3	4	5	○
Staff is service-oriented	1	2	3	4	5	○

Please share with us your experience with other Club programs and services.

	Aware of		Have Tried		Will Try		Not Interested	
	Yes	No	Yes	No	Yes	No	Yes	No
Pilates								
Individual	○	○	○	○	○	○	○	○
Group Allegro	○	○	○	○	○	○	○	○
Group Mat	○	○	○	○	○	○	○	○
Personal Fitness Training								
Individual	○	○	○	○	○	○	○	○
Group	○	○	○	○	○	○	○	○
Bay Sport								
Physical Therapy	○	○	○	○	○	○	○	○
Executive Physical Exam	○	○	○	○	○	○	○	○
Cholesterol Screening	○	○	○	○	○	○	○	○
Complimentary Injury Check	○	○	○	○	○	○	○	○

	Aware of		Have Tried		Will Try		Not Interested	
	Yes	No	Yes	No	Yes	No	Yes	No
Adult Swim Classes								
Individual	○	○	○	○	○	○	○	○
Group	○	○	○	○	○	○	○	○
Nutrition Consultation w/Dietician	○	○	○	○	○	○	○	○
Yoga Classes	○	○	○	○	○	○	○	○
Gymnasium								
Basketball Leagues	○	○	○	○	○	○	○	○
Badminton Individual Lessons	○	○	○	○	○	○	○	○
Badminton Group Lessons	○	○	○	○	○	○	○	○
Social/Athletic								
Golf outings	○	○	○	○	○	○	○	○
Club seminars	○	○	○	○	○	○	○	○
Club parties	○	○	○	○	○	○	○	○
Electronic Funds Transfer	○	○	○	○	○	○	○	○

(Automatic payment from your checking account)

The following questions are for classification purposes only:

Gender: _____Male   _____Female   Age: _____   Please indicate the year you joined DC: _____

How many visits to the Club do you make during a typical week? _____

What time of day do you most frequently utilize the Club? _____before 9:00am   _____9–12:00pm   _____12:00–4:00pm
_____4:00–8:00pm   _____8:00pm–close

What type of membership do you have?   _____Individual   _____Family   _____Racquet   _____Fitness

Please circle your two most preferred methods for the Club to communicate with you about programs and events.

Special Mailing   Statement Insert   Email   Sports Desk Bulletin
Club Bulletin Boards/Posters   Newsletter   DC Website   Activity Information Center

What one improvement would make visiting the Club a significantly better experience for you?
_____
_____

Please share any additional comments you may have.
_____
_____

Optional: We may wish to contact you about a comment or suggestion that you've made.

Name: _____   Member number: _____

Email address: _____

Thank you for your comments! Please return your completed survey by _____

Appendix Q
Sample Corporate Sales Checklist

Step 1   <u>Decide What It Is You Are Going To Sell</u>

_____ Memberships
_____ Brown bags
_____ Seminars
_____ HRAs
_____ Testing

Step 2   <u>Develop A Presentation Package That Can Be Used During Any Initial Contacts</u>

_____ Industry data on savings achieved
_____ Pamphlet and/or sheet on services
_____ Club brochure
_____ Business cards
_____ Generic Sales Presentation

Step 3   <u>Target Your Companies</u>

_____ Companies already using Club or with Member in the Club
_____ Local Chamber business listing
_____ Utilize specific criteria outlined in handbook and prioritize!

Step 4   <u>Learn All You Can About The Companies</u>

_____ Interviews with Members
_____ Check with PR departments
_____ Library
_____ Chamber information

Step 5   <u>Decide What It Is You Want To Accomplish With Your First Contact</u>

_____ Make a sale
_____ Get an appointment to introduce your services
_____ Get them to visit the club

Step 6   <u>Getting the First Appointment</u>

_____ Get current Member to arrange Appointment
_____ Write a short letter as outlined
_____ Include with you letter a nice reminder item (book, etc.)
_____ Make sure you will follow-up with a call; give day and
time period (Tuesday through Thursday)
_____ Make the follow-up phone call.
_____ Send a thank you after scheduling appointment
_____ Follow-up regularly and include small gift

Step 7   <u>The First Appointment: Make It Work For You</u>

_____ Get them to the Club if you can
_____ Bring a generic presentation package
_____ Make sure you bring your homework on the company
_____ Arrive early

       _____ Bring a partner
       _____ Keep presentation short and to the point
       _____ Get a commitment for a next step
       _____ Listen for needs

Step 8   <u>Immediate Appreciation Is A Hallmark Of Any Appointment</u>

      _____   Send a brief handwritten thank you upon returning to the Club
      _____   Express appreciation for their time and let them know when your proposal will arrive

Step 9   <u>Get Your Proposal In The Person's Hands</u>

      _____   Customize your proposal and include

- Executive Summary
- Services/products you will provide
- Delivery system for services
- Timetable
- Benefits
- List of clients
- List of Members who work for that company
- Fees and schedules

      _____   Deliver your proposal in person. Try to hand it to the person who makes the decision.
      _____   Send proposal only if delivering in person is impossible. Your proposal must be accompanied by a cover that outlines your next step, including date(s) of follow-up.

Step 10 <u>Follow-Up Your Proposal With A Call</u>

      _____ Allow two or three weeks before you call
      _____ Find out their feelings toward the proposal
      _____ Answer any questions
      _____ Try to schedule an appointment
      _____ Continue to follow-up

Step 11 <u>Taking Your Proposal To An Agreement</u>

      _____   Make your next appointment effective by being prepared for further questions
      _____   Realize that you may have to make additional presentations before signing
      _____   Have an agreement prepared ahead of time in the event you have a chance to sign
      _____   Realize it might take six to twelve months to finalize

Step 12 <u>Service the Sale</u>

      _____ Deliver what you promise
      _____ Provide regular feedback to the company
      _____ Maintain contact with company representatives
      _____ Perform evaluation of their services

Appendix R
Selected Health/Fitness Industry Programming Practices

The programs featured in this appendix are examples of programming that has been conducted successfully in various clubs in the health/fitness industry.

❑ **4th of July Member Classic**

I. Program Overview
- 5K & 1 mile races through community

II. Program Specifics

A. Program Goals:
- Gain exposure for the club in the community; the local paper includes articles on it which can lead to new members and revenue leads
- Promote wellness in the club; help increase retention

B. Equipment/Facility Needs:
- 5K & 1 mile courses, timing system, pace vehicle

C. Number of Members/Guests Participating:
- 140—50% of which were members

D. Marketing/Promotion Actions:
- Running magazines
- Newsletter/e-mail blasts
- Past-participants
- Banners & fliers throughout the community and club
- Registration at www.active.com

E. Fee Charged:
- $18/$16/$13 (per member)
- $18/$16/$13 (per guest)

F. Number of Staff Involved:
- 7-10 staff involved

III. Revenue & Expense = Profitability

A. Program Revenues:
- # of participants: 140
- Revenue per participant (fee): Approximately $15 per person
- Sponsorship: Donated food items and $1000
- Total revenues: $3,410

B. Program Expenses:
- Marketing promotions: $100
- Supplies: $50
- Awards: Trophies for the overall winner and for each age division; T-shirts, food, and drinks after the race for participants—$900 total
- Payroll (average time & average payroll dollars): $200
- Total expenses: $1,250

C. Program Net: $1,850

IV. The Keys That MADE IT WORK
- Good advertising using websites and running magazines

- Flexible staff—staff takes pride in gaining exposure for the club
- Good location for course—private gated community
- Active community—relatively young community with health conscience people
- Past successes—runners enjoy the race and return each year

❏ 5k Club

I. Program Overview
This club was designed to take the hassle out of running in 5K races. We pick certain 5K races to run every month and advertise the 5K throughout the club. Members are able to register for the race here at the club and can charge the registration fee to their membership account. We pick up the race packets for them and make them available at the pro shop five days before the race. After each race on Saturday mornings, members that participated come back to the club for breakfast. This program gets great reception because it's easy for members to participate in the races and it gives them a chance to meet other members interested in running.

II. Program Specifics
A. Program Goals:
- Achieve member-to-member connections through 5K race and breakfast participation
- Make it convenient for the members to participate in 5K races that support community events and charities

B. Equipment/Facility Needs:
- Club dining facility

C. Number of Members/Guests Participating:
- 15-20 people per race

D. Marketing/Promotion Actions:
- Each 5K that we participate in is posted in the club newsletter
- Different 5K club fliers for each race are posted throughout the club
- Message on hold phone system advertising the 5K club

E. Fee Charged:
- Members are charged $5 above the cost of the race registration. This club does not generate a lot of revenue, but it is a great retention tool.

F. Number of Staff Involved: 2

III. Revenue & Expense = Profitability
A. Program Revenues:
- # of Participants: About 15-20 members
- Revenue per Participant (fee): $5
- Sponsor dollars (if any): $0
- Total revenues: $5 per person

B. Program Expenses:
- Marketing promotions: We print fliers in-house and post throughout the club. We also put information in the newsletter and on the message on hold system
- Supplies: $5 per person covers the food cost for the breakfast that we serve after each race
- Total expenses: $5 per person

C. Program Net:
- Program does not generate any revenue but rather serves as a member retention tool

❏ After-School Activity Camp

I. Program Overview
- A fun-filled day of outdoor activities, arts, crafts, and lunch for the kids.

II. Program Specifics

A. Program Goals:
- Gain recognition in community
- Grow membership
- Generate revenue – generated $85,000 in first year

B. Equipment/Facility Needs:
- Areas for activities: Open field, swimming pool, basketball court, etc.

C. Number of Members/Guests Participating:
- About 150 different children participate in some degree; 80% are children of members

D. Marketing/Promotion Actions:
- Local neighborhood paper
- Folders at the local elementary school
- Fliers/e-mail blasts
- Personal phone calls
- Newsletter

E. Fee Charged:
- $115/$145 (per member)
- $145/$195 (per guest)

F. Number of Staff Involved: 2-8 people involved

III. Revenue & Expense = Profitability
A. Program Revenues:
- # of participants: 150
- Revenue per participant (fee): $115-$195
- Sponsor dollars (if any): Food items are donated
- Total revenues: $85,000

B. Program Expenses:
- Marketing Promotions: $200 for local paper
- Supplies: Food/art supplies = $1,000/yr
- Payroll * (average time & average payroll dollars): $42,000/yr.
- Total Expenses: $43,000/yr.

C. Program Net: $42,000

IV. The Keys That MADE IT WORK
- The hard work of our youth program coordinator who takes pride in his work
- Flexible, consistent staff
- Great promotions—mail database has helped a great deal
- Active community—a young working community with lots of young kids
- Location—elementary school target market is nearby

❏ Anniversary Gala

I. Program Overview

In November 2001, the Club hosted a gala in celebration of the 20th anniversary of the club. For the occasion, we had eight sports celebrities serve on an honorary committee as well as the Stanley and the Grey Cup on hand. The club invited approximately 4,000 people (including current & past members and the business community at large). Over 1,900 invitees attended the event that was featured live on KRDS (TV) with a lot of publicity provided via the press for days both before and after the event.

II. Program Specifics

A. Program Goals:
- Generate membership leads through exposure to the club
- Generated press for the club

B. Equipment/Facility Needs:
- A stage, sound system, giant screens, bars, DJ, coat check/racks, decoration, red carpet, outside light system, limo, etc.

C. Number of Members/Guests Participating: 1,900

D. Marketing/Promotion Actions:
- Traditional invitations, e-mail invitations and a media kit were produced and sent delivered. Posters, banners were prominent throughout the club
- Follow-up phone calls to all guests, members, and media
- Sponsored gift to everyone (sponsored by Roots). Business cards were collected for door prizes (and for follow-up of course).
- Along with their gift they received a guest pass, and an invitation to "Save $150.00 on Initiation Fees!"
- Link to a referral program in December, January, and February

E. Fee Charged: $0

F. Number of Personnel Involved: Approximately 50 people (staff and volunteers)

III. Revenue & Expense = Profitability

A. Program Revenues:
- # of participants: 1,900
- Revenue per participant (fee): $0—but we had at least 85 tours linked to the event, and approximately 50 new members signed-up in the following months ($50,000).
- Sponsor dollars (if any): Over $30,000 in money and supplies, and another $100,000 in free media publicity
- Total revenues: $50,000 to date

B. Program Expenses:
- Marketing promotions: $5,000
- Supplies: $15,000
- Awards: 0
- Payroll (average time & average payroll dollars): $2,000 (with over 40 volunteers)
- Total Expenses: $20,000

C. Program Net: $30,000 to date

IV. The Keys That MADE IT WORK

- The unique positioning of the club in this market place
- The strong names on the honorary committee
- Our contact list of sponsors and suppliers and VIP's
- Very strong, creative visuals
- Staff working on making it happen

❑ Birthday Parties & Sleepovers

I. Program Overview

Birthday parties and sleepovers at the club are a huge success due to the careful planning and an enthusiastic team to execute the parties. We cater to every party need and provide a high-energy party that all will remember. We are as flexible as the member needs us to be and always set out to offer the best Member service possible.

II. Program Specifics

A. Program Goals:
- To offer a party that both the parents and kids will remember forever. To cater to all member needs and be as flexible as possible, without losing the profit margin
- To constantly reevaluate the party structure and consistently offer the best parties possible

B. Equipment/Facility Needs:
- Party room with decorations—gift table, food table, soft seating area for parents
- A cozy and high-energy party atmosphere

C. Number of Members/Guests Participating:
- 15 - 20 children; 2 - 6 adults - birthday parties
- 20 -120 children; 25 adults – sleepovers

D. Marketing/Promotion Actions:
- Fliers around the club. Information in the newsletter
- Targeted Girl Scouts—promoted through direct contact with troop leaders
- Word of mouth
- Parties in a visible location for self-promotion
- Discounts in newsletter for parties

E. Fee Charged:
- $20 to $35 per person, depending on the type of party (A $300 facility fee is assessed for sleepovers)

F. Number of Staff Involved:
- 1 – 5 depending on the size of the party and the number of participants

III. Revenue & Expense = Profitability

A. Program Revenues:
- # of participants - Birthday party (minimum of 10 participants), sleepovers (minimum of 15 participants), adults (1-25 participants)
- Revenue per participant (fee): $20-$35/ per person
- Total revenues: Varies, based on the size of the party

B. Program Expenses:
- Marketing promotions: Paper cost
- Supplies equipment costs: all products for party—paper products, décor, food

- Awards: $0
- Payroll: Average $7 per hour, per extra person—3-4 hours for birthday parties; 13 hours for sleepovers
- Total expenses: Between $50 and $100 per birthday party and from $600 - $800 for sleepovers

C. Program Net:
- Varies; usually about a 50-60% profit for both types of programs. Most of the sleepover revenue is generated during hours we are usually closed.

IV. The Keys That MADE IT WORK

- PROMOTION
- Enthusiastic extra personnel to work every party
- Planner with the resources to handle all party needs
- Planning and preparation
- Flexibility

❑ Boxing Night

I. Program Overview: Amateur boxing night; 10 bouts – 3 minutes each; roast beef dinner; awards

II. Program Specifics

A. Program Goals:
- Sell out the event
- Ensure that participants get their money's worth

B. Equipment/Facility Needs:
- Boxing ring
- Awards and trophies
- Referees
- Physician on standby

C. Number of Members/Guests Participating:
- 200 participants total (including guests)

D. Marketing/Promotion Actions:
- Found a sponsor (La Queue de Cheval)
- Posters
- Billing statement stuffer
- Word of mouth advertising
- Staff promotion

E. Fee Charged:
- $50 per member or $60 per table
- 8 people per table; 20 tables

F. Staff Involved:
- F&B staff, logistics staff, maintenance.

III. Revenue & Expense = Profitability

A. Program Revenues:
- # of participants - 160

- Revenue from Fees: $12,000
- Sponsor dollars (if any): $1,000
- Total revenues: $13,000

B. Program Expenses:
- Supplies: $3,500
- Awards: $500
- Payroll: $720
- Total expenses: $4,720

C. Program net: $8,280

IV. The Keys That MADE IT WORK
- Good concept
- Strong marketing and visuals
- Fits within the club's environment
- Teamwork
- Flawless execution

❑ Cross-Training Challenge

I. Program Overview
To offer a fun, current, and educational approach to group exercise.

II. Program Specifics

A. Program Goals:
- To encourage members to cross-train throughout the club
- Increase group-exercise participation

B. Equipment/Facility Needs:
- Dumbbells, bands, tubing, steps, spin bikes, mats, jump ropes, medicine balls

C. Number of Members/Guests Participating:
- 120 sign-ups; 86 participants

D. Marketing/Promotion Actions:
- Prizes
- Posters
- Word of mouth
- Professionalism
- Fliers

E. Fee Charged: None

F. Staff Involved: All group-exercise staff (approximately 25)

III. Revenue & Expense = Profitability

A. Program Revenues:
- Sponsor dollars: $500 for prizes

B. Program Expenses:
- Awards (t-shirts) $500
- Total expenses $500

C. Program Net: $0

IV. The Keys That MADE IT WORK
- Staff & participant enthusiasm
- Following current trends
- Education of staff
- Teamwork
- Prizes

❑ Fibromyalgia Seminar

I. Program Overview
We teamed up with our physical therapy staff to produce a seminar on fibromylagia. The staff brought in a physician to speak on the subject and the club supplied wellness professionals from different areas, including massage, personal training, yoga, and aquatics.

II. Program Specifics
A. Program Goals:
- Educate members and guests concerning fibromyalgia
- Provide an opportunity to give relief to those afflicted by symptoms of this syndrome
- Generate revenue (future and immediate) for the club in potential Membership growth and through non-member class enrollment

B. Equipment/Facility Needs:
- Large group-exercise room and seven tables, 35-40 chairs

C. Number of Members/Guests Participating:
- Approximately 20 members/20 guests came to the seminar. Three people signed up for the water therapy class (12 sessions for $40.00). Ten people requested to be contacted about membership.

D. Marketing/Promotion Actions:
- Sign on the marquee
- Pass out interest sheets (e.g., who would be interested in...)
- Fliers mailed to everybody who replied to interest sheets
- Club newsletter article
- Promotional pamphlets placed in strategic locations throughout the club, at public places, and other affiliated health offices

E. Fee Charged: $0

F. Number of Staff Involved:
- One personal trainer, one massage therapist/yoga instructor, four physical therapists

III. Revenue & Expense = Profitability

A. Program Revenues:
- # of participants: 35
- Revenue per participant (fee): $0
- Sponsor dollars (if any): $0
- Total revenues: Three people signed-up for the class we offered in conjunction with the seminar (water therapy Class) $120.00 + 10 leads for membership.

B. Program Expenses:
- Marketing Promotions: One ream of paper for fliers
- Supplies $0
- Awards: $0
- Payroll: 1-hour meetings at lunch and outside lunch prep time, 20 hrs. @ avg. of 10.00 per hour
- Total expenses: $206

IV. The Keys That MADE IT WORK

- Dedicated health and wellness professionals with a genuine concern for the
- participants
- Ability of fitness staff to work with physical therapy staff to reach target market
- Being aware of the membership growth opportunity provided through marketing this type of seminar to non-members. If and when they join, these new members are then already aware of some of the services we offer that can help them as an individual.
- Recording/polling interests of the participants at the seminar allows us to find out if they want the club to contact them with further information about membership.
- Partnering local healthcare professionals with personal trainers, massage therapists, etc. Many people are asked by their physicians/physical therapists to maintain lifestyle changes but are left on their own to find a medium to accomplish this. By bringing this seminar to our club, we market ourselves attractively as a place where these people can help facilitate a change in their lives and have a positive experience in an inviting environment.

❑ Fitness Holiday

I. Program Overview
A holiday-style program emphasizing healthy living. Included are many activities (indoor and outdoor) that exercise and educate the client. In addition, there is also a daily cooking course complete with a chef where clients learn how to prepare healthy, delicious meals.

II. Program Specifics
A. Program Goals:
- Provide clients with a healthy week of exercise and diet
- Educate clients on healthy living
- Everything should be fun and social

B. Equipment/Facility Needs:
- A chalet rental in Whistler, Canada. All exercise equipment such as bikes, skis, extra would be rented.

C. Number of Members/Guests Participating: 12 clients

D. Marketing/Promotion Actions:
- Signage throughout the club
- Articles and advertisement in newsletter
- Informational seminars
- Encouragement from personal trainers

E. Fee Charged: $4,500 per week

F. Staff Involved: Two fitness staff and chef

III. Revenue & Expense = Profitability
A. Program Revenues
- # of Participants: 12
- Revenue per participant (fee): $4,500
- Total revenues: $54,000

B. Program Expenses
- Marketing promotions: $1,000
- Supplies; accommodations and rentals: $15,000
- Flights: $9,000
- Payroll (average time & average payroll $): $5,000
- Total Expenses: $30,000

C. Program Net: $24,000

IV. The Keys That MADE IT WORK
- Great idea
- Organization
- Quality staff
- Great location

❑ Hell Week is Back Again

I. Program Overview
A program not for the weak of mind or body—Hell Week is Back Again! This military boot camp-style class, lead by our top instructor, challenges anyone who dares to take it. Each participant is take to their limit and loves it. The week is made up of five mornings each with 1-hour workout sessions. Workouts are group-oriented and physically challenging. Each workout begins with a 2-3 mile jog, followed by a total-body workout. The end of "Hell Week" ends with 15-20 minutes of games and other team activities. All participants receive a "Hell Week" T-shirt. There is a $40 charge for this "Mission Impossible!" Proceeds benefit St. Jude's Children's Hospital.

II. Program Specifics
A. Marketing/Promotion Actions:
- Fliers entitled, "Hell Week is Back Again!" were made and placed strategically throughout the fitness center.
- A large poster was made featuring a picture of the instructor in full military fatigues and face paint with the slogan;—"We Want You!"—placed in the reception area.
- All fitness specialists were asked to suggest this class to their clients.
- Featured in our monthly newsletter

B. Fee Charged: $40 per member

III. Revenue & Expense = Profitability

A. Program Revenues: Total revenues $600

B. Program Expenses: Total expenses $410

C. Program Net: $190

❑ **Introduction to Hot Stone Therapy**

I. Program Overview

Hot stone therapy has become extremely popular in the spa/massage marketplace. The use of heated basalt lava stones allows for a therapeutic, yet profoundly relaxing massage. The introduction of this service to members has expanded the club's scope of massage services it provides. Where members may have gone elsewhere to receive this service previously, they now are now able to enjoy (and pay for access to) Hot Stone Therapy at SMC.

II. Program Specifics

A. Program Goals:
- Expand clubs massage services, appeal to a wider scope of members
- Create a volume and rate variance above and beyond past budgets

B. Equipment/Facility Needs:
- Existing rooms are used. Additions include roasters, stones, and cleaning supplies.

C. Number of Members/Guests Participating:
- Out of the total number of massages over the last month, hot stone therapy has been utilized by 3% of members taking advantage of massage program.

D. Marketing/Promotion Actions
- Signage and fliers
- Mini - demonstrations with hot stones to membership and staff
- Front-desk staff prompting members when they call for an appointment

E. Fee Charged: $ 85 (member), $ 95 (guest)

F. Number of Staff Involved:
- Initially one therapist; subsequently, four therapists will be able to provide service.

III. Revenue & Expense = Profitability

A. Program Revenues:
- Total revenues: $850

B. Program Expenses:
- Total expenses: $414

C. Program Net:
- After payroll, the club has broken even after just 10 sessions.

IV. The Keys That MADE IT WORK
- Increased availability by therapists
- Education and exposure to new service
- Quality, consistent service

Appendix S
Program Best Practices Benchmark Form

Club Name:_____ Contact Name:_____

Telephone:_____ Fax:_____

Email:_____

I.   Program Title:

II.   Program Overview (limit one paragraph):

III.   Program Specifics

    A.   Program Goals:

    B.   Equipment/Facility Needs:

    C.   Number of Members/Guests Participating (if personal training list # sessions weekly and % of total membership)

D.   Marketing/Promotion Actions (list specific actions you took to market the program and sign-up of participants

1.	
2.	
3.	
4.	
5.	

E.   Number of Staff Involved

IV.   Revenue & Expense = Profitability

Revenues		Expenses & Net	
# Participants		Payroll	
Fee Charged		Commissions	
Revenue from Fees		Other Expenses	
Other Revenue (sponsor)		Total Expenses	
Total Revenue		Program Net	

V.   The Five Keys That MADE IT WORK

1.	
2.	
3.	
4.	
5.	

Please attach any marketing materials or related materials used in delivering and marketing your program.

Appendix T
Selected Risk Management Forms*

Club Name
Authorization for Release of Protected Health information

I, _____, hereby authorize _____
to release the following health information:

```



```

and forward it to the following person/facility:

Name or person or facility: _____

Address (street, city, state and zip code):

```



```

Phone #: _____   Email: _____

This information is for the purpose of:

```



```

This authorization is in effect until _____, when it expires.

I understand that by signing this authorization:

- o I authorize the use or disclosure of my individually identifiable health information as described above for the purpose listed. I understand that authorization is voluntary.
- o I understand the notice of Privacy Practices provides instructions should I choose to revoke my authorization.
- o I understand that if the organization I have authorized to receive the information is not a health plan or health care provider, the released information may no longer be protected by federal privacy regulations.
- o I understand that I have the right to receive a copy of this authorization.
- o I understand that I am signing this authorization voluntarily and that treatment, payment, or eligibility for my benefits will not be affected if I do not sign this authorization.

I DECLARE UNDER PENALTY OF PERJURY THAT THE INFORMATION ON THIS FORM IS TRUE AND CORRECT.

SIGNATURE: _____   DATE: _____

---

*Because the selected risk management forms in this appendix can represent a form of legal document, before using them legal counsel should review them concerning their application to state and local laws, which can vary from location to location.

IDENTIFYING INFORMATION

_____ Copy of identification attached.

Type of identification: _____
(e.g. driver's license, birth certificate, passport, federal ID card, managed care card, etc.)

Number on identification: _____

IF NO IDENTIFICATION IS ATTACHED, YOUR SIGNATURE MUST BE NOTARIZED.

Notarized by: _____

On: _____

Notary Public Number: _____

NOTARY MUST STAMP IN THE SPACE PROVIDED

ACTIVITY RELEASE AND INDEMNITY AGREEMENT - ADULT

THIS RELEASE AND INDEMNITY AGREEMENT ("Release") is made by the undersigned adult (the "Participant"), to release and indemnify _____, a _____ corporation, its parent company, affiliated or subsidiary companies, and all their respective officers, directors, agents, contractors, employees, heirs, successors, and assigns (collectively, the "Club"), as set forth below.

1. **Activity**. Participant, on Participant's own behalf and on behalf of the other members of Participant's family, including Participant's spouse, parents, children, heirs, and assigns, (singularly and collectively referred to as "Participant") hereby grants to the Club this full release and indemnification as consideration in exchange for permitting Participant to participate in the following athletic or physical activity which may utilize Club premises and/or equipment (the "Activity"): _____.

Participant is entering into this Release after (i) having viewed or having had the opportunity to view Club premises and/or equipment; (ii) if there is an instructor, having reviewed or having had the opportunity to review the instructor's qualifications; (iii) having had the scope of the services and/or the associated risks explained to Participant; and/or (iv) having had an opportunity to ask questions regarding the services and/or the risks associated with the Activity.

2. **Release and Indemnity**.

   • **PARTICIPANT IS VOLUNTARILY PARTICIPATING IN THE ACTIVITY WITH FULL KNOWLEDGE, UNDERSTANDING AND APPRECIATION OF THE RISKS OF INJURY INHERENT IN ANY PHYSICAL EXERCISE, MASSAGE OR THERAPY PROGRAM, PHYSICAL ACTIVITY OR ATHLETIC ACTIVITY AND EXPRESSLY ASSUMES ALL RISKS OF INJURY AND EVEN DEATH WHICH COULD OCCUR BY REASON OF PARTICIPANT'S PARTICIPATION.**

   • **PARTICIPANT RELEASES CLUB FROM ANY LIABILITY AND AGREES NOT TO SUE CLUB WITH RESPECT TO ANY CAUSE OF ACTION FOR BODILY INJURY, PROPERTY DAMAGE, OR DEATH OCCURRING TO PARTICIPANT AS A RESULT OF PARTICIPATING IN THE ACTIVITY.**

   • **PARTICIPANT HEREBY ASSUMES FULL RESPONSIBILITY FOR RISKS OF BODILY INJURY, PROPERTY DAMAGE OR DEATH TO PARTICIPANT DUE TO THE ORDINARY NEGLIGENCE OR GROSS NEGLIGENCE OF THE CLUB AND THE ORDINARY NEGLIGENCE, GROSS NEGLIGENCE, OR WILLFUL MISCONDUCT OF ANY THIRD PARTY INCLUDING OTHERS PARTICIPATING IN THE ACTIVITY.**

   • **PARTICIPANT AGREES TO INDEMNIFY, DEFEND, AND HOLD HARMLESS, AT PARTICIPANT'S SOLE COST, THE CLUB FROM ANY AND ALL CLAIMS ARISING OUT OF PARTICIPANT'S PARTICIPATION IN THE ACTIVITY.**

   • **ALL PERSONAL PROPERTY BROUGHT TO THE ACTIVITY, IS BROUGHT AT THE SOLE RISK OF PARTICIPANT AS TO ITS THEFT, DAMAGE, OR LOSS.**

3. **Medical**. Participant consents to emergency medical care and transportation in order to obtain treatment in the event of injury to Participant as the Club may deem appropriate. This Release extends to any liability arising out of or in any way connected with the medical treatment and transportation provided in the event of an emergency.

4. **Severability**. Participant expressly agrees that the terms of release and indemnity contained herein are intended to be as broad and inclusive as is permitted by the laws of the state in which Club operates its business. Any provision or portion of this Release found to be invalid by the courts having jurisdiction shall be invalid only with respect to such provision or portion. The offending provision or portion shall be construed to the maximum extent possible to confer upon the parties the benefits intended thereby. Said provision or portion, as well as the remaining provisions or portion hereof, shall be construed and enforced to the same effect as if such offending provision or portion thereof had not been contained herein.

PARTICIPANT HAS READ AND VOLUNTARILY SIGNS THIS RELEASE AND INDEMNITY AGREEMENT.

PARTICIPANT:

_____

Signature

_____

Printed Name

_____

Date

ACTIVITY RELEASE AND INDEMNITY AGREEMENT - MINOR

THIS RELEASE AND INDEMNITY AGREEMENT ("Release") is made by the undersigned adult, as parent or legal guardian (the "Representative") of the below listed minor(s) (the "Participant"), to release and indemnify _____, a _____ corporation, its parent company, affiliated or subsidiary companies , and all their respective officers, directors, agents, contractors, employees, heirs, successors, and assigns (collectively, the "Club"), as set forth below.

1. **Activity**. Representative, on Participant's behalf and on behalf of the other members of Representative's family, including Representative's spouse, parents, children, heirs, and assigns, (singularly and collectively referred to as "Representative") hereby grants to the Club this full release and indemnification as consideration in exchange for permitting Participant to participate in the following athletic or physical activity which may utilize Club premises and/or equipment (the "Activity"): _____.

Representative, on Participant's behalf, is entering into this Release after (i) having viewed or having had the opportunity to view Club premises and/or equipment; (ii) if there is an instructor, having reviewed or having had the opportunity to review the instructor's qualifications; (iii) having had the scope of the services and/or the associated risks explained to Participant; and/or (iv) having had an opportunity to ask questions regarding the services and/or risks associated with the Activity.

2. **Release and Indemnity**.

   - REPRESENTATIVE PERMITS PARTICIPANT TO PARTICIPATE IN THE ACTIVITY WITH FULL KNOWLEDGE, UNDERSTANDING AND APPRECIATION OF THE RISKS OF INJURY INHERENT IN ANY PHYSICAL EXERCISE PROGRAM, MASSAGE OR THERAPY PROGRAM, PHYSICAL ACTIVITY OR ATHLETIC ACTIVITY AND EXPRESSLY ASSUMES ALL RISKS OF INJURY AND EVEN DEATH WHICH COULD OCCUR BY REASON OF PARTICIPANT'S PARTICIPATION.

   - REPRESENTATIVE RELEASES CLUB FROM ANY LIABILITY AND AGREES NOT TO SUE CLUB WITH RESPECT TO ANY CAUSE OF ACTION FOR BODILY INJURY, PROPERTY DAMAGE, OR DEATH OCCURRING TO PARTICIPANT AS A RESULT OF PARTICIPATING IN THE ACTIVITY.

   - REPRESENTATIVE HEREBY ASSUMES FULL RESPONSIBILITY FOR RISKS OF BODILY INJURY, PROPERTY DAMAGE OR DEATH TO PARTICIPANT DUE TO THE ORDINARY NEGLIGENCE OR GROSS NEGLIGENCE OF THE CLUB AND THE ORDINARY NEGLIGENCE, GROSS NEGLIGENCE, OR WILLFUL MISCONDUCT OF ANY THIRD PARTY INCLUDING OTHERS PARTICIPATING IN THE ACTIVITY.

   - REPRESENTATIVE AGREES TO INDEMNIFY, DEFEND, AND HOLD HARMLESS, AT REPRESENTATIVE'S SOLE COST, THE CLUB FROM ANY AND ALL CLAIMS ARISING OUT OF PARTICIPANT'S PARTICIPATION IN THE ACTIVITY.

   - ALL PERSONAL PROPERTY BROUGHT TO THE ACTIVITY, IS BROUGHT AT THE SOLE RISK OF PARTICIPANT AS TO ITS THEFT, DAMAGE, OR LOSS.

3. **Medical**. Representative on Participant's behalf, consents to emergency medical care and transportation in order to obtain treatment in the event of injury to Participant as the Club may deem appropriate. This Release extends to any liability arising out of or in any way connected with the medical treatment and transportation provided in the event of an emergency.

4. **Severability**. Representative expressly agrees that the terms of release and indemnity contained herein are intended to be as broad and inclusive as is permitted by the laws of the state in which Club operates its business. Any provision or portion of this Release found to be invalid by the courts having jurisdiction shall be invalid only with respect to such provision or portion. The offending provision or portion shall be construed to the maximum extent possible to confer upon the parties the benefits intended thereby. Said provision or portion, as well as the remaining provisions or portion hereof shall be construed and enforced to the same effect as if such offending provision or portion thereof had not been contained herein.

REPRESENTATIVE HAS READ AND VOLUNTARILY SIGNS THIS RELEASE AND INDEMNITY AGREEMENT.

PARTICIPANT(S):

REPRESENTATIVE:

_____
Printed Name

_____
Signature

_____
Printed Name

_____
Printed Name

_____
Printed Name

_____
Date

Cardiovascular Health Pre-Activity Screening

For each of the following questions, please place a check by each item that has direct application to you..

_____   Age: Men>45   Women>55

_____   Family History: MI or sudden death before 55 years of age for father or other first degree male
                            Relative or 65 years of age for mother or female first degree relative.

_____   Cigarette Smoker: (Current or have quit in the previous 6 – months)

_____   Dyslipidemia: Blood cholesterol>200 mg/dl
            (one or more of the   LDL cholesterol>130 mg/dl
            Following)   HDL<40 mg/dl
                                       LDL/HDL ratio>3 to 1
                                       Triglycerides>150

_____   Hypertension: Blood Pressure – systolic ≥ 140 or diastolic ≥90
                                        on blood pressure medication.

_____   Impaired Fasting Glucose: Fasting glucose ≥ 100 or presence of diabetes

_____   Sedentary lifestyle: Do not participate in at least 30 minutes of moderate physical
                                       activity at least 3x a week.

_____   Obesity: BMI > 30,
                                       Waist circumference > 102 cm for men and > 88 cm for women

Place a check the appropriate category that applies to this indivudal.

_____   **Low Risk:**   Men < 45 years of age and women < 55 years of age who are asymptomatic and have no more
                                than one risk factor as indicated above..

_____   **Moderate Risk:**   Men > 45 years of age and women > 55 years of age or those who have two or more
                                risk factors as indicated above.

_____   **High Risk:**   Individuals with one or more symptoms of cardiovascular disease or known cardiovascular,
                                metabolic or pulmonary disease.

Any individual classified as either moderate risk or high risk needs to receive a physician's clearance prior to
participating in a program of structured physical activity.

** Physician's Note Required**   Date Contacted: _____

Emergency Medical Authorization
Adult

I hereby give consent, in the event I am incapacitated and unable to provide such consent and approval for a situation requiring medical attention and action for the administration of any treatment or care deemed necessary, and my designated representative, _____ can not be reached in a reasonable period of time to extend such consent and approval on my behalf for attention and action for the administration of any treatment and/or care deemed necessary for the listed above by Dr. _____, or any of his/her associates, the preferred physician, or Dr. _____, or any of his/her associates, the preferred dentist, or in the event the appropriate preferred physician, dentist or other identified healthcare professional is not available, by another qualified physician, dentist or healthcare professional; and the transfer of myself to _____ hospital, the preferred hospital, or any hospital reasonably accessible.

This authorization does not cover non-emergency medical situations or non-emergency major surgery unless the opinions of at least two other licensed physicians, dentists or healthcare professionals concurring in the necessity of such emergency medical action are obtained prior to the performance of such emergency medical action/surgery and unless all reasonable attempts to obtain my approval and in the event I am incapable of providing such approval then efforts to contact my designated representative have been exhausted, defining such period for non-emergency medical action/surgery as 24 hours.

The following information is being released by me in the event that the physician, dentist, healthcare professional or hospital is unable to access my medical history;

Allergies:

Medications:

Physical limitations/restrictions:

Other critical information (e.g. blood type, health conditions, etc.):

Insurance coverage:

Insurance provider		Policy number	

I the undersigned, hereby agree appoint and constitute the club, and its duly authorized representative(s), namely _____, for the period of _____, 20____, through and including _____, 20____, and do hereby authorize them to obtain any x-ray examination, anesthesia, medical or surgical diagnosis or treatment, and hospital care to be provided for me in the event I am unable to provide approval and my designated representative can not be reached for approval in a reasonable period of time, under the general and special supervision, and on the advice of a licensed physician, dentist, or other qualified health care professional acting under their supervision.

Signature: _____

Name (print): _____

Club representative (witness) signature: _____

Club representative name (print): _____

Date: _____   State of _____

                                  Country of _____

Club Name
Incident Report Form

I. General Incident Information

Month Day Year Time of Incident	Club Member	Club Name:
A.M. P.M.	_____ Yes _____ No	Club Location:

	First M.I. Last	Hospital/EMS or Physician Notified?
Name of Injured Person:		_____ Yes _____ No
Street Address:		Name of Caller: _____
		Time of Initial Call: _____
		Time of any Follow-Up Calls: 1. _____
State/City/Zip:		2. _____ 3. _____
		Time of EMS arrival: _____
Phone #'s:		Time of EMD departure: _____
		Hospital taken to: _____
Email address:		Name of EMS contact: _____

II. General Description of the Incident

Description of Incident:

_____

_____

_____

_____

Bleeding related injury?   _____ Yes _____ No

Visible injury?   _____ Yes _____ No

Not outwardly noticeable injury, but person expressed pain?   _____ Yes _____ No

If an eye injury, was eye wear/protection being worn?   _____ Yes _____ No

III. Incident Details, including Club Response to the Incident

Description of the injury/injuries:	Description of club response/first aid:

IV. Responder, Supervisor and Witness Information

First Responder (name):

Responders position/title;

CPR certified? _____ Yes _____ No   AED certified? _____ Yes _____ No

First Aid certified? _____ Yes _____ No

Signature:

Manager on Duty (name):

Manager on Duty position/title:

CPR certified? _____ Yes _____ No   AED certified? _____ Yes _____ No

First Aid certified? _____ Yes _____ No

Signature:

Witness (name):

Witness address: _____

Witness phone: (B) _____   (H) _____   (C) _____

Witness email: _____   Signature: _____

Witness (name):

Witness address: _____

Witness phone: (B) _____   (H) _____   (C) _____

Witness email: _____   Signature: _____

V. Details on Location of Incident

1. Specific location: _____ fitness center _____ studio _____ gymnasium

_____ pool _____ tennis court _____ locker rooms

_____ spa _____ lobby/circulation area

_____ children's area _____ steam/sauna/whirlpool (circle)

_____ outside

2. Please describe the conditions of the environment during the time of the incident (e.g. was it a wet surface, was it extremely hot, etc.)

3. Other comments

VI. Miscellaneous

1. Did the police investigate? _____ Yes _____ No   If yes, please give name, rank and contact information on the lines below.

Name: _____   Rank: _____

Contact phone number: _____

2. Did another agency investigate (fire department, etc.) _____ Yes _____ No
If yes, please give name, rank and contact information on the lines below.

Name: _____   Rank: _____

Contact phone number: _____

Report submitted by: _____   Signature: _____

Date and time submitted: _____

Please make multiple copies, including one for the person's file, the club's incident files, the insurer and the individual involved in the incident.

Appendix U
Suggested References

- *2002 Profiles of Success; IHRSA's Industry Data Survey of the Health and Fitness Club Industry.* Compiled by the International Health, Racquet & Sportsclub Association and Industry Insights, Inc. Boston, MA. 2002.

- *2003 Profiles of Success; IHRSA's Industry Data Survey of the Health and Fitness Club Industry.* Compiled by the International Health, Racquet & Sportsclub Association and Industry Insights, Inc. Boston, MA. 2003.

- *2004 Profiles of Success; IHRSA's Industry Data Survey of the Health and Fitness Club Industry.* Compiled by the International Health, Racquet & Sportsclub Association and Industry Insights, Inc. Boston, MA. 2004.

- *2007 Profiles of Success; IHRSA's Industry Data Survey of the Health and Fitness Club Industry.* Compiled by the International Health, Racquet & Sportsclub Association and Industry Insights, Inc. Boston, MA. 2007.

- *2010 Profiles of Success; IHRSA's Industry Data Survey of the Health and Fitness Club Industry.* Compiled by the International Health, Racquet & Sportsclub Association. Boston, MA. 2010.

- *Sportsclub2008 IHRSA Asia Pacific Market Report: The Size and Scope of the Health Club Industry.* Compiled by the International Health, Racquet & Sportsclub Association and Deloitte. Boston, MA. 2008.

- *2008 IHRSA European Market Report: The Size and Scope of the Health Club Industry.* Compiled by the International Health, Racquet & Sportsclub Association and Deloitte. Boston, MA. 2008.

- *2008 IHRSA Global Report: The State of the Health Club Industry.* Compiled by the International Health, Racquet & Sportsclub Association. Boston, MA. 2008.

- *2010 IHRSA European Market Report: The Size and Scope of the Health Club Industry.* Compiled by the International Health, Racquet & Sportsclub Association and Deloitte. Boston, MA. 2010.

- *2010 IHRSA Global Report: The State of the Health Club Industry.* Compiled by the International Health, Racquet & Sportsclub Association. Boston, MA. 2010.

- *22 Immutable Laws of Branding: How to Build a Product or Service into a World Class Brand.* Al Reis and Laura Reis. Harper Collins. New York. 1998.

- *A Study of Consumer Attitudes Toward Physical Fitness and Health Clubs.* American Sports Data, Inc. Hartsdale, NY. 2002.

- *A Study of Former Health Club Members.* Conducted for IHRSA by American Sports Data, Inc. Hartsdale, NY. 1998.

- *ACSM's Health/Fitness Facility Standards and Guidelines.* 4th Edition. Steve Tharrett and James A. Peterson. Human Kinetics. Champaign, IL. 2012.

- *AED Position Paper.* ClubCorp Internal Document. Dallas, TX. 2002.

- *"Best of HBR on Leadership; It Is Hard Being Soft."* Harvard Business Review. Boston, MA. 2001.

- *Beyond the Universe.* Bill Pearl. Bill Pearl Enterprises, Inc. Agni Press. New York. 2003.

- *Building Membership Best Practices.* IHRSA Publication. Boston, MA. 2000.

- *ClubCorp Athletic Operations Manual.* ClubCorp Internal Document. Dallas, TX. 1998.

- *ClubCorp Standards of Operation for Athletics and Tennis.* ClubCorp Internal Document. Dallas, TX. 2003.

- *Discovering the Soul of Service.* Leonard Berry. The Free Press. New York. 1999.

- *Employee Compensation and Benefits Survey Results for the Commercial Health and Fitness Industry.* IHRSA and Industry Insights. Boston, MA. 2006.

- *The Experience Economy.* Joseph Pine, II, and James Gilmore. Harvard Business School Press. Boston, MA. 1999.

- *Fitness American Style: A Look at How and Why Americans Exercise.* Prepared for IHRSA by Roper Starch Worldwide. Boston, MA. 2001.

- *2005 Guidelines for Cardiopulmonary Resuscitation and Emergency Cardiovascular Care.* International Consensus on Science Part III: Adult Basic Life Support. Circulation 2005. American Heart Association in collaboration with International Liaison Committee on Resuscitation. Dallas, TX. 2005.

- *Health and Fitness Club Review.* Granville Baird Ltd. London, England. 2000.

- *IHRSA/ASD Health Club Trend Report (1987-2003).* American Sports Data, Inc. Hartsdale, NY. 2004.

- *2003 IHRSA Global Report: State of the Health Club Industry.* Compiled by the International Health, Racquet & Sportsclub Association. Boston, MA. 2003.

- *2004 IHRSA Global Report: State of the Health Club Industry.* Compiled by the International Health, Racquet & Sportsclub Association. Boston, MA. 2004.

- *2005 IHRSA Global Report: State of the Health Club Industry*. Compiled by the International Health, Racquet & Sportsclub Association. Boston, MA. 2005.

- *2005 IHRSA European Market Report: The Size and Scope of the Health Club Industry*. Compiled by the International Health, Racquet & Sportsclub Association. Boston, MA. 2005.

- *IHRSA's Guide for Health Club Operators: How to Prevail in Competitive Markets*. John McCarthy. International Health, Racquet & Sportsclub Association. Boston, MA. 2006.

- *IHRSA's Guide to Lenders and Investors*. 2nd edition. IHRSA. Boston, MA. 2004.

- *ISPA 2004 Consumer Trends Report*. Complied and prepared by the International Spa Association and the Hartman Group, Inc. Lexington, KY. 2004.

- *ISPA 2008 Global Consumer Study*. Commissioned by the International Spa Association, Lexington, Kentucky. Prepared by Research International. 2008.

- *ISPA 2010 U.S. Spa Industry Study*. Commissioned by the International Spa Association, Lexington, Kentucky. Prepared by Price Waterhouse Cooper. 2010.

- *Karoake Capitalism: Daring to Be Different in a Copycat World*. Jonas Ridderstrale and Kjell A. Nordstrom. Praeger Publishers. Westport, CT. 2005.

- *King of Clubs: Grow Rich in More Than Money*. Robert Dedman with Debbie Deloach. Taylor Publishing. Dallas, TX. 1999.

- *Leadership and the One-Minute Manager*. Ken Blanchard, Patricia Zigarmi, and Drea Zigarmi. William Morrow and Company, Inc. New York. 1985.

- *Legal Aspects of Preventative and Rehabilitative Exercise Programs*. 2nd Edition. Herbert and Herbert. Professional Reports Corporation. Canton, OH. 1989.

- *Legends of Fitness*. Stephen Tharrett, Frank O'Rourke, and James A. Peterson. Healthy Learning, Monterey, California. 2011.

- *Marketing Health and Fitness Services*. Richard Gerson. Human Kinetics. Champaign, IL. 1989.

- *Marketing for Results: A Common Sense Approach for Health Clubs*. Brenda Abdilla. CBM Books. Fort Washington, PA. 1996.

- *Marketing Outreach Techniques for Clubs*. Management Vision, Inc. Internal Document. New York. 2002.

- *Muscletown USA*. John Fair. Pennsylvania State University Press. University Park, PA. 1999.

- *Opening a Spa*. Melinda M. Minton. Minton Business Solutions. Fort Collins, CO. 2002.

- *Programming Best Practices*. ClubCorp Internal Document. Dallas, TX. 2003.

- *Raving Fans*. Ken Blanchard and Sheldon Bowles. William Morrow and Company, Inc. New York. 1993.

- *Spa Industry Survey*. Conducted and prepared by Price Waterhouse Coopers for the International Spa Association. Lexington, KY. 2002.

- *Sports Club Bell Notes*. ClubCorp Internal Document. Dallas, TX. 2003.

- *Sports and Fitness Programming Manual*. ClubCorp Internal Document. Dallas, TX. 1999.

- *The ACE Fitness and Business Forms Handbook*. Stephen Tharrett. Healthy Learning. Monterey, CA. 2006.

- *The Health/Fitness Club Operator's Guide to Recruiting and Retaining Great Employees*. Stephen Tharrett. Healthy Learning, Monterey, CA. 2007.

- *The One Minute Manager Builds High Performing Teams*. Ken Blanchard, Don Carew and Ernie Parisi-Carew. William Morrow and Company. New York. 1990.

- *The Seven Habits of Highly Effective People*. Stephen Covey. Fireside Publishing. New York. 1989.

- *Trends in Physical Fitness Behavior* (1987-2002). American Sports Data, Inc. Hartsdale, NY. 2003.

- *Uniform System of Accounts for the Health, Racquet & Sportsclub Industry*. Copyrighted by the Educational Institute of the American Hotel and Motel Association. Lansing, MI. 1998.

- *Why and Where People Exercise*. An IHRSA study conducted by American Sports Data, Inc. Hartsdale, NY. 1995.

- *Why People Quit*. An IHRSA Study conducted by American Sports Data, Inc. Hartsdale, NY. 1998.

- *Why People Stay: Health Club Member Retention Research and Best Practices*. IHRSA Publication. Boston, MA. 2000.

- *Winning the Retention Battle: Parts One through Four*. Conducted by the Fitness Industry Association and Leisure Industry Week with assistance from Gladstone MRM. London, England. 2001.

Stephen J. Tharrett, MS, is currently the owner and president of Club Industry Consulting, a global consulting business established in 2006 and based in the U.S. Tharrett is also a partner in Club Intel, a recently formed company that is focused on providing the global club industry with insight, inspiration, and impact revolving around the emotional power of a brand and its ability to establish a powerful base of advocates and fans. From 2008 to 2010, Tharrett served as the Chief Executive Officer for the Russian Fitness Group, a privately held health/fitness club company that was, at the time, the largest in Russia.

Prior to forming Club Industry Consulting in 2006, Tharrett had a 20-plus-year career with ClubCorp, a billion-dollar private club company based in Dallas, Texas, where he served in several roles, ranging from director of athletics to senior vice president for athletics, golf and tennis, as well as serving on the company's leadership cabinet and business planning committee.

Tharrett is the author or co-author of three other management textbooks: *The Health/Fitness Club Operator's Guide to Recruiting and Retaining Great Employees*, *The ACE Fitness and Business Forms Handbook*, and *Legends of Fitness: The Forces, Influencers, and Innovations That Helped Shape the Fitness Industry*. Tharrett is also the co-editor of ACSM's *Health/Fitness Facility Standards and Guidelines, Fourth Edition*. Tharrett has three new books coming out in 2012. He is a former president of IHRSA, having served as president of the international association from 1996–1997.

James A. Peterson, Ph.D., FACSM, is a sports medicine consultant who resides in Monterey, California. A fellow of the American College of Sports Medicine, he was a faculty member at the United States Military Academy at West Point from 1971 to 1990. From 1990 to 1995, he served as the director of sports medicine for StairMaster Sports/Medical Products, Inc. He has written or co-authored over 80 books and more than 200 articles on a variety of sports, health, and wellness topics. He holds two FDA-approved patents on back pain management measures. Since 1997, he has been a contributing editor to *ACSM's Health & Fitness Journal* ("Take 10" column). He served as the co-editor of the second, third, and fourth editions of *ACSM's Health/Fitness Facility Standards and Guidelines*. He has appeared on several national television shows, including ABC's Good Morning America, the CBS Evening News, and ABC's Nightline. Since 1992, he has served as a fundraiser for the Make-A-Wish Foundation®. Jim and his wife, Susan, have been married for over 40 years.

About the Authors